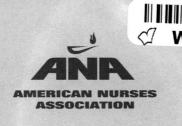
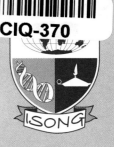

GENETICS AND ETHICS IN HEALTH CARE

New Questions in the Age of Genomic Health

RITA BLACK MONSEN

DSN, MPH, RN, FAAN
EDITOR

American Nurses Association
Silver Spring, MD • 2009

Library of Congress Cataloging-in-Publication Data

Genetics and ethics in health care : new questions in the age of genomic health/
edited by Rita Black Monsen.
     p. ; cm.
   Includes bibliographical references and index.
     ISBN-13: 978-1-55810-263-7 (softcover : alk. paper)
     ISBN-10: 1-55810-263-9 (softcover : alk. paper)
   1. Medical genetics--Moral and ethical aspects. 2. Nursing ethics. 3. Nursing ethics—
Cross-cultural studies. I. Monsen, Rita Black. II. American Nurses Association.
III. International Society of Nurses in Genetics.
   [DNLM: 1. Genetics, Medical—ethics—United States. 2. Delivery of Health Care—
ethics—United States. 3. Genetic Predisposition to Disease—United States. 4. Genetic
Privacy—ethics—United States. 5. Health Policy—United States. 6. Informed
Consent—ethics—United States. 7. Nurse's Role—United States. QZ 50 G32805 2009]
   RB155.5.G4615 2009
   174.2'96042—dc22

                                                                          2008044243

The opinions in this book reflect those of the authors and do not necessarily reflect positions or policies of the American Nurses Association. Furthermore, the information in this
book should not be construed as legal or other professional advice.

Published by Nursesbooks.org
The Publishing Program of ANA

American Nurses Association
8515 Georgia Avenue, Suite 400
Silver Spring, MD 20910-3492
1-800-274-4ANA
http://www.nursesbooks.org/

The ANA is the only full-service professional organization representing the interests of the nation's 2.9
million registered nurses through its 54 constituent
member nurses associations, its 23 organizational affil-
iates serving 330,000 members of national nursing
specialty organizations, and its workforce advocacy
affiliate, the Center for American Nurses. The ANA
advances the nursing profession by fostering high
standards of nursing practice, promoting the rights of
nurses in the workplace, projecting a positive and realistic view of nursing, and by lobbying the Congress
and regulatory agencies on health care issues affecting
nurses and the public.

Page and cover design: Laura C. Johnson, Grammarians, Inc., Washington, DC
Editorial team: Rosanne O'Connor Roe and Eric Wurzbacher
Copyediting: Steven A. Jent, Denton, TX ⌐ *Proofreading:* Ashley Mason, Atlanta, GA
Indexing: Estalita Slivoskey, Ellendale, ND
Composition: Laura C. Johnson, Grammarians, Inc.
Printing: McArdle Printing, Inc., Upper Marlboro, MD

ISBN-13: 978-1-55810-263-7   SAN: 851-3481   2.5M   12/08

First printing December 2008.

CONTENTS

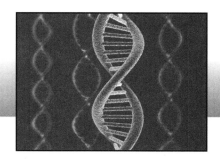

PROLOGUE

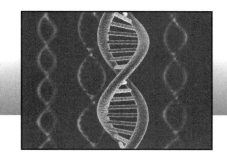

Genetics and Genomic Health Care:

The Mission and Aims of the National Human Genome Research Institute and Its Potential Impact on Clinical Practices

Dale Halsey Lea, MPH, RN, CGC, APNG, FAAN
Jean F. Jenkins, PhD, RN, FAAN
National Human Genome Research Institute
National Institutes of Health

How many ideas have

there been in history

that were unthinkable

ten years before they

appeared?

⟶ Fyodor Dostoyevsky

The National Institutes of Health (NIH), a part of the U.S. Department of Health and Human Services, is the primary Federal agency for conducting and supporting basic and clinical research. For over a century, the NIH has played a leading role in advancing clinical health care by supporting evidence-based research in disease prevention as well as research priority areas such as causes, treatment, and cures for common and rare diseases. NIH research affects the health of individuals, families, and communities throughout the lifespan and around the world.

The Human Genome Project—the international research effort that has identified the location and sequence of all human genes—was the culmination of the history of genetics research, which began in 1911 with mapping the genes of the fruit fly (Drosophila melanogaster). The National Human Genome Research Institute (NHGRI), established in 1989, led the National Institutes of Health contribution to the Human Genome Project, which was completed in 2003 with the publication of the full and complete sequence of the human genome. As noted by Francis Collins, director of NHGRI, the genome can be thought of as a book with many uses.

> It's a history book—a narrative of the journey of our species through time. It's a shop manual, with an incredibly detailed blueprint for building every human cell. And it's a transformative textbook of medicine, with insights that will give healthcare providers immense new powers to treat, prevent and cure disease. (NHGRI 2008b)

NHGRI has provided financial support to scientists at universities throughout the United States. Their research has contributed to our understanding of basic and structural genomics, which has the potential to revolutionize health care. The next steps in furthering this mission include three major themes: genomics to biology, genomics to health, and genomics to society (Collins and Guttmacher 2003). Results of this ongoing research are transforming approaches to screening, diagnosing, and treating human disease. As a result, genetic technologies and genetic information are becoming integral to clinical decision-making and treatment.

In recognition of the significant implications for individuals and society for having the detailed genetic information made possible by the Human Genome Project, NHGRI created an Ethical, Legal, and Social Implications (ELSI) research program in 1990 as an integral part of the U.S. Human Genome Project. ELSI is devoted to the analysis of the ethical, legal, and social implications of new genetic information and knowledge, and the development of policy options for public consideration. ELSI focuses on four research priorities of concern to all healthcare professionals and the public: privacy and fairness of use and interpretation of genetic information; responsible clinical integration of genetic technologies; issues surrounding genetics research; and public and professional education about these issues.

To ensure the responsible use of genetic information, ELSI has provided funding and management for research grants and education projects, including nursing education and research, at institutions throughout the United States. ELSI funding has been instrumental for genetics nursing workshops, research, and policy projects such as the conference and report of the Expert Panel on Genetics and Nursing (HRSA

2000). It has also funded nursing research of social issues in genetics and genomics such as individual, family, and cultural responses to new genome technologies and information.

Within NIH, NHGRI has taken a leading role in ensuring that healthcare professionals and the public have access to and education about genome research and its implications. In 2003, NHGRI created the Education and Community Involvement Branch (ECIB) to create education and community involvement programs to engage the public in understanding genomics and the accompanying ethical, legal, and social issues. ECIB leads NHGRI's public education efforts, and advises the NHGRI director and senior staff on public education and community involvement. The branch initiates, develops, implements, and evaluates education and community involvement programs to engage the public in understanding genomics and its implications for health and society. Education programs inform the public of the latest advances in genomics, and support the dissemination of information to teachers, students, and consumers. The goal is to empower the public with knowledge and tools to use genetic information and technology to improve and maintain optimal health (NHGRI 2008a).

NHGRI recognizes that nurses are at the interface of the translation of genomic research into clinical practice, and that nurses are already caring for individuals and families who have a specific genetic condition or genetic component to their health and disease. NHGRI, therefore, has provided significant help to nurses to gain the genetic knowledge and clinical expertise needed to provide care in the genomic era.

Two examples of this support are the nursing textbooks, *Nursing Care in the Genomic Era: A Case-Based Approach* and *Essential Nursing Competencies and Curricula Guidelines for Genetics and Genomics*. In the former, Francis Collins, Director of NHGRI, and Alan Guttmacher, Deputy Director, explain:

> As health professionals with a tradition of patient-oriented care, nurses must play a key role in both developing and applying these and many other aspects of genomic health care. Indeed, unless nursing plays a key role in genomics, the genomic era will fail to live up to its promise. And, unless genomics plays a key role in nursing, the nursing profession will fail to live up to its promise. (Jenkins and Lea 2005, p. xiv)

Essential Competencies was created by nursing leaders in genetics with the support of NHGRI among other federal agencies. The document defines essential genetic and genomic competencies for all registered nurses. Genetic and genomic competencies are viewed as integral to the practice of all nurses regardless of academic preparation, practice setting, role, or specialty. These professional competencies include:

- Demonstrating in practice "the importance of tailoring genetic and genomic information and services to clients based on their culture, religion, knowledge level, literacy, and preferred language."
- Advocating "for the rights of all clients for autonomous, informed genetic and genomic-related decision-making and voluntary action."

In the professional practice domain, competencies include the registered nurse's obligation to identify "ethical, ethnic/ancestral, cultural, religious, legal, fiscal, and societal issues related to genetic and genomic information and technologies." Competencies, with NHGRI support, has now been endorsed by 44 nursing and other patient care organizations (Jenkins, Calzone, Lea, and Prows 2006).

This monograph provides significant information that helps you prepare to provide competent care in the genomic era. Nurses are critical in taking a lead role when working with state, federal, and international health agencies, and in providing guidance to individuals, families, communities, and health systems regarding genetics technologies, services, and related social issues. Issues such as privacy and confidentiality and informed consent are of concern to the consumer and the nurse (Cassells, Jenkins, Lea, Calzone, and Johnson 2003). This book offers nurses important information and guidance on these and other ethical and policy issues related to genetics and genomics. Such knowledge further enhances nursing's expertise and full participation in the design of healthcare services that adequately consider policy when providing genomic health care.

References

Cassells, J. M., J. Jenkins, D. H. Lea, K. Calzone, and E. Johnson. 2003. An ethical assessment framework for addressing global genetic issues in clinical practice. *Oncology Nursing Forum* 30: 383–390.

Collins, F. S., E. D. Green, A. Guttmacher, and M. S. Guyer. 2003. A vision for the future of genomics research: A blueprint for the genomic era. *Nature* 422 (24): 835–847.

Health Resources and Services Administration (HRSA). 2000. *Expert panel on genetics and nursing: Implications for education and practice.* Washington, DC: HRSA.

Jenkins, J., K. Calzone, D. H. Lea, and C. Prows. 2008. *Essential nursing competencies and cur-ricula guidelines for genetics and genomics.* http://www.nursingsociety.org/aboutus/Documents/geneticscompetency.pdf (accessed October 7, 2008).

Jenkins, J., and D. H. Lea. 2005. *Nursing care in the genomic era: A case-based approach.* Sudbury, MA: Jones & Bartlett Publishers.

National Human Genome Research Institute (NHGRI). 2008a. *Education and community involvement branch.* http://www.genome.gov/11008538 (accessed October 7, 2008).

———. 2008b. *An overview of the Human Genome Project.* http://www.genome.gov/12011238 (accessed Octover 7, 2008).

INTRODUCTION

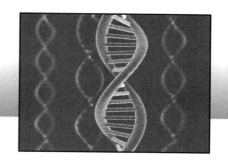

Genetics and Ethics in Nursing: New Questions in the Age of Genomic Health

Rita Black Monsen, DSN, MPH, RN, FAAN

This text is intended for nurses and nursing students, but is likely to be useful to others in the health professions, the life sciences, philosophy, ethics, and the humanities. The aim of this monograph is to bring forward the new questions associated with advances in genetics technology and genomic health care now proliferating across our nation and the world. My original idea was to open a forum of conversations that would explore what new issues and implications come before us when revolutionary new diagnostics and therapeutics begin to appear, some not completely developed. By this I mean that we may be offering testing for genetic mutations or treatments for gene-based health problems without totally understanding and anticipating the possible harms or undesirable effects that may accompany them.

In addition, I wished to provide a showcase for voices that we do not often encounter in our literature, voices from communities of color: diverse religious and ethnic communities that are all around us but seldom appear in our science-based discussions of genomic health care. We do hear from these communities, but often only when we seek out their views and recommendations. Often, their perspectives are not included in policy-making and legislative proposals that indeed affect all of our people, and populations in many other parts of the world.

While we could not include representative contributions from all of the major cultural groups, we have attempted to present a cross-section of religious and ethnic groups. This effort was made in view of the role that the International Society of Nurses in Genetics has made to invite participation by nurses in our global community. In addition, the American Nurses Association has supported, and in some instances led, efforts to educate nurses as they provide care across cultural lines and in concert with diverse providers and consumers here and abroad.

In many ways, these new questions about genetics and genomics in human life present dilemmas with no good answers. They are similar to the many ethical questions we have seen over our lifetimes in healthcare arenas. In their similarity, they may engender conversations that call us to consider the basic principles of ethics and morality and the meaning of health and quality of life in the twenty-first century. Are these principles still relevant? Can we cast the questions that arise out of genetics and genomic health care in terms of goodness or appropriate comportment as we practice our chosen profession and serve others? One valuable guide, the code of ethics of the American Nurses Association, will always continue to frame our thoughts and actions as these questions arise with new discoveries in genetics and genomics that are revolutionizing our definitions of health, illness, and cure.

This text will include some basic discussion of the biochemical and molecular phenomena as components of genes, genetic material, and chromosomes, but we have not attempted to present detailed technical explanations that require a significant understanding of molecular biology. The reader is encouraged to seek additional information, and perhaps tutorial assistance, to enhance their knowledge of basic cell physiology. Four valuable online sources of in-depth information are the website of the National Coalition for Health Professional Education in Genetics (www.nchpeg.org), the Genetics Home Reference (http://ghr.nlm.nih.gov), the National Genetics Education Development Centre (http://www.genetic seducation.nhs.uk/), sponsored by the National Health Service in the United Kingdom, and Australia's Centre for Genetics Education (http://www. genetics.com.au/). Additional resources can be explored at the Genetics Home Reference website (http://ghr.nlm.nih.gov/ghr/resource/education), where the interested reader can find a wide variety of information for professional, academic, and lay audiences.

This book is about what we have accomplished at this point in the history of humanity's quest to understand the causal factors in health and illness. The prologue has already introduced the reader to the center of genetics and genomics in healthcare delivery—the National Human Genome Research Institute at the National Institutes of Health—and its role in conducting research and funding projects that reveal the contribution of genes to human health.

Finally: while this book has been made possible by experiences with the many clinicians and teachers who practiced with me as well as all of the authors, it is important to say at the beginning that the identities of all of the patients and families mentioned in this monograph have been modified to protect their anonymity.

About This Book

Part 1. Genetics, Genomics, and Ethics: Basic Considerations

Part 1 presents the significant documents and groups that govern nursing practice in working with patients and families who have genetic concerns: the American Nurses Association (ANA) code of ethics and the description of the scope and standards for nurses in genetics. The essential role of policy development at the national level composes the chapter on the work of the Department of Health and Human Services Secretary's Advisory Committee on Genetics, Health, and Society. A basic discussion of ethics and the principles that guide healthcare providers introduces some of the new developments in healthcare technology and what dilemmas may now be challenging us. There is a chapter on informed consent and how it promotes greater understanding of gene-based testing and therapies among patients and families.

This section also discusses implications for human life: our understanding of identity and the legacies that we pass on to our offspring. We close with cautions about the use of genetic and genomic discoveries; and the dangers of commercial exploitation of individuals, families, and communities as genetic technologies proliferate in agriculture, health care, and athletics. We are most concerned, finally, with the possibility of inadequate preparation of healthcare professionals to utilize gene-based diagnostics and therapeutics appropriately for the improvement of health and quality of life of entire societies.

Part 2. Religious and Cultural Perspectives of Communities and Societies

Part 2 presents perspectives from communities that represent large population segments whose religious and cultural allegiances are integral to the experience of family life and making health decisions. While not all major groups have been included, a diverse selection of voices is presented. These chapters are included to provide a glimpse into the thinking and decision-making patterns seen in several religious and cultural traditions, some not directly discussing genomic technologies. They may be helpful as we collaborate with peoples from diverse cultural and religious communities to inform them about their options with regard to genetic and genomic health.

Part 3. Applications of Genetics and Genomics in Health Care

Part 3 discusses selected applications of genetic and genomic technologies, particularly the current patterns of mutational testing that are widely available today, in areas affecting children and those with known risks of cancer, Huntington's disease, and cystic fibrosis. Again, while not all highly prevalent genetic conditions are presented, a selection of the major health problems that affect millions of Americans as well as millions across the globe do appear here.

While these chapters present the more common tests, the reader should know that additional mutational analyses are being transferred from the laboratory to the clinical setting. One of the most rapidly advancing areas of research is expected to broaden our understanding of the appearance of such population-level causes of morbidity and mortality as heart disease, cancer, and diabetes. We are moving quickly to the place in our history when we will be able to study the interplay of several genes as well as environmental factors that result in conditions of health and illness.

Part 4. Case Studies in Genetics and Ethics

Part 4 concludes the book with several case studies that illustrate what families face in specific circumstances that involve genetics, genetic testing, and the care of family members who are affected with a genetic condition. We can get a glimpse of the burdens associated with gene mutations that may spread through families and that have the potential to affect many future generations.

Acknowledgements

I am most appreciative of the support of Rosanne O'Connor Roe, the manager of Nursesbooks.org, the Publishing Program of the American Nurses Association, editor and project manager Eric Wurzbacher, and Laura Johnson, designer and compositor of Grammarians, Inc.

Additional Informational Resources

- *Genetics Home Reference* is the National Library of Medicine's web site for consumer information about genetic conditions and the genes or chromosomes related to those conditions. http://ghr.nlm.nih.gov/

- *National Coalition for Health Professional Education in Genetics* (NCHPEG) is a coalition of organizations and individuals promoting health professional education and access to information about advances in human genetics. http://www.nchpeg.org/

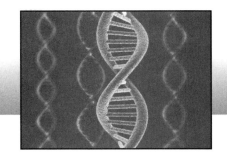

CODA

Genetics and Genomics in Historical Context

A Brief History of the Early Days of Clinical Genetics

Margaret Abbott, MPH, BS, RN

The Genetics Clinic at the Johns Hopkins Hospital was established in 1957. The staff consisted of the Medical Director, Fellows in Genetics (physicians in specialized training), two caseworkers, and me.

My first order of business was the ascertainment of patients for the new clinic. The method was by review of medical records of patients affected with dwarfism and patients affected with selected heritable disorders. The cost of patient visits was covered by grant funds.

On the appointment date the two case workers and I monitored the patients' progress and their accompanying families, explaining the routine. I maintained a patient file including clinical data sent to referring physicians. Additionally, I had my own research on longevity (Hawkins, Murphy, & Abbey, 1965).

Genetic counseling was strictly the responsibility of the MD Fellows in Genetics. I attended the one-to-one genetic counseling sessions with patients and families and contributed to clarification information they had received.

Reference

Hawkins, M. R., Murphy, E. A., & Abbey, H. (1965, July). The familial component in longevity: A study of the offspring of novogenarians, I. Methods and preliminary report. *Bulletin of the Johns Hopkins Hospital* 117, 24–36.

How Far We Have Come

Rita Black Monsen, DSN, MPH, FAAN

Ms. Abbot speaks of one the very earliest programs in clinical genetics in the United States and in the world, one that provided services with an interdisciplinary team of professionals. She began this part of her career at a time when the state of the science was one that had only recently accepted the correct number of chromosomes (46) in the cell nuclei of humans (Tjio & Levan, 1956).

In the 1960s, academic health sciences centers throughout the world developed and expanded genetics programs and public health agencies began to offer genetic screening to prevent such disabling conditions as phenylketonuria and congenital hypothyroidism among newborns. In the 1970s, greater precision in diagnosing gene-based illness came with molecular biology and cytogenetic technologies. Nurses, social workers, and genetic counselors were being given greater responsibilities for family interviews, development and analyses of pedigrees, and delivery of counseling services.

Today, academic centers and the biotech industry cooperate to delineate the causes and, where possible, gene-based therapeutics to explain and treat heritable conditions. In addition, we are able to define the roles of multiple genes and environmental factors that lead to conditions that affect larger segments of populations such as heart disease, cancer, diabetes, and certain disorders of mental health.

Ms. Abbott practiced with Victor McKusick, MD, widely recognized as the "father" of clinical genetics. Her work spans the latter half of the 20th century when genetic technologies proliferated and enabled medical professionals across the world to offer understanding of and, in many instances treatment for, illnesses that had been a matter of conjecture for most of human history.

Reference

Tjio, J. H., & Levan, A. (1956). The chromosome number of man. *Hereditas* 42, 1–6.

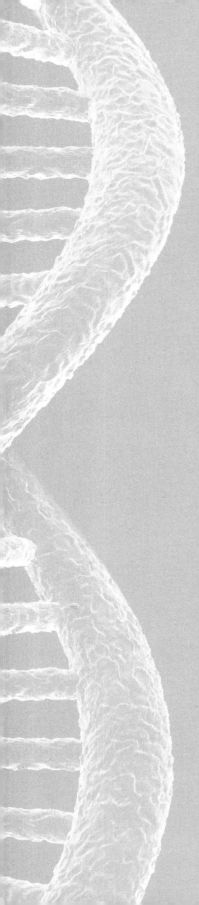

PART 1

Genetics, Genomics, and Ethics: Basic Considerations

We open this monograph with examining and discussing some overarching topics that inform a major subtext of whole work: the level of preparation of healthcare professionals to utilize gene-based diagnostics and therapeutics appropriately for the improvement of health and quality of life of entire societies. Included, then, in this section are the ethical beliefs and assumptions of the nursing community, the major efforts toward public policy-making (especially at the national level), and the basic tenets of ethics in health care today. We provide a discussion of the central decision challenge for the use of genetic and genomic technologies in health care by individuals and families: the informed consent.

As well, this section addresses some of the implications for human life: our understanding of identity and the legacies that we pass on to our offspring. We consider the meaning of genetic information in our lives, in our understanding of the human experience, and in the implications for family life across generations. Lastly, we discuss some of the many possible dangers that attend genomic advances, including associated discrimination and commercialization as well as the responsibilities of professionals for their appropriate use.

PART 1 ⌒ CONTENTS

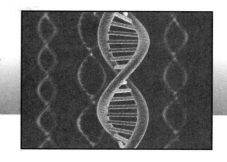

CHAPTER 1

The ANA Code of Ethics

Laurie Badzek, JD, MSN, RN, LLM, NAP

Nurses are at the forefront of providing care for patients. Genetic information focuses on individual genes in the genome. Genomic information focuses on all genes in the genome interacting. Nurses are increasingly expected to use genetic and genomic information when providing care for patients. Nurses recognize and respond to the revolutionary changes that occur in providing health care. The American Nurses Association (ANA), and, more specifically, the Center for Ethics and Human Rights (the Center), have been involved in the development, promotion, and dissemination of genetic and genomic information because ANA recognizes the impact genomic information has on patient care. ANA and its Center have been leading the way in the genomic revolution for more than a decade.

In the early 1990s when human genome mapping was in its infancy, ANA was surveying nurses to elicit information about the use and storage of genetic information. The data from the survey was reported in a seminal document entitled *Managing Genetic Information: Implications for Nurses* (Scanlon and Fibison 1995). The document identified four key areas for practice with ethical implications linked to the Code of Ethics. The key areas discussed by Scanlon and Fibison were informed consent, privacy and confidentiality, veracity, and non-discrimination. The outcome of that initial project launched ANA and specifically the Center into a decade of assisting nurses with the management of genetic information that continues even today.

Following the initial project on managing genetic information, ANA partnered with the Genome Institute at the National Institute of Health and the American Medical Association to seek funding to secure a grant to begin the work that resulted in the National Coalition for Health Professional Education in Genetics (NCHPEG). Today, NCHPEG is the premier resource for health information and an active organization in promoting and improving genetic and genomic health information for health professionals in all disciplines. National nursing organizations comprise the largest health profession membership in NCHPEG. Other examples of early ANA leadership include ANA's recognition of genetics as an area of nursing specialty through credentialing and standards. ANA worked collaboratively with the International Society of Nurses in Genetics (ISONG) to develop and disseminate information on Nursing and Genetics. The ANA continues to have a strong collaborative relationship with ISONG.

Constituent members of the ANA have been active in creating and passing resolutions related to genetics and cloning that similarly span the decade. In 1999 and 2003, the ANA House of Delegates approved statements relating to genetics education and therapeutic and reproductive applications of genetics. In 2000, ANA developed a position statement on "human cloning by means of blastomere splitting and nuclear transplantation" (ANA 2000). Most recently, the ANA Center for Ethics and Human Rights Advisory Board appointed for 2006–2008 began a review of the 2000 human cloning position statement.

The ANA through its Governmental Affairs department (GOVA) has continuously monitored federal legislation related to genetics and genomics. As needed, GOVA has made the positions of ANA members known to federal legislators. Legislation related to medical record privacy issues, mobility and health insurance, and stem cell research are the most notable examples of proposed federal legislation requiring ANA vigilance, monitoring, and input.

Most recently, in 2005 ANA supported and assisted in consensus building around the development of *Essential Core Competencies and Curricula Guidelines for Genetics and Genomics* (Jenkins et al. 2006). In both 2005 and 2006, ANA hosted at its headquarters the consensus and strategic planning meetings for the Core Competencies. Nurses from national organizations across the United States attended the 2005 meeting to finalize the competencies; in 2006 their goal was to develop a strategic plan for implementation of the competencies.

Core Competencies address professional responsibilities and practice intended to guide the design of educational experiences for students and practicing nurses. The underlying premise of the document can be linked to the ethical obligation of the nurse to be competent in practice and to use the ANA Code of Ethics for Nurses (ANA 2001) to guide practice. As strategies for implementation of the Core Competencies are developed and familiarity with genetics and genomic information in nursing practice increases, the Code of Ethics and knowledge of its provisions and interpretive statements will be helpful to nurses as they encounter new practice questions.

The Code of Ethics is intended to be a dynamic document and not a relic (Fowler 1999). The ethical foundations within the Code can be traced to the same fundamental values and commitments found within the writings of Florence Nightingale and her Nursing Pledge (Nightingale 1860). Nightingale's Nursing Pledge is recognized as the earliest code of nursing ethics in modern nursing. Although the ethical foundations are unchanged, the social context in which we view them continually changes as advances in medicine and nursing practice occur. The first formal Code of Ethics was adopted by the ANA delegation in 1950. The Code of Ethics has seen many revisions but none as comprehensive as the process that resulted in the current document. The Code of Ethics is not negotiable and can only be changed by formal processes with the ANA (ANA 1994).

The revolution around genetic information will likely increase the number and intensity of ethical questions and challenges. The current Code of Ethics says nothing specifically about genetics, but rather serves as the foundational document for ethical nursing practice within the profession. The document provides a framework for nurses when faced with an ethical decision. A future revision of the Code of Ethics may well address genetic and genomic science, given that this revision is projected to be the basis for effective health care in the future.

The Code of Ethics consists of nine provisions accompanied by interpretive text. The provisions (See Table 1–1) can be divided into three parts:

- Fundamental values and commitments of the nurse
- Boundaries of duty and loyalty
- Duties beyond individual patient encounters

Each of the three parts can provide direction to nurses as they navigate the ethical challenges or dilemmas related to genetic and genomic advances in health care.

The three provisions (Provisions 1, 2, and 3) focus on the fundamental values and commitments of the nurse. These provisions primarily relate to human dignity, the worth of persons, the commitment of the nurse to the patient whether the patient

TABLE 1–1
The Provisions of the Code of Ethics for Nurses

1. The nurse, in all professional relationships, practices with compassion and respect for the inherent dignity, worth and uniqueness of every individual, unrestricted by considerations of social or economic status, personal attributes, or the nature of health problems.

2. The nurse's primary commitment is to the patient, whether an individual, family, group, or community.

3. The nurse promotes, advocates for, and strives to protect the health, safety, and rights of the patient.

4. The nurse is responsible and accountable for individual nursing practice and determines the appropriate delegation of tasks consistent with the nurse's obligation to provide optimum patient care.

5. The nurse owes the same duties to self as to others, including the responsibility to preserve integrity and safety, to maintain competence, and to continue personal and professional growth.

6. The nurse participates in establishing, maintaining, and improving healthcare environments and conditions of employment conducive to the provision of quality health care and consistent with the values of the profession through individual and collective action.

7. The nurse participates in the advancement of the profession through contributions to practice, education, administration, and knowledge development.

8. The nurse collaborates with other health professionals and the public in promoting community, national, and international efforts to meet health needs.

9. The profession of nursing, as represented by associations and their members, is responsible for articulating nursing values, for maintaining the integrity of the profession and its practice, and for shaping social policy.

(ANA 2001)

is an individual, a family, or a community, and the promotion of health and safety in the health care environment. The guidelines for practice (informed consent, privacy and confidentiality, veracity, and non-discrimination) identified by Scanlon and Fibison (1995) were connected to the fundamental values and commitments of the nurse located in the first three provisions of the Code of Ethics. Respect for human dignity is the "fundamental principle that underlies all of nursing practice"..."irrespective of the nature of the health problem" (Code of Ethics, §1.1, §1.3). As genetic and genomic information provide more specific information about the uniqueness of individuals and the potential for health risks and diseases, respect for persons without consideration of their current or future health status will take on new meaning for nurses. The right to self-determination and other patient rights will similarly expand as patients consider not only genetic testing decisions but also gene therapy or gene manipulation to avoid negative health states.

The advancement of genetic and genomic science already has nurses asking questions about their commitment to the "identified patient" and the difficulties that arise in "addressing patient interest [and determining] recognition of the patient's place in the family or other network of relationship" (Code of Ethics, §2.1). The ability to utilize a process of decision-making within the context of the Code of Ethics will become increasingly necessary as nurses rationalize their ethical decisions and actions.

Current concerns around privacy and confidentiality, as well as, the storage, retrieval, and use of patient information will likely yield to increasing pressures to find new mechanisms to assure protections in this area. New concerns about easily transportable electronic medical records, data chips and cards, and the ability of our nation to support and protect a national data set of patient records are questions with ethical implications that must be answered. The duties of the nurse in protecting patient information and making disclosures will become more complex ethical decisions as the knowledge and relationship of personal genetic information between relatives is understood. Since the duties of the nurse around confidentiality are not absolute, decisions about modifications in order to protect the patient, other innocent parties, and in circumstances of mandatory disclosure for public health reasons (ANA Code of Ethics §3.2) will become multifaceted, requiring more nursing knowledge and judgment in determining the boundaries of duty and loyalty.

ANA Code of Ethics Provisions 4, 5, and 6 address the nurse's boundaries of duty and loyalty. Nurses are accountable and responsible for providing optimal care. The nurse's obligation to provide optimal care is subject to an ever-increasing knowledge base. Accountability and responsibility imply that the nurse is competent and making judgments using knowledge, education, and skill. The introduction of genetic and genomic information into the practice setting is projected to impact almost every disease and health condition except perhaps trauma. The application of genetic and genomic knowledge to practice will be essential, thus, effectively expanding the areas of nursing knowledge, responsibility, and accountability.

When practice changes the incorporation of new knowledge is necessary to maintain competence. "Educational resources should be sought by nurses and provided by institutions to maintain and advance the competence of nurses" (Code of Ethics, §4.3). The commitment of nurses to lifelong learning (Code of Ethics, §5.2) will enable nurses to obtain the knowledge and skill needed to manage the impact of increasing genomic information on patient care. The established Core Competencies for nurses in genetics and genomics serve as a baseline for the development of curricula for initial education and continuing education for nurses.

Increasing genetic and genomic science will also impact the health care environments where nurses practice. Nurses will have responsibilities in the establishment of policies that assure organizational structures support nursing practice and promote patient rights. "Organizational changes are [often] difficult to accomplish and may required persistent efforts over time" (Code of Ethics, §6.3). Nurses will need to engage in individual and collective action to assure that nursing practice environments keep pace with rapidly changing science and inherent ethical issues.

Nursing duties beyond individual patient encounters are described in the final three provisions of the Code of Ethics for Nurses (Provisions 7, 8, and 9). Advancing health and retaining the value of nursing to society is the responsibility of every nurse. Nurses, both individually and collectively, should participate in the policy decisions related to changes brought about by the integration of increased genetic and genomic information in patient care. The public trusts nurses and expects nurses to assist them as they navigate the health care system. The role of nurses as advocates and educators of the public will increase as the health care environment becomes more complicated with additional information. Concerns around the use of genetic and genomic information, such as, access, privacy, quality, cost, and impact on culture, that threaten the provision of ethical health care make policy discussions and nursing participation in those discussions of paramount importance. Nurses' participation in broad discussions around genetics and genomics, beyond the level of the individual patient, will assure improved health care for all persons.

Nurses speak with the strongest voice when they speak collectively and with consensus. The expression of the values and ethics of the profession are reviewed and confirmed through professional associations (Code of Ethics, §9.2). The establishment of Core Competencies is an example of how nurses through their organizations are defining educational goals and responsibility for the profession. More than 25 national nursing associations endorsed the Core Competencies, giving credibility to their significance. Further reflection and ultimately action on how nursing will implement these educational criteria will define how nurses maintain the integrity of the profession. Envisioning the inclusion of genetic information gathered by nurses along with the family history and initial assessment is only a fragment of what the future might hold in terms of new practices.

Engaging in the science of genetics and genomics "through the ongoing development of nursing knowledge derived from nursing theory, scholarship, and research in order to guide nursing actions" (Code of Ethics, §9.2) will result in evidence-based nursing practice. Nurses should not shy away from, but rather should embrace the opportunity to participate in and gain understanding about the newest scientific discoveries that will revolutionize patient care. Nursing organizations through their participation in the work of NCHPEG are creating the foundation of information needed for health professional knowledge in genetics. Diagnosis, disease management, and drug therapy are among the areas of health care that are anticipated to change as a result of the unfolding science of the human genome. Ultimately, the goal of the profession is to reshape nursing practice based on evidence to benefit the health care of all persons.

A profession by its very definition is a body defined by a code of ethics. Although the current Code of Ethics for Nurses does not make not specific reference to genetics, the applicability of the Code of Ethics to genetics and genomics is apparent in all areas defined by the document. The Code of Ethics assures patients that nurses will provide quality care and advocate for patients when the issues presented by the rapidly advancing science of genetics and genomics arise. Nurses, cognizant of the potential for threats to patient rights, are engaging in a dialog to better understand the ethical issues and be prepared to resolve issues that arise in practice. Nurses are working collaboratively with their colleagues in the other health professions to adapt to and prepare for the practice changes resulting from advances in genetic and genomic science. Collectively and collaboratively with their interdisciplinary colleagues, nurses are engaging in educational efforts that identify areas of educational competence and strategies that will assist nurses and other health providers as we traverse the impact of new scientific knowledge on patient care. Nurses, who are at the forefront of patient care, must be active participants of change not only at the bedside, but also in communities and larger forums that will result in shaping our nation's future health care.

References

American Nurses Association. 1994. *Position statement: The nonnegotiable nature of the ANA code of ethics for nurses with interpretive statements.* http://www.nursingworld.org/MainMenu Categories/HealthcareandPolicyIssues/ANAPositionStatements/EthicsandHumanRights/ prtetcode14446.aspx (accessed September 16, 2008).

———. 2000. *Position statement: Human cloning by means of blastomere splitting and nuclear transplantation.* http://www.nursingworld.org/MainMenuCategories/Healthcareand PolicyIssues/ANAPositionStatements/EthicsandHumanRights/prtetclone14445.aspx (accessed September 16, 2008).

———. 2001. *Code of ethics for nurses with interpretive statements.* Silver Spring, MD: Nursesbooks.org.

Fowler, M. 1999. Relic or resource? The code for nurses. *American Journal of Nursing* 99 (3): 56–57.

Jenkins, J., K. Calzone, D. H. Lea, and C. Prows. 2008. *Essential nursing competencies and curricula guidelines for genetics and genomics.* http://www.nursingsociety.org/aboutus/ Documents/geneticscompetency.pdf (accessed October 7, 2008).

Nightingale, Florence. 1860. *Notes on nursing: What it is and is not.* Harrison & Sons: London. (Edition used: 1969. New York: Dover.)

Scanlon, C., and W. Fibision. 1995. *Managing genetic information: Implications for nurses.* Washington, DC: American Nurses Publishing.

CHAPTER 2

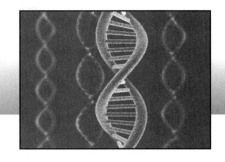

Integrating Ethical Guidelines with Scope and Standards of Genetics and Genomics Nursing Practice

Karen Greco, PhD, RN, ANP

Since the initial publication of *Standards of Nursing Practice* by the American Nurses Association in 1973 (also available as an appendix in ANA 2004), nurses have been bound by the standards that guide their professional practice. Nurses are also bound by the scope and standards of the specialty in which they practice and codes of ethics that guide professional behavior. Few nurses understand why these documents are important and how they relate to each other and to nursing practice. This article will define the scope and standards of genetics and genomics nursing practice and discuss how codes of ethics for nurses serve to provide a guiding framework for carrying out the practice of genetics and genomics nursing outlined in the scope and standards of practice.

Increased access to genetic information and technology brings with it a host of ethical challenges. For example, how can nurses maintain an individual's genetic privacy by keeping genetic information confidential and still honor their duty to inform family members of potential risk for an inherited disease that could cause harm without medical intervention? How can nurses support patient autonomy and at the same time ensure no harm to the patient if patients want to pursue unregulated direct-to-consumer DNA testing through the Internet? These issues are not unique to genetics nurses and other genetics healthcare specialists. All nurses have a role in the management of genetic information and are therefore affected by ethical issues such as these. As the public continues to become more aware of genetic and genomic contributions to health and disease, nurses will be even more on the front lines addressing genetics- and genomics-related questions and the ethical issues that go with them.

Codes of Ethics for Nurses

All nurses are bound by a professional code of ethics, such as *Code of Ethics for Nurses with Interpretive Statements* (2001) and ICN Code of Ethics for Nurses (ICN 2006). Codes of ethics for nurses serve to provide a guiding framework for carrying out the practice of nursing outlined in the scope and standards of practice. Ethics codes give a framework for nurses' standards of conduct and assist nurses in translating standards into action (ICN 2006). They also help translate ethical principles such as autonomy, beneficence, confidentiality, fidelity, informed consent, justice, privacy, and veracity into behaviors expected of nurses as they practice nursing.

An ethical code offers an ordered series of key principles to guide practitioners, put forth by an authoritative professional organization (Olick 2004). Codes of ethics make explicit the goals and values of the profession and serve as moral principles that guide nurses' behavior and decisions (ANA 2004). Ethical codes provide a framework to set the ethical standards for the profession and serve as a tool for nurses to use in ethical analysis and decision-making (ANA 2004).

The core of ANA's *Code for Nurses with Interpretive Statements* are nine fundamental ethical provisions to guide ethical behavior and decision making for professional nurses. Each principle has several subcategories with one or more paragraphs that serve as interpretive statements, which describe how nurses can implement these principles. *ICN Code of Ethics for Nurses* is a briefer document listing four categories under which general standards of ethical conduct are organized: Nurses and People, Nurses and Practice, Nurses and the Profession, and Nurses and Co-Workers. For example, "The nurse ensures that the individual receives sufficient information on which to base consent for care and related treatment" is one of the principles listed under "Nurses and People" (ICN 2006, 4). There are no interpretive statements, and this document is much more general. The ANA document is much more specific and comprehensive, and includes the integration and application of ethical principles such as respect for human dignity, protecting confidentiality, self-determination, informed consent, and safeguarding privacy. In genetics nursing the ANA code of ethics may be more useful for the practicing nurse because of the additional content. For example:

> *Provision 3.* The nurse promotes, advocates for, and strives to protect the health, safety, and rights of the patient.

> *3.1 Privacy.* The nurse safeguards the patient's right to privacy. The need for health care does not justify unwanted intrusion into the patient's life. The nurse advocates for an environment that provides for sufficient physical privacy, including auditory privacy for discussions of a personal nature and policies and practices that protect the confidentiality of information.

What Are Standards and Why Do We Need Them?

Standard setting and the accompanying self-regulation are primary attributes of a profession. Professional standards of practice for nursing help measure competency and provide definition and structure to the practice of nursing (Townes and Cook 2001). According to the American Nurses Association, "standards are authoritative statements by which the nursing profession describes the responsibilities for which its practitioners are accountable" (ANA 2004, 1).

Standards of practice also have legal implications which nurses need to understand. When standards for acceptable professional behavior are defined, nurses who do not meet these standards are potentially liable for negligence (Powell 2003). In medical negligence litigation the courts decide whether or not a healthcare professional's conduct in a particular instance falls below an acceptable "professional standard of care" (Rosenbaum 2003). Scope and standards of nursing practice are documents by which nurses can be judged in a court of law. Nurses also need to be aware of legislation affecting standards of nursing practice because Federal law supersedes both state law and professional standards. For example, standards or no standards, nurses have a legal obligation under federal law to follow the HIPAA (Health Insurance Portability and Accountability Act, enacted by Congress in 1996) privacy requirements (45CFR46) before sharing or discussing protected health information (PHI) with a family member, even a spouse (Muller and Flarey 2004).

Professional standards need to be broad to encompass a wide range of activities, and flexible enough to still be applicable as the profession evolves and changes over time (C. Bickford, personal communication, January 19, 2005). Standards are "living guidelines" (Muller and Flarey 2004, 255) and need to take into account the changing nature of health care and nursing practice so that the document remains applicable to changing practice and does not become easily outdated. The leadership of a profession is responsible for regularly examining, questioning, revisiting, and revising standards of practice (Muller and Flarey 2004).

Determining the Scope of Nursing Practice

The scope of nursing practice describes "the *who, what, where, when, why,* and *how* of nursing practice" and provides the boundaries of nursing practice and who can practice it (ANA 2004, 1). The International Society of Nurses in Genetics (ISONG) scope of practice refers to "a range of nursing functions and abilities that are differentiated according to level of practice, role of the nurse, and work setting" (ISONG and ANA, 1998, 97). According to the International Council of Nurses, "scope of practice is defined within a legislative regulatory framework, and communicates to others the roles, competencies, and the professional accountability of the nurse" (ICN 2000). The scope of practice parameters are a framework to guide nursing practice and are complemented by professional codes of ethics, nursing practice standards, and the legislative or regulatory framework in which the nurse practices. For example, in the United States the nurse practice act for each state influences what activities or functions the nurse is allowed to perform in that state. Similarly, different countries have regulations defining the scope of nursing practice. Scope and standards of nursing practice flow from the definition of nursing practice and represent the essence of what nurses do. "Ethics guide scope through an individual ability to accept and manage consequences, in accordance with safe standards of practice" (Klein 2005).

Evolution of Genetics Nursing Practice as a Specialty

Nurses have been involved in genetic counseling and education since the 1960s, when nurses provided services to children with genetic disorders and their families. In 1984 a small group of nurses practicing in genetics formed the Genetics Nursing Network, which later became ISONG. In 1988, ISONG was incorporated as a nursing specialty organization dedicated to fostering the scientific and professional growth of nurses in human genetics worldwide (ISONG 2007). ISONG is the official professional organization of nurses in genetics in the United States and also represents genetics nurses worldwide. In 1997 ISONG worked with ANA to establish genetics nursing as an official specialty of nursing practice. This was followed by the publication of the scope and standards of clinical genetics nursing practice as a collaborative effort between the ANA and ISONG (ISONG and ANA, 1998). See Table 2–1 for this timeline.

TABLE 2–1
Milestones in Genetics Nursing Practice

1960s   Nurses publishing about the nurse's role in genetics and conducting genetics research.

1984   Genetics Nursing Network formed (later became ISONG).

1988   International Society of Nurses in Genetics (ISONG) incorporated.

1997   Genetics Nursing designated an official nursing specialty by American Nurses Association.

1998   *Statement on the Scope and Standards of Genetics Clinical Nursing Practice* published by ISONG and ANA.

2001   ISONG approved formation of the Genetic Nursing Credentialing Commission (GNCC).

2001   Credentialing of the first Genetics Advanced Practice Nurses (APNG).

2002   GNCC goes online at www.geneticnurse.com, develops a logo, and is incorporated.

2002   Credentialing of the first Genetic Clinical Nurses (GCN).

2007   *Genetics and Genomics Nursing: Scope and Standards of Practice* published by ISONG and ANA.

Scope and Standards of Genetics and Genomics Nursing Practice

ANA is responsible for defining the scope and standards of practice for the nursing profession as a whole in the Unites States. ISONG, as the nursing specialty organization representing genetics nurses, is responsible for defining and establishing the scope of professional nursing practice in genetics as a specialty nursing practice. ISONG has been the leader in defining genetics nursing practice, establishing scope and standards of practice for genetics nurses, and providing resources and support to establish credentialing for genetics nurses based on these standards of practice.

Through ISONG's efforts, in 1997 ANA established genetics nursing as an official nursing specialty. This was followed by publication of *Statement on the Scope and Standards of Genetics Clinical Nursing Practice* by ISONG and ANA in 1998, a landmark accomplishment for genetics nursing as a specialty practice. This document defined the parameters of genetics nursing practice, influenced genetics education programs, and served as the foundation for credentialing of genetics nurses. The roles and practice of nurses in genetics have evolved and expanded since the publication of the original scope and standards of clinical genetics nursing practice. In addition, ANA made significant revisions to the scope and standards of practice with publication of the 2004 *Nursing: Scope and Standards of Practice,* including a new template for standards documents created by nursing specialty organizations. ISONG, in collaboration with ANA, has created a new document entitled *Genetics and Genomics Nursing: Scope and Standards of Practice* (2007) that reflects current genetics nursing practice based on this more general ANA template. The purpose of the new scope and standards document is to define the parameters of genetics nursing practice at both basic and advanced practice levels.

This latest revision is different from the 1998 *Scope and Standards of Genetics Clinical Nursing Practice* in several key areas. The 2007 document reflects the evolution and expansion of genetics nursing and represents all areas of genetics nursing practice, including non-clinical roles such as education, research, and administration. Its language better reflects ISONG's presence as an international organization rather than an organization with international members. ANA recognizes that ISONG is an international organization and the scope and standards of genetics nursing practice may be adopted globally or serve as a foundation for scope and standards of genetics nursing practice in countries outside the United States.

The scope and standards of genetics nursing practice has also been revised to better reflect current nursing practice. For example, recent genetic and technology advances are helping us better understand how genetic changes affect human variation as well as the development of common diseases such as cancer, heart disease, Alzheimer's disease, and diabetes that are prevalent in adults (Greco 2003). Scientific discoveries have advanced clinical capabilities for diagnosing and treating rare single gene disorders, and increased our ability to predict susceptibility to many common diseases such as cardiovascular and autoimmune diseases, Alzheimer's disease, cancer, and diabetes through genetic testing. This expanding knowledge continues to affect how genetics services are defined and delivered (ISONG and ANA 2007). These changes also carry with them new ethical challenges such as the privacy and confidentiality of genetic information, and informed consent related to genetic testing, genetic research, and other genetics services.

Scope and Standards of Practice as a Foundation for Credentialing of Nurses in Genetics

ISONG perceived the importance of recognizing genetics nursing competency and formed a credentialing committee in 1999, which created a mechanism to promote credentialing of genetics nurses. Genetics nurses needed credentialing in order to establish competency in genetics and have their expertise recognized. From the ISONG scope and standards of genetics nursing practice, the credentialing committee compiled a list of competencies and associated measures for credentialing genetic nurses at the masters and baccalaureate level (Cook et al. 2003; Monsen 2005). In 2002, the Genetic Nursing Credentialing Commission (GNCC) was created as an organization separate from ISONG to oversee the credentialing of nurses in genetics in the United States. Credentialing for genetics nurses is based on a portfolio of accomplishments documenting the nurse's genetics expertise. Clinical competency is demonstrated by submitting case histories that show the nurse's ability to apply genetics knowledge according to the scope and standards of genetics nursing practice (Greco and Mahon 2001). These case histories also need to show the nurse's ability to address relevant ethical issues. This is an example of how standards of practice and ethical guidelines can be used to demonstrate clinical competence.

Scope of Genetics and Genomics Nursing Practice

The *Who* of Genetics Nursing Practice

In the scope of genetics and genomics nursing practice, genetics nurses are defined at the basic level and advanced level. These levels of practice can be distinguished by education, professional experience, practice focus, specific roles and functions, and certification or credentialing. Basic level genetics nurses are registered nurses who routinely provide genetics services to individuals, families, groups, communities, or populations. Nursing practice is evolving so all registered nurses will be providing basic level genetics services. There is also an expanded knowledge base for specialty practice.

- Basic level genetics nurses are expected to have either formal genetics clinical experiences through their entry level nursing preparatory programs or on-the-job training in their specified role under the supervision of a professional trained in genetics.
- Genetics nurses practicing at the advanced practice level must have a graduate degree in nursing, have completed graduate level genetics course work, and maintain current genetics knowledge through participation in continuing education and other activities. (ISONG and ANA 2007).

The definitions of genetics nurse and genetics nurse in advanced practice in the scope and standards of genetics and genomics practice are not identical to those used by GNCC in determining eligibility for credentialing of nurses in genetics. The GNCC credential is limited to nurses practicing in clinical genetics settings and does not include nurses in non-clinical roles, whereas the scope and standards of practice applies to genetics and genomics nurses in both clinical and non-clinical roles.

The scope of practice for genetics nurses in advanced practice is broader than the scope of practice for basic level genetics nurses. For example, genetics nurses in advanced practice can provide genetic counseling (ISONG and ANA 1998, 2007). "Genetic counseling provides patients with information about their condition and helps them make informed decisions" (National Human Genome Research Institute 2007).

The *What* of Genetics Nursing Practice

The *what* of genetics nursing practice encompasses the definition of genetics nursing and what nurses do as they care for the genomic health of individuals, families, communities, and populations. The definition of genetics nursing practice is based on the scope of nursing practice as defined by ANA (2004). The definition of genetics nursing practice in the revised scope of genetics nursing practice is as follows:

Genetics nursing is the protection, promotion, and optimization of health and abilities, prevention of illness and injury, alleviation of suffering through the diagnosis of human response, and advocacy in the care of the genomic health of individuals, families, communities, and populations. This includes health issues, genetic conditions, diseases or susceptibilities to diseases which are caused or influenced by genes in inter-action with other risk factors that may require nursing care (ISONG and ANA 2007).

The *Where* of Genetics Nursing Practice

Genetics nurses practice in a variety of healthcare and other settings which include but are not limited to: hospitals and their affiliated clinics; academic medical centers and universities; regional genetic centers; ambulatory and primary healthcare facili-ties; industrial, community, and school health settings; state and federal agencies; private industry, including clinical and biotechnology laboratories and pharmaceuti-cal companies; managed healthcare organizations; and healthcare recipient and provider insurance organizations. As genetic services continue to emerge in a greater variety of settings, especially primary care settings, the need for genetics nurses will similarly expand (ISONG and ANA 2007).

The *Why* and *How* of Genetics Nursing Practice: The Interface with Ethics

The *why* of genetics nursing practice goes back to the definition of genetics nursing, which is to protect, promote, and optimize health and abilities, prevent illness and injury, alleviate suffering, and advocate for the genomic health of individuals, fami-lies, communities, and populations. The *how* goes back to what nurses do as they engage in this process.

The *how* and *why* are primary areas where ethics interfaces with standards of nursing practice since ethics guide nurses' behavior. Under the ANA code of ethics (ANA 2001) autonomy, or self-determination, is the philosophical basis for informed con-sent in health care. "Patients have a moral and legal right to determine what will be done with and to their own person" (Provision 1.4). The standards of nursing prac-tice support this concept of autonomy expressed in the code by having standards that include involving the patient in holistic data collection, validating diagnoses or issues with the patient, and involving the patient in formulating expected outcomes (ANA 2004).

Here are a couple of examples of how beneficence (the responsibility to do good) and nonmaleficence (the responsibility to do no harm) are addressed in the code of ethics. The code of ethics addresses nonmaleficence by stating that the nurse has a responsibility to be vigilant to safeguard and protect the patient, and report and handle any unethical, incompetent, illegal, or impaired practice in the employment setting that may jeopardize the patient, the nurse, or others. For example, if a nurse were to observe genetic test results being copied from a patient chart to be sent to the patient's insurance company along with routine billing information without the patient's specific written consent, the nurse would have an ethical and legal obligation to intervene.

The code of ethics also says the nurse has a responsibility to maintain standards of professional practice (ANA 2001). By maintaining standards of professional nursing practice the nurse will be competent in his/her practice and able to carry out nursing care that benefits the patient. This is also another example of how the code of ethics and professional standards of practice work together.

The Ethics Standards in the Scope and Standards of Genetics Nursing Practice

Standards of genetics nursing practice follow the format of ANA's *Nursing: Scope and Standards of Practice* (2004) and consist of two sections: standards of practice and standards of professional performance. The standards of practice consist of six standards:

- Assessment
- Diagnosis
- Outcomes identification
- Planning
- Implementation
- Evaluation

The standards of professional performance consist of these nine standards:

- Quality of practice
- Practice evaluation
- Education
- Collegiality
- Collaboration
- Ethics
- Research
- Resource utilization
- Leadership

The ethics standard, reproduced as Table 2–2 on page 24, states "The genetics nurse employs ethical provisions in all areas of practice" (ISONG and ANA 2007). This is followed by the first measurement criterion, which states that the genetics nurse is guided by a code of ethics such as *Code of Ethics for Nurses with Interpretive Statements* (ANA 2001) or *ICN Code of Ethics for Nurses* (2000). Again, the professional standards of practice and code of ethics are related. The ANA code of ethics states that the nurse safeguards the patient's right to privacy and has a duty to maintain the confidentiality of information (ANA 2001). The ethics standard of performance criterion 3 states that the genetics nurse "maintains patient confidentiality within legal and regulatory parameters."

Each standard of genetics nursing practice includes measurement criteria for all genetics nurses and additional measurement criteria for genetics nurses in advanced practice. Again this follows the format of the ANA standards. Because genetic counseling is defined as an advanced practice skill, the ethics standard includes the following advanced practice criterion: "The genetics nurse in advanced practice addresses ethical issues related to the provision of genetic counseling services such as: informed consent, confidentiality, autonomy, and beneficence."

Wording in the standards for genetics nursing practice is intentionally broad and not intended to list every ethical situation that may occur in genetic nursing practice. For example, measurement criterion 9 for the ethics standard states that the genetics nurse "addresses ethical issues related to genetic information." This statement is general enough to apply as genetics nursing practice evolves, yet still covers any current situation in the nurse's practice that involves ethical issues related to genetic information, such as the privacy of genetic information, confidentiality of genetic test results, or informed consent for genetic research.

Summary

Standards of nursing practice help measure competency, provide definition and structure to the practice of nursing and describe the responsibilities for which nurses are accountable (ANA 2001). Professional standards need to be broad to encompass a wide range of activities and flexible enough to still be applicable as the profession evolves (C. Bickford, personal communication, January 19, 2005). Standards need to take into account the changing nature of health care and nursing practice so that they do not rapidly become outdated.

All nurses are bound by a professional code of ethics which makes explicit the goals, values, and obligations of the nursing profession (ANA 2001). A code of ethics provides a framework for nurses to use in ethical analysis and decision making and sets

TABLE 2–2
Standard 12, Ethics

The genetics nurse employs ethical provisions in all areas of practice.

Measurement Criteria:

The genetics nurse:

- Is guided by a code of ethics for nurses such as *Code of Ethics for Nurses with Interpretive Statements* (ANA 2001), ICN Code of Ethics for Nurses (2006), or a relevant national code of ethics.

- Provides care and services in a manner that preserves and protects the client's autonomy, dignity, and rights.

- Maintains client confidentiality within legal and regulatory parameters.

- Serves as a client advocate assisting clients in developing skills for self-advocacy.

- Maintains a therapeutic and professional client–nurse relationship within appropriate professional role boundaries. This also includes, but is not limited to, faculty–student, researcher–participant, and supervisor–subordinate relationships.

- Demonstrates a commitment to practicing self-care, managing stress, and connecting with self and others.

- Contributes to resolving ethical issues of clients, colleagues, or systems as evidenced in such activities as participating on ethics committees.

- Identifies ethical dilemmas in clinical practice and uses resources in formulating ethical responses.

- Addresses ethical issues related to genetics information.

- Participates in formulating guidelines about the ethical considerations of new and existing genetics services and technology.

- Reports illegal, incompetent, or impaired practices.

- Participates on multidisciplinary and interdisciplinary teams that address ethical risks, benefits, and outcomes.

- Informs administrators or others of the risks, benefits, and outcomes of programs and decisions that affect healthcare delivery.

(continued)

TABLE 2–2
Continued

Additional Measurement Criteria for the Genetics Nurse in Advanced Practice:

The genetics nurse in advanced practice:

- Informs the client of the risks, benefits, and outcomes of healthcare regimes such as genetic testing.
- Addresses ethical issues related to the provision of genetic counseling services, such as informed consent, confidentiality, autonomy, and beneficence.
- Participates in efforts to address ethical issues such as ethics committees and institutional review boards (IRBs).

the ethical standards for the profession (ANA 2004). Codes of ethics for nurses serve to provide a guiding framework for carrying out the practice of nursing outlined in the scope and standards of practice. Nurses have a responsibility to be familiar with and understand the implications of the scope and standards that define the parameters of nursing practice and the codes of ethics that guide professional behavior and decisions.

References

American Nursing Association (ANA). 1973. *Standards of nursing practice.* Kansas City, MO: American Nurses Publishing.

———. 2001. *Code of ethics for nursing with interpretive statements.* Washington DC: Nursesbooks.org.

———. 2004. *Nursing: Scope and standards of practice.* Silver Spring, MD: Nursesbooks.org.

Cook, S. S., R. Kase, L. Middelton, and R. B. Monsen. 2003. Portfolio evaluation for professional competence: Credentialing in genetics for nurses. *Journal of Professional Nursing* 19 (2): 85–90.

Greco, K. E. 2003. Nursing in the genomic era: Nurturing our genetic nature. *MEDSURG Nursing* 12 (5): 307–312.

Greco, K. E., and S. M. Mahon. 2001. Genetics nursing practice enters a new era with credentialing. *Internet Journal of Advanced Nursing Practice* 5 (2). http://www.ispub.com/ostia/index.php?xmlFilePath=journals/ijanp/vol5n2/genetics.xml (accessed October 7, 2008).

International Council of Nurses. 2006. *The ICN code of ethics for nurses.* http://ethics.iit.edu/codes/coe/int.council.nurses.2006.html (accessed October 7, 2008).

International Society of Nurses in Genetics (ISONG). 2007. Home page. http://isong.org (accessed October 7, 2008).

International Society of Nurses in Genetics (ISONG)/American Nurses Association (ANA). 1998. *Statement on the scope and standards of genetics clinical nursing practice.* Washington D.C.: American Nurses Publishing.

———. 2007. *Genetics and genomics nursing: Scope and standards of practice.* Silver Spring, MD: Nursesbooks.org.

Klein, T. A. 2005. Scope of practice and the nurse practitioner: Regulation, competency, expansion, and evolution. *Topics in Advanced Practice Nursing eJournal* 5 (2). http://www.medscape.com/viewprogram/4188 (accessed October 7, 2008).

Monsen, R. B. 2005. *Genetics nursing portfolios: A new model for credentialing.* Silver Spring.: Nursesbooks.org.

Muller, L. S., and D. L. Flarey. 2004. Consent for case management: Using the CMSA standards of practice. *Lippincott's Case Management* 9 (6): 254–256.

National Human Genome Research Institute. 2007. *Talking glossary.* http://www.genome.gov/glossary.cfm?key=genetic%20counseling (accessed October 7, 2008).

Olick, R. S. 2004. Ethics in public health. Codes, principles, laws, and other sources of authority in public health. *Journal of Public Health Management and Practice* 10 (1): 88–89.

Powell, S. K. 2003. Standards of practice for case managers: The bottom line. *Lippincott's Case Management* 8 (3): 97.

Rosenbaum, S. 2003. The impact of United States law on medicine as a profession. *Journal of the American Medical Association* 289 (12): 1546–1556.

Townes, J., and P. R. Cook. 2001. Standards of practice: A measure of competence. *Home Healthcare Nurse* 19 (6): 383–386.

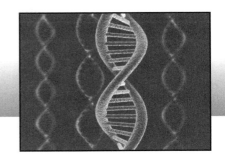

CHAPTER 3

Shaping Genetic Policy: The United States Initiatives

Agnes Masny, MSN, MPH, RN, CRNP

Introduction

With the completion of the Human Genome Project we now have a better understanding of the molecular cause and modification of specific diseases or conditions. Genetic technologies that accompany these discoveries are helping to predict who may be at risk for disease, to analyze gene interactions that modify disease, to establish clinical guidelines for diagnoses and prognoses of disease, to identify genes associated with diseases, and to screen newborns for disease. These new discoveries and technologies promise to provide genetic information about our family, our society, changing the life of every United States citizen. But how will these discoveries reach every American? How will they come to be used for good and not harm? Public health policy shapes the answer to this question.

Genetics Policy Development in the Context of Health Policy

Any new health discovery carries with it the potential of good or harm to the individual or society. Government oversight helps provide direction to influence legislation or judicial action that affects the allocation or regulation of specific goods to achieve benefits for society (Longest 2002). Strictly speaking, appropriate allocation and regulation of resources is the goal of all public health policy. The completion of the Human Genome Project and the multitude of genetic and genomic discoveries following the sequencing of the human genome have driven current health policy regarding genetics. This, in turn, has created public demand for genetic technologies and services and subsequent public concern about privacy, discrimination, access, stigmatization, and misuse of genetic information. Therefore genetic health policy must address the scientific and ethical challenges of genetic testing and technologies.

Policy in the United States is determined by the interaction of the executive, judicial and legislative branches of government and the public reaction to laws and policy. Public concern and civil suits may help to initiate a policy response at the executive or legislative level, such as the protections for the disabled provided by the Americans with Disabilities Act (ADA) of 1990. Or the accumulation of legal cases may draw attention to the need for legislative protections at the state or federal level. In 1996, the Health Insurance Portability and Accountability Act (HIPAA) was a legislative response to employees' concerns about losing health insurance after changing jobs or becoming unemployed.

Another approach to policy development is executive oversight of issues that affect the public. The Department of Health and Human Services (DHHS), one of the 15 executive departments, provides protection for the health and welfare of all Americans and access to essential human services. Although these departments fall under the executive branch of government, they influence legislation, policy, and national guidelines. Specifically, DHHS is responsible for many of the regulatory, programmatic, and financial aspects of the healthcare system and plays a key role in the planning, delivery, and financing of health care. DHHS programs are administered by 11 operating divisions, including 8 agencies in the Public Health Service and 3 human service agencies (agencies and divisions are listed online at http://www.hhs.gov/about/whatwedo.html/).

One of the roles of the executive departments is to advise the president on current policy and legislative actions, policy research, evaluation, and economic analysis of issues that the department oversees. Additionally, Public Law 92–463 of the Public Health Services Act provides for department heads to form and use advisory committees. This executive approach to policy formation has been widely used to address genetic issues. DHHS has provided a forum for expert discussion and public review of genetic issues through two of its advisory committees, the Secretary's Advisory Committee on Genetic Testing (SACGT), convened from 1998 to 2002, and the Secretary's Advisory Committee on Genetics Health and Society (SACGHS), convened in 2002 and actively meeting at this printing. Recommendations from these advisory committees have also helped to guide the secretary of DHHS in making policy recommendations (see Table 3–1).

TABLE 3–1
U.S. Genetic Policy Initiatives

1991	Ethical, Legal, and Social Issues (ELSI)	Program of the Human Genome Project to study ethical and social issues emerging from use of genetic information.
1995	Task Force on Genetic Testing	Charged by ELSI to make recommendations for safe and effective genetic tests.
1998	Secretary's Advisory Committee on Genetic Testing (SACGT)	Recommended by Task Force on Genetic Testing and chartered by Secretary of Health and Human Services (HHS) Donna Shalala to develop oversight measures for safe and effective genetic testing.
2002	SACGT	Disbanded by President George W. Bush.
2002	Secretary's Advisory Committee on Genetics, Health and Society (SACGHS)	Chartered by HHS Secretary Tommy Thompson for two years to study and advise secretary on broad range of genetic and genomic applications in health care and society.
2004	SACGHS	Has charter renewed for two years.

Ethical Considerations Regarding Genetics Prompts Government Response

Ethical concerns were recognized early as a potential impact of the Human Genome Project. These issues included confidentiality, genetic test accuracy, the burden of genetic knowledge for the individual, and the misuse of genetic information leading to discrimination or stigmatization. (Botkin 1990; Juengst 1997/1998). The Department of Energy (DOE) and the National Institutes of Health (NIH) also recognized these concerns and devoted 5% of the Human Genome Project budget to study the ethical, legal, and social issues arising from clinical use of genetic information. The Ethical, Legal and Social Issues (ELSI) program identified several topics for study and oversight, including how genetic information would be used, how genetic information affects members of a family or a community, privacy, confidentiality, patenting, access to personal sequence data by insurance companies, potential for job discrimination based on personal sequence data, and the prospects for genetic screening, therapy, and engineering.

In 1995, the Committee to Evaluate the Ethical, Legal and Social Implications Program of the Human Genome Project was charged with reviewing the work of the Joint NIH and DOE working group of ELSI. In turn, the committee charged a Task Force on Genetic Testing to review genetic testing in the United States and to make recommendations to ensure the development of safe and effective genetic tests. In its final report the Task Force on Genetic Testing identified four major areas of concern: "(1) the way in which tests are introduced into clinical practice; (2) the adequacy and appropriate regulation of laboratory quality assurance; (3) the understanding of genetics on the part of healthcare providers and patients; and (4) the continued availability and quality of testing for rare diseases" (NHGRI 1997). Although the task force recommended the establishment of a process for genetic test development and review, it did not specify changes in existing laboratory reviews to incorporate new genetic tests (Holtzman 1999). Thus, the formation of an advisory committee to the secretary of DHHS was recommended by the NIH-DOE Task Force on Genetic Testing and the Joint NIH-DOE Committee to evaluate the ELSI program of the Human Genome Project. These groups pointed out the need for public policy development in helping national leaders deal with the benefits and challenges of genetic testing and its corresponding information.

Secretary's Advisory Committee on Genetic Testing (SACGT)

Responding to the joint recommendations of the Task Force on Genetic Testing and the NIH-DOE committee, DHHS, under the directorship of Secretary of Health and Human Services Donna Shalala, chartered the SACGT in June of 1998. DHHS requested that SACGT build on the work of the task force to assess whether current programs for ensuring the accuracy and effectiveness of genetic tests were satisfactory. This assessment required consideration of the potential benefits and risks (including socioeconomic, psychological, and medical harms) to individuals, families, and society. If, after assessment and public consultation, further measures were deemed necessary, SACGT was further charged to recommend oversight measures for genetic tests.

SACGT was primarily charged with assessing oversight of genetic tests, but the training and education of healthcare providers and the promotion of greater public understanding of genetics were also key areas for policy consideration. Public consultation was a key strategy for SACGT; genetic public policy needed the input of a wide range of stakeholders. Therefore, attempts to gather public input included requests for public comment in the Federal Register, mailings to professional organizations, opportunities to provide public comments during meetings, and specially convened public meetings to gather the public's perspective on genetic testing limitations, benefits and risks, and the accessibility of genetic tests to diverse populations (SACGT 1999).

Secretary's Advisory Committee on Genetics Health and Society (SACGHS)

With a change in administration in 2002, the SACGT was disbanded. In September 2002, Secretary of Health and Human Services Tommy Thompson chartered a new advisory committee to continue the discussion and deliberations on the ethical and social issues raised by advances in genetics. SACGHS was charged with a range of functions including:

> assessing how genetic technologies are integrated into health care and public health; studying the clinical, ethical, legal, and societal implications of genetic applications, such as pre-implantation diagnosis and emerging technological approaches to clinical testing; identifying opportunities and gaps in research and data collection efforts; exploring the use of bioterrorism; examining patent policy and licensing practices for their impact on access to genetics technologies; analyzing uses of genetic information

in education, employment, insurance, including health disability, long-term care, and life, and law, including family, immigration, and forensics; and serving as a public forum for discussion of emerging scientific, ethical, legal, and social issues raised by genetic technologies. (DHHS 2002)

Early deliberations of SACGHS recognized that the scope of the committee's work included both genetics and genomics. Whereas genetics focuses one or a few germlines—inherited or acquired mutations in the genome associated with a specific diseases or conditions—genomics focuses on a large number of genes in the genome as they interact with endogenous and exogenous factors impacting health and disease (SACGHS 2006; Guttmacher, Collins, and Drazen 2004). Discussions and recommendations of SACGHS regarding genetic tests and services were expressly intended to cover future uses of genetic and genomic technologies.

Initially health professionals objected that attention to recommendations already made from the SACGT would be diluted or lost in the broad range of issues proposed for SACGHS (Michaels, Bingham, Boden, Clapp, Goldman, Hoppin, et al. 2002). However, SACGHS has tried to incorporate the previous work and advice of SACGT into its own. Furthermore, SACGHS has made attempts to identify critical issues. Early meetings included informational presentations designed to provide the committee with an understanding of the issues encompassed in its charter and the background needed to identify and prioritize issues. For example, leading experts reviewed existing and emerging directions in genetic technologies and their clinical and public health applications; the financing of genetic technologies in the U.S. healthcare system; and future directions in genetics and genomics research, to name a few. After hearing from experts SACGHS appointed an advisory committee to design a prioritization process, by which they arrived at twelve genetic/genomic technologies and services:

- Access
- Coverage and reimbursement
- Direct-to-consumer marketing
- Genetic discrimination
- Genetic education and training
- Genetic exceptionalism (treating genetic information as distinct from medical information and requiring special consideration)
- Large population studies
- Oversight of genetic testing
- Patents and access
- Pharmacogenomics

- Public awareness
- Vision statement

The committee organized the priority issues into four categories (see Figure 3–1):

- High-priority issues that warrant more in-depth study,
- High-priority issues that can be addressed in a relatively straightforward way or with short-term action plans,
- High-priority issues requiring only monitoring, and
- Overarching issues that should be considered within the context of deliberations and recommendations for all issues.

FIGURE 3–1
SACGHS Categories of Genetics/ Genomics Priority Issues in Health Care

Overarching Issues, Shaping Deliberations for All Priority Issues

↓   ↓   ↓

ACCESS   PUBLIC AWARENESS   GENETIC EXCEPTIONALISM

HIGH PRIORITY ISSUES FOR

IN-DEPTH STUDY	SHORT-TERM ACTION AND MONITORING	MONITORING
• Coverage and Reimbursement of Genetic Technologies and Services	• Genetic Discrimination	• Patents and Access
• Large Population Studies	• Education and Workforce Training	• Oversight of Genetic Tests
• Pharmacogenomics	• Vision Statement	
• Direct-to-Consumer Marketing of Genetic Tests		

(SACGHS 2004a)

The priority issues and their policy considerations, with the exception of public awareness and the vision statement, are discussed below. These priority issues are abridged from *A Roadmap for the Integration of Genetics and Genomics into Health and Society* (SACGHS 2004a) and can be viewed in their entirety online. The issues of public awareness and a vision statement pertain to all the other priority areas, but by themselves do not raise specific ethical concerns.

Access to Genetic Technologies

Barriers to the accessibility of genetic technologies can prevent patients and consumers from fully benefiting from genetic services and advances in genetics. Both SACGT and SACGHS recognized the importance of populations having access to genetic research and technologies. The cost of genetic testing and services as well as insurance coverage were identified as potential barriers to access.

Policy Considerations

- The federal government places a high priority on access to health care.
- Many issues in genetics have an access component. Access provides a context to consider all priority issues.
- Barriers to and disparities in access are issues endemic to the entire healthcare system, and because genetics is integrated in numerous medical disciplines, efforts to address specific aspects of access throughout the healthcare system may be difficult and better addressed by a legislative body with a broader mandate.

Policy Efforts

Several SACGT efforts were directed to explore the financial barriers to access as well as disparities in access to genetic testing services. SACGT formed an Access Working Group and contributed to a Coverage and Reimbursement Issue Brief. The work group also held a town meeting on disparities in access to genetic testing. Since SACGHS identified access to genetic technologies as an overarching issue, this priority issue became a recurrent theme for all the other issues. Further details on SACGT's and SACGHS's efforts are found under "Coverage and Reimbursement."

Coverage and Reimbursement of Genetic Technologies

Decisions made by public and private health plans about coverage and reimbursement influence the quality and cost of health care. Coverage and reimbursement also influences individuals' access to providers, services, procedures, and tests. Eighty-five percent of Americans have some health insurance through individual, employer-based plans or public insurance programs such as Medicare and Medicaid. Therefore, health insurance coverage and reimbursement to genetic technologies is a key factor in access to services and health outcomes.

For the most part, coverage decisions, including those for genetic technologies, are made by private insurers on a case-by-case basis or by a formal coverage policy that is applicable to all plan holders. Most formal policies include criteria for coverage, such as the presence of evidence-based risk factors (e.g., symptoms, family history) or that the results will influence treatment decisions.

Policy Considerations

- Medicare payments are important, as they establish the upper limit of what Medicaid can pay for the same service and may provide the basis on which private healthcare payers determine payment amounts.

- By law, Medicare cannot cover screening tests done in the absence of signs, symptoms, or personal history of disease.

- Most health plans provide coverage for preventive service. Genetic tests, on the other hand, are not generally covered.

- The Clinical Laboratory Fee Schedule is established by the Centers for Medicare and Medicaid Services (CMS) and determines Medicare's payment amounts for laboratory tests including genetic tests.

- Because the U.S. healthcare financing system is complex and involves numerous stakeholders, recommendations on coverage and reimbursement need to target all sectors: federal agencies and programs (e.g., CMS/Medicare, Agency for Healthcare Research and Quality, Health Resources and Services Administration, Federal Employee Health Benefit Plan, military health plan), state agencies and programs (e.g., Medicaid), and the private and professional sectors.

- Recommendations aimed at federal programs may be effective based on SACGHS's placement within DHHS and its advisory role to the secretary of DHHS.

- Recommendations calling for changes in the Medicare statute would require congressional approval.

Policy Efforts

The SACGT heard about practices and policies for reimbursement for genetic tests and services including various types of public and private insurance, e.g., Medicare, Medicaid, managed care, and indemnity insurance. SACGT drafted a report on coverage and reimbursement for genetic testing services that included recommendations on research to support evidence-based coverage and reimbursement decisions. However, final action was not taken on this report since the SACGT's charter was not renewed. Nonetheless, SACGT efforts helped promote the subsequent development of the Evaluation of Genomic Application in Practice and Prevention Project (EGAPP) that is systematically evaluating genomic applications (CDC 2004).

SACGHS picked up the issue of coverage and reimbursement as a priority area needing in-depth study and completed its own report (SACGHS 2006), which can be accessed online. Two recommendations from the SACGHS for the secretary of HHS included:

- Genetic tests with a preventive component should be considered specifically with respect to the benefit they could offer the populations they serve. Private payers would do well to make their own coverage determination about preventive tests and services rather than follow Medicare's lead.
- The secretary should assign an appropriate group to develop a set of principles for deciding which tests should be covered. The criteria should clarify the existing analytical and clinical validity, clinical utility of tests, and any gaps in evidence (SACGHS 2006).

Direct-to-Consumer Marketing

Concerns have been raised about direct-to-consumer (DTC) advertising of genetic tests and products, both in health care and in non-health-related areas. In addition, even greater concern has been raised about direct access to genetic tests and products. The advertising and sale of medical services and products directly to consumers has become a common and generally accepted practice. The average consumer lacks the background to critically evaluate marketers' claims. Direct access to genetic technologies raises other concerns because their complex nature often necessitates careful interpretation by well-trained health professionals. The Food and Drug Administration (FDA) and the Federal Trade Commission (FTC) both have roles in protecting consumers from false and misleading advertisements in the healthcare arena. FTC has primary jurisdiction for truth in advertising of foods (including supplements) and over-the-counter drugs and devices. FDA maintains jurisdiction over the labeling and advertising of prescription drugs. Also, FDA has jurisdiction over suspected cases of misrepresentation in advertising or labeling for over-the-counter drugs and devices.

Policy Considerations

- Consumers are entitled to health information that balances benefits against the risk of harm.

- Consumers expect to take an active role in their healthcare decisions. DTC marketing can help consumers gather information and discuss it with their healthcare provider.

- DTC advertising can lead to inappropriate requests for tests and medications.

- Direct harm may be caused by invalid tests, testing when not indicated, and inaccurate or misleading test results which can lead to inappropriate or harmful therapeutic choices and undermine the public's trust in genetic technologies.

- Consumers have direct access to non-health-related genetic testing (e.g., paternity, ancestry testing).

- Is there a need for a broader regulatory system to protect the public and ensure that they are receiving accurate information?

Policy Efforts

SACGT compiled a report (2000) which recommended that current FDA and FTC regulations be enforced in the area of genetic test promotion and marketing. SACGT also held a session on FDA and FTC regulations governing the labeling, promotion, and advertising of medical devices.

SACGHS followed the guidance of SACGT and also recommended enhanced collaboration between the FDA and the FTC in monitoring direct-to-consumer advertising for genetic tests. SACGHS encouraged relevant DHHS agencies to analyze the public health impact of such marketing and direct access to genetic tests. DHHS agencies and the FTC took steps to respond to these suggestions. Two inter-agency work groups have been formed to help monitor claims made by companies advertising genetic tests on the Internet and to evaluate the public health impact of direct-to-consumer marketing of genetic tests. The first work group, composed of staff from FTC, FDA, CDC, and NIH, is providing a forum for DHHS agencies to collaborate with FTC in the assessment of the scientific accuracy of claims made by companies advertising genetic tests on the Internet. The second work group, composed of representatives from FDA, CDC, NIH, and the Health Resources and Services Administration (HRSA), is exploring mechanisms for collecting data on the public health impact of direct-to-consumer marketing of genetic tests. Both of these efforts will benefit greatly from the collective resources and expertise of CDC, FDA, HRSA, and NIH (SACGHS 2004b).

Genetic Discrimination

As genetic technologies move from discovery into mainstream clinical medicine, they have the potential to greatly improve human health and the health status of the population. However, there are concerns that patients are not taking advantage of genetic services or participating in genetic research studies because of fears that they may be discriminated against based on genetic information. Although very few actual cases of genetic discrimination in health insurance and employment have been documented, perceptions persist that such discrimination is occurring or will occur in the future.

Policy Considerations

- SACGHS made recommendations on the need for federal protections and expressed support for the Genetic Information Nondiscrimination Act (GINA) proposed in the House (H.R. 493) and in the Senate (S. 358). These bills— passed into law in May 2008—proposed protection for all Americans from the misuse of genetic information in employment and health insurance decisions (GINA 2008; NHGRI 2008).

- Further recommendations in this area could be premised on the passage of federal genetic non-discrimination legislation or, failing passage, other policy approaches.

- Would federal genetic nondiscrimination law interact with existing law in the areas of health insurance, employment and discrimination? Statutes in these areas, including the Americans with Disabilities Act (ADA), the Health Insurance Portability and Accountability Act (HIPAA), and the Employee Retirement Income Security Act, are complex and their relatedness has not been fully tested.

- Federal law in this area could be construed as taking a genetic exceptionalist approach, which asserts the uniqueness of genetic information and its impact on individuals and families. (This approach is discussed later in this chapter on pages 42–43.) Its enactment may be informative about whether exceptionalism influences public perceptions of genetic determinism (the view that genes are solely responsible for physical and behavioral attributes), utilization of genetic services, and participation in genetic research. In a society that tends to embrace genetic determinism, a law that is exceptionalist in nature may serve to solidify that belief.

- Federal law may assuage the fear stemming from genetic determinism by protecting against the possibility of harm. However, no research to date has been done on specific state or federal laws to assess their impact on beliefs about genetic determinism.

Policy Efforts

SACGT wrote two letters on the subject of genetic discrimination, one to Secretary Shalala in April of 2000 and one to Secretary Thompson in May of 2001. The first letter expressed SACGT's concern over public misgivings about the potential for the misuse of genetic information and pointed out that these worries could lead to underutilization of beneficial genetic tests. Recognizing the potential harm from the use of genetic testing technologies, the committee expressed support for federal legislation to prohibit discrimination on the basis of genetic information in both employment and health insurance. SACGT believed that legislation would simultaneously prevent misuse of genetic information and ease fears about genetic discrimination.

SACGHS, in its first action as a committee, sent a letter to Secretary Thompson citing similar concerns expressed by SACGT and gave support for the Senate's bill prohibiting genetic discrimination in health insurance and employment. To garner further support for anti-discrimination legislation, SACGHS gathered key stakeholders' perspectives on the issue including consumers, health professionals, insurers, and employers. In October 2004, public testimony from patients and the public made it very clear that fears of potential misuse of genetic information deterred individuals from genetic testing, and that this fear, rather than best medical practice, shaped healthcare decisions. SACGHS compiled the following to drive home the weight of this issue:

- Over 300 pages of the public's comments regarding genetic discrimination (SACGHS, 2004c)
- A summary record on DVD of the October 2004 public testimony (SACGHS, 2005)
- An analysis of the adequacy of current law protecting against genetic discrimination (Lanman, 2005). This analysis was commissioned by SACGHS with the assistance of the Department of Justice, Department of Labor, Equal Employment Opportunity Commission, and, within the Department of Health and

Human Services, the Office for Civil Rights and Centers for Medicare and Medicaid Services.

This analysis concluded that no federal laws directly or comprehensively address the issues raised by the use of genetic information. Other conclusions also highlighted the substantial gaps in the current laws that could lead to confusion for consumers, insurers, and employers, as well as the potential for costly litigation.

In due course, the Genetic Information Nondiscrimination Act of 2008 was signed into law on May 21, 2008 after having been passed by the Senate unanimously and the House of Representatives 414 to 1.

Genetics Education and Training of Health Professionals

Our increasing understanding of the role of genetics and genomics in human health and disease is expected to yield more targeted approaches to health care and public health. Because of the interdisciplinary nature of genetics, a wide range of health professionals will need training in genetics to achieve optimal use of genetic technologies and ensure the appropriate integration of genetic knowledge into the healthcare and public health systems. Currently, health professionals are not sufficiently trained and educated in genetics to meet these goals, and efforts are lacking both during professional education and training and throughout clinical practice.

Policy Considerations

- Appropriate education in genetics and genomics is crucial to ensure the effective and efficient integration of genetic and genomic technologies and services into clinical and public health practice and to ensure equitable access.

- Published literature shows that there remain inadequacies in provider knowledge about genetics and the ability to implement this knowledge in clinical practice. Gaps in nursing genetic education and training were well defined by a report on experts on genetics and nursing (Health Resource and Services Administration 2000).

- The federal government may have a role in facilitating the translation of genetics into practice, but not necessarily in developing guidelines, curricula, or educational tools that might more appropriately be under the purview of health education professionals through funding and leadership.

- The federal government already takes a lead role in the funding of the education of healthcare professionals through programs authorized under Title VII and Title VIII of the Public Health Service Act, which can serve as a mechanism for encouraging change.

Policy Efforts

SACGT formed a work group to identify gaps or areas in need of improvement regarding genetics education of health professionals. SACGT staff assigned to the Education Work Group also undertook extensive fact-finding and analysis in the area of genetics education and training of health professionals, and presented findings to the committee in August 2001. Over the next two years, the work group convened a roundtable and organized a policy conference to gather the perspectives of the public and leaders in health education and practice. Topics included the challenges of incorporating genetics into the education of health professionals and ways to address problem areas and gaps. The work group was in the process of developing a report when SACGT's charter was not renewed.

SACGHS also took up the issues surrounding genetics education, training, and workforce. A working group conducted surveys and interviews with health professional organizations including medical, nursing, public health, dental, and allied health professional organizations to assess the need for genetics and genomic education and training. The findings confirmed the previous gaps in education as well as the need to broaden the focus of education and training to incorporate genomics and the need for clinically applicable educational models to allow for effective integration of genetic and genomics into practice, such as family history tools or web-based practice tools. SACGHS issued a Resolution on Genetics Education and Training of Health Professionals (SACGHS 2004d) in June 2004, that urged DHHS to actively incorporate into its policies and programs the philosophy that genetic information should be treated as part of the spectrum of health information and viewed as an integral part of the practice of all health professionals.

Further recommendations urged DHHS agencies to work with state, federal, and private organizations (e.g., the National Coalition for Health Professional Education in Genetics) to support the development and dissemination of practice models showing the applicability of genetics and genomics. Other recommendations that directly affected nursing were the support of federal programs for faculty training in genetics and genomics and collaboration with relevant professional organizations to incorporate genetic and genomic information into accreditation, licensure, and certification processes.

Genetic Exceptionalism

Genetic exceptionalism is the concept that genetic information is inherently unique, should receive special consideration, and should be treated differently from other medical information. According to this perspective, genetic information is special for a number of reasons:

- It is a unique identifier.
- It is heritable and shared through generations.
- It has relevance to family members.
- It can be predictive of future disease.
- It can, and has been, used to stigmatize and discriminate;.
- It can be sensitive and have psychological impacts.

Others hold that other types of medical information share these characteristics (e.g., HIV status can be sensitive, stigmatizing, and relevant to family members) and thus genetic information should not be treated differently from other medical information. The questions that center around this debate include the following:

- Is genetic information inherently unique?
- If genetic information is inherently unique, do its qualities warrant special attention?
- Should our public policies be premised on genetic exceptionalism?
- Does the idea of genetic exceptionalism serve a social good that should be advanced through laws and institutions?
- Is there an alternative concept that would allow the special features of genetic information to be acknowledged without necessitating a genetic exceptionalist approach?

Policy Considerations

- The challenge of effectively defining genetic versus non-genetic information for public policy purposes needs to be met.
- If genetic information were categorized as either highly sensitive or not sensitive, there would be debate about what information should be placed into each category and who should decide this.

- The physical separation of genetic from non-genetic information may be so complicated and costly as to actually interfere with the delivery of effective, high-quality care.

- These requirements may further frustrate attempts by healthcare practitioners to provide optimal care to their patients and may impede the sharing of relevant medical information.

- Adopting a genetic exceptionalist approach in law and policy may serve to reinforce the flawed perception of genetic determinism, a concept that inappropriately endows genetics with absolute power.

- Rejecting the genetic exceptionalist approach raises concerns about inadequate protection of genetic information, which may cause people to withhold information from healthcare providers or forgo genetic services altogether.

- As a pluralistic society, the United States favors making policy by an incremental approach. For this reason, a possible advantage of the genetic exceptionalist approach might be incremental progress on systematic examination of issues such as access to health care.

Policy Efforts

SACGT was mindful of the concerns about policy based on genetic exceptionalism, but did not carry out a formal study of its conceptual underpinnings, pros and cons, or societal and public policy implications. SACGHS considered genetic exceptionalism an overarching issue that would affect the deliberations of other issues. Attempts were made to use the context of genetic exceptionalism to balance adequate protections with the clinical integration of genetics and genomics into practice.

Large Population Studies

A number of countries around the world have undertaken national population studies that capitalize on the findings of the Human Genome Project to further study genetic variability within and across populations and to provide associations with this variability and common disease. The United States has no such large-scale cohort study specifically designed to further investigate the relationship between environmental factors, genetic markers, and common disease. The potential benefits of a national population study are identification of major susceptibility factors (genetic and environmental) for common diseases of public health consequence in the United States; determination of the true population risk of genetic variants; elucidation of the effect of environmental factors on disease; and identification of gene–gene and gene–environment interactions of major consequence.

Policy Considerations

- Is a large population study the most effective way to study gene environment interactions and their association with disease?

- Will the results of a large population study reduce health disparities by identifying targeted treatments for specific populations or worsen disparities through lack of access to the study's findings or clinical applications?

- Will the results have social implications for the understanding of race and group identity or increase the potential for stigmatization?

- How will recruitment and consent be obtained while maintaining appropriate protection against coercion?

- What is the role of the federal government in such a study, and are there obstacles that would make it especially difficult in the United States (e.g., the lack of a universal healthcare system or the lack of a uniform electronic medical record system)?

Policy Efforts

SACGT did not explore policy questions relevant to large population cohort studies aimed at advancing knowledge of the role of genetic variation in common, complex diseases. SACGHS established a task force to gather information about policy issues related to such a study. At the October 2005 meeting, SACGHS heard from members of the scientific and ethics community. Additionally, SACGHS discussed the NIH exploratory overview of how a U.S. population study could be designed and conducted (SACGHS 2005). SACGHS's role in this priority area was to help identify policy issues related to a large population study. The task force identified the following areas for further discussion:

- Strategies for public engagement to ensure a representative sample.

- Need for national and international collaboration to foster the usefulness of socio-demographic, epidemiologic, and genetic data.

- Guidelines for intellectual property rights from the study findings and ways to guarantee scientific access to the data.

- Strategies for notification of clinically significant study results to participants while ensuring confidentiality and privacy of participants.

At the October 2005 meeting, SACGHS decided there was significant reason for DHHS to support a large population study. The committee organized fact-finding and consultations with key stakeholders and issued a report (SACGHS 2007) on policy issues raised by such a study. The complete report can be accessed online.

Oversight of Genetic Technologies

FDA, CMS, CDC, and FTC all have roles in the oversight of the development, use, and marketing of genetic technologies. CMS certifies laboratories that provide health-related genetic testing to patients through the Clinical Laboratory Improvement Amendments (CLIA); CLIA certification ensures the analytical validity of health-related laboratory tests, but not their clinical validity. Oversight of genetic testing in non-health-related areas is largely the province of the private sector or professional organizations; the federal government does not have a role in regulating the availability of non-health-related genetic tests. As a result, laboratories may also offer unvalidated non-health-related genetic testing. FTC could take action against laboratories making false advertising claims about genetic tests, but it has not yet used its authority. Clinical laboratories that conduct genetic tests without oversight through CLIA must be identified and brought into CLIA compliance.

Policy Considerations

- There is consensus about the need for enhanced oversight of genetic tests. However, there is still debate about the most appropriate oversight mechanism for genetic tests and the laboratories that perform them.

- Proponents of oversight propose greater involvement of FDA. Opponents argue that laboratory development of genetic tests is a part of the medical practice of laboratory physicians and that while it has a role in ensuring the safety of medical devices, FDA is prohibited from interfering with the practice of medicine.

- Establishing clinical validity of genetic tests takes significant time and could slow the development of new genetic tests or cause laboratories to stop offering them.

- Strengthening the CLIA regulations might be a way to achieve enhanced oversight, while others believe that current CLIA regulations are sufficient and that additional regulations would burden laboratories doing genetic tests.

- CMS takes a flexible approach in certifying small academic research laboratories and provides technical assistance to laboratories seeking certification, but many laboratories conducting rare disease testing still believe that CLIA regulations are difficult and costly to meet.

- Do current regulatory mechanisms provide a balance between access, safety, competition, and independence of medical practice?

Policy Efforts

SACGT reviewed the oversight of genetic testing, including multiple levels of public consultation. The committee concluded that oversight was warranted for all genetic tests because of gaps in the existing federal oversight measures, the rapidly evolving nature of genetic tests, their anticipated widespread use, and extensive concerns expressed by the public about their potential for misuse or misinterpretation. The committee's report (SACGT 2000) recommended that the FDA should regulate genetic tests provided as laboratory services using a flexible approach to prevent the development of new tests. Expansion of CLIA regulations was proposed to incorporate specific provisions for genetic testing laboratories. The committee additionally urged the Secretary to provide DHHS agencies with sufficient resources to oversee genetic tests, including test review, enhanced CLIA oversight of testing laboratories, coordinated data collection, and information dissemination.

SACGT began a categorization scheme to classify genetic tests according to the level of risk and the level of review needed. The committee ultimately decided that no methodology would be able to distinguish high-risk tests. However, the FDA found SACGT's work identifying data elements critical to the evaluation of genetic tests to be most useful and modified these elements to help with device reviews.

The committee considers oversight a high-priority issue and is monitoring developments in this area, including calls for stronger regulation of genetic testing such as the Genetics and Public Policy Center's white paper submitted to CMS (Murphy, Javitt, and Hudson 2005). SACGHS also supports the work of the CDC's Office of Genomics and Disease Prevention through the Evaluation of Genomic Application in Practice and Prevention Project (EGAPP) developing a database with the evidence-based information on clinical experience with genetic tests (CDC 2004).

Patents and Access

Patents promote innovation by creating an incentive to disclose inventions publicly through the granting of exclusive rights for a limited period. Typically, disclosure of an invention spurs competitors to refine the underlying art and ideas or to find a better means to the same end. This is true of DNA-based inventions as well as any other. However, according exclusive rights to an invention limits future use of that invention and licensing fees add costs to biomedical research and to the healthcare system. In recent years, concerns have emerged that gene patents and licensing practices may be inhibiting research and blocking the development and performance of genetic testing services by clinical laboratories.

Policy Considerations

- U.S. courts have made it clear that inventions involving genes and genetic technologies are patentable subject matter.

- Do patent and licensing policies affect research in genetics and access to clinical genetic technologies in unique ways?

- How do patents protect the rights to intellectual property and encourage research investment without hindering access to scientific discovery that may be used for improvements in health care?

Policy Efforts

Both SACGT and SACGHS identified the issue of gene patenting as a policy concern that affects accessibility of genetic technologies. SACGT recommended further study by appropriate experts to determine whether certain gene patenting and licensing processes impair access. SACGHS made this issue a high priority for monitoring and established a task force on gene patents and licensing practices to further explore the work of the National Academy of Sciences (NAS 2005), available online.. SACGHS continues to study gene patents and the use of gene licensing by federal and private sectors in order make further recommendations regarding gene patent policy.

Pharmacogenomics

Individuals may respond differently to drugs because of differences in genetic makeup or the unique genetic features of the disease being treated. Genes play a role in how patients react to drugs and how effective they are. Pharmacogenomic testing may offer more individualized medicine: identification of genetic determinants may help to apply the appropriate pharmaceutical interventions—drug targets, drug transporters, and drug metabolizing enzymes—to patients based on the molecular nature of their disease and their genetic makeup. Pharmacogenomics is also being applied in the identification of new targets for drug development and in the evaluation of candidate drugs in the laboratory and in clinical drug trials.

Policy Considerations

- Pharmacogenomic tests may be expensive and may increase the cost of drugs and drug development.
- How will the clinical validity and utility of pharmacogenetic tests be established?
- Determining the role of genetic variation in common disease and its treatment will require the statistical power of large cohorts (see large population studies).
- Will pharmacogenomics promote or hinder access to new drugs in specific populations?
- Will the government require pharmacogenomic reassessment of existing drugs?
- What federal oversight is needed to determine the evidence that pharmacogenomic testing will improve healthcare outcomes, costs, and quality?
- How will the government monitor unintended adverse consequences, such as increasing healthcare costs and health disparities or creating orphan diseases (rare diseases or those effecting a subgroup of the population, which lead pharmaceutical companies to question the expense of research for small potential sales)?
- Pharmacogenomics may have unforeseen social impacts; for example, current notions of race and ethnicity may be challenged by pharmacogenomic data.

Policy Efforts

SACGT did not specifically look at pharmacogenomics; however, its recommendations on oversight of genetic testing apply to the development of pharmacogenomic tests. SACGHS heard from experts in the field of pharmacogenomics in June 2005. A task force on pharmacogenomics was then appointed to identify key issues for SACGHS deliberation. This committee identified four major areas for possible policy recommendations:

- research and development;
- infrastructure for data standards, regulation, and surveillance of safety and uptake of pharmacogenomic tests;
- integration of pharmacogenomics into clinical practice; and
- the ethical, legal, social, and economic issues of pharmacogenomics.

SACGHS recognized that the potential uptake of pharmacogenomics could be achieved if an ethical, regulatory, and legal framework helped to guide this integration. At this writing, SACGHS was preparing a report for the DHHS secretary which would address:

- the impact of pharmacogenomics on the use of race or ethnicity in tailoring drug treatments, with an emphasis on preventing stigmatization and discrimination;
- access to clinical trials in diverse populations;
- the costs or cost savings from tailored pharmaceuticals;
- allocation of resources for new innovations (e.g., CMS interpretation of Medicare Part D coverage of pharmacogenomic tests);
- changes in the informed consent process whereby potential informational harms and group harms (e.g., stigmatization of groups) would be addressed in pharmacogenomic research studies; and
- assurance of privacy and confidentiality.

Conclusions

The work of the Secretary's Advisory Committee on Genetic Testing and the Secretary's Advisory Committee on Genetics, Health, and Society illustrates the ways that public policy can address the ethical challenges of integrating genetic and genomic advances into society. The initiatives described here are public and professional efforts to help shape a national policy. These are initial steps of executive oversight in shaping public policy. The policy process requires further executive and legislative commitment and action to safeguard the public and ensure that all U.S. citizens will reap the benefits of genetic and genomic technologies.

References

Botkin, J. R. 1990. Ethical issues in human genetic technology. *Pediatrician* 17: 100–107.

Centers for Disease Control and Prevention (CDC). 2004. *Evaluation of genomic applications in practice and prevention (EGAPP): Implementation and evaluation of a model approach.* http://www.cdc.gov/genomics/gtesting/egapp.htm (accessed October 7, 2008).

Department of Health and Human Services (DHHS). 2002. *Charter: Secretary's advisory committee on genetics, health, and society.* http://www4.od.nih.gov/oba/sacghs/SACGHS_charter.pdf (accessed October 7, 2008).

GINA 2008. (Genetic Information Nondiscrimination Act of 2008; HR 493). http://frwebgate.access.gpo.gov/cgi-bin/getdoc.cgi?dbname=110_cong_bills&docid=f:h493enr.txt.pdf (accessed October 7, 2008).

Guttmacher, A., F. S. Collins, and J. M. Drazen. 2004. *Genomic medicine: Articles from the New England Journal of Medicine.* Baltimore MD: Johns Hopkins University Press.

Health Resources and Services Administration (HRSA). 2000. *Report of the expert panel on genetics and nursing: Implications for education and practice.* Washington, DC: HRSA.

Holtzman N.A. 1999. Promoting safe and effective genetic tests in the United States: Work of the task force on genetic testing. *Clinical Chemistry* 45 (5): 732–738.

Juengst, E.T. 1997/1998. Caught in the middle again: Professional ethical considerations in genetic testing for health risks. *Genetic Testing* 1 (3): 189–200.

Lanman, R.B. 2005. *An analysis of the adequacy of current law in protecting against genetic discrimination in health insurance and employment.* http://www4.od.nih.gov/oba/sacghs/reports/legal_analysis_May2005.pdf (accessed October 7, 2008).

Longest, B. 2002. *Health policymaking in the United States.* 3rd ed. Chicago: Health Administration Press.

Michaels, D., E. Bingham, L. Boden, R. Clapp, L. R. Goldman, and P. Hoppin, S. Krimsky, C. Monforton, D. Ozonoff, and A. Robbins, 2002. Advice without dissent. *Science* 298: 703.

Murphy, J., G. Javitt, and K. Hudson. 2005. *Creating a genetic testing specialty under CLIA: What are we waiting for?* Baltimore, MD: Genetics and Public Policy Center, Johns Hopkins University. http://www.dnapolicy.org/pub.reports.php?action=detail&report_id=25 (accessed October 7, 2008).

National Academy of Sciences (NAS). 2005. *Reaping the benefits of genomic and proteomic research: Intellectual property rights, innovation, and public health.* Prepublication. Washington, DC: National Academies Press. http://books.nap.edu/openbook.php?isbn=0309100674 (accessed October 7, 2008).

National Human Genome Research Institute. (NHGRI) 1997. *Promoting safe and effective genetic testing in the United States.* http://www.genome.gov/10002393 (accessed October 7, 2008).

———. 2008. Genetic Information Nondiscrimination Act: 2007–2008. http://www.genome.gov/24519851 http://www.genome.gov/10002393 (accessed October 7, 2008)

Secretary's Advisory Committee on Genetics Health and Society (SACGHS). 2004a. *A roadmap for the integration of genetics and genomics in society: A report on the study priorities of the Secretary's Advisory Committee on Genetics, Health and Society.* http://www4.od.nih.gov/oba/sacghs/reports/reports.html (accessed October 7, 2008).

———. 2004b. *Direct-to-consumer marketing of genetic tests.* The Secretary's Advisory Committee on Genetics, Health and Society Letter to the Secretary of Health and Human Services. http://www4.od.nih.gov/oba/sacghs/reports/reports.html (accessed October 7, 2008).

———. 2004c. *Public perspectives on genetic discrimination: September 2004–November 2004.* http://www4.od.nih.gov/oba/sacghs/reports/reports.html (accessed October 7, 2008).

———. 2004d. *Resolution of the Secretary's Advisory Committee on genetics, health and society on genetics education and training of health professionals.* http://www4.od.nih.gov/oba/sacghs/ reports/reports.html (accessed October 7, 2008).

———. 2005. *Perspectives on genetic discrimination.* http://www4.od.nih.gov/oba/SACGHS/ reports/reports.html#discrimination (accessed October 7, 2008).

———. 2006. *Coverage and reimbursement of genetic tests and services: Report of the Secretary's Advisory Committee on Genetics, Health and Society.* Washington, DC: Department of Health and Human Services.

———. 2007. *Policy issues associated with undertaking a new large U.S. populations cohort study of genes, environment and disease.* http://www4.od.nih.gov/oba/sacghs/reports/SACGHS_ LPS_report.pdf (accessed October 7, 2008).

Secretary's Advisory Committee on Genetic Testing (SACGT). 1999. *About SACGT: Secretary's Advisory Committee on Genetic Testing.* http://www4.od.nih.gov/oba/sacgt/aboutsacgt.htm (accessed October 7, 2008).

———. 2000. *Enhancing the oversight of genetic tests: Recommendations of SACGT.* http://www4. od.nih.gov/oba/sacgt/reports/oversight_report.pdf (accessed October 7, 2008).

CHAPTER 4

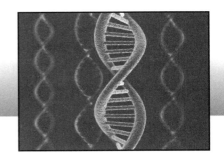

Ethics and Genetics in the Twenty-first Century

Chris Hackler, PhD

Traditional Principles of Bioethics: Evolving in the Twentieth Century

There is a long history of thought about the ethical dimensions of the healthcare professions. The famous Oath of Hippocrates, dating from around the fourth century BCE, contains a clear statement of the idea that physicians should always keep the patient's welfare foremost in mind and refrain from any harm or injustice to the patient or family. This idea, that the primary ethical obligation of the health professions is to serve the best interests of the patient, remained the polestar of medical ethics throughout ancient and medieval times. The biblical story of the Good Samaritan was told as a metaphorical expression of the role of the beneficent physician. As nursing developed as a profession, it also looked to the image of selfless and beneficent service as the professional ideal.

The prominence of this ideal as the summation of professional ethical wisdom lasted well into the previous century. A number of events in mid-century, however, stimulated a renaissance of reflection about the ethical values that should guide the health professions. Developments in both medical research and medical treatment (including technologies) raised questions about the sufficiency of the Principle of Beneficence, as it came to be known.

Medical Research:
Ethical Challenges and Developments

After World War II the world learned about horrific experiments that were carried out on Jews, prisoners of war, and other captive populations by Nazi doctors. Similar experiments were conducted by Japanese doctors on their captive populations, but it was during the Nuremberg war crimes trials that the world first learned of such brutal practices in the name of medical science. The experiments were generally intended to gain knowledge useful to the German war effort, but the most basic rights and interests of the coerced subjects were systematically ignored. Individuals were forced to endure agonizing and degrading treatment and then killed when they were no longer useful. Social utility had always been the justification for medical experimentation, but the excesses of the Nazi doctors made exceedingly clear that other human values of even greater importance could be, and had been, sacrificed in the name of the social good.

At home, as the American public learned, these basic values had sometimes been ignored as well. A number of unethical experiments were exposed in the late 1960s, culminating in the revelation in 1972 that a study of untreated syphilis had been conducted by the U.S. Public Health Service for decades in a group of black males in rural Alabama (Katz et al. 2007). It was apparent that the subjects had little idea of the purpose of the study, that deception had been used to recruit and retain them in the study, and that experimental procedures had been represented as therapeutic. In response to these revelations, Congress established in 1974 the National Commission for the Protection of Human Subjects of Biomedical and Behavioral Research to study the ethics of research and to recommend ways to protect the rights of research subjects (President's Council on Bioethics 2008). The commission formulated three principles of ethics that should guide research with human subjects.

First, research should be undertaken only if it holds reasonable promise of benefit to either the individual subject or to future patients. It is wrong to subject individuals to risk or even to inconvenience if the knowledge to be gained is trivial. The Principle of Beneficence echoes the traditional Hippocratic ethic, though it adds the dimension of benefiting other people as well.

In order to counterbalance and check potential justification by good results alone, the commission added the Principle of Respect for Persons. Potential subjects of research should be treated as rational agents with their own goals and the ability to deliberate about how to achieve those goals. It would be wrong for researchers to ignore, discount, or sacrifice the interests of potential subjects in order to acquire knowledge, no matter how beneficial it might be to others. Respecting the autonomy of individuals means giving them adequate information about the research study, then allowing them to make their own free choices about participation. Of course, some individuals lack full capacity to decide for themselves, and respecting them as persons requires protecting their interests.

The third consideration that the Commission said should guide research is the Principle of Justice. Both the risks and the benefits of research should be spread evenly over all groups in a society. No group (for example, minorities, poor people, or rich people for that matter) should bear disproportionate burdens in advancing medical knowledge, nor should they reap disproportionate benefits (President's Council on Bioethics 2008).

Medical Treatment and Technologies: Ethical Challenges and Further Changes

Rapid advancement of medical technology in the second half of the twentieth century presented the public with a number of new ethical puzzles. Organ transplantation, especially the possibility of cardiac transplantation, forced us to reconsider our traditional definition of death. In addition, new life-sustaining technologies were able to support biological life well beyond the irreversible loss of cerebral function.

Public concern about restraints on the use of medical technology became more pressing through the 1970s and 1980s. The President's Commission for the Study of Ethical Problems in Medicine and Biomedical and Behavioral Research was mandated by Congress in 1978 to study issues raised by the new technology. They issued influential reports on a number of topics, including defining death, making health-care decisions, foregoing life-sustaining treatment, and of special relevance to this volume, genetic engineering, and genetic screening and counseling (President's Council on Bioethics 2008).

As a prelude to their work, the commission articulated three ethical principles that would guide their deliberations, building on the prior work of the 1974 research commission. The first principle was *well-being*: promoting the overall best interests of everyone involved. The commission recognized that patient well-being should be primary, but that the well-being of others, including family, caregivers, and the larger community, is also ethically relevant. The second principle was *self-determination or autonomy*. Respecting this principle means giving patients information about their condition and about possible choices, and honoring the choices that patients make. It also means safeguarding their privacy. The third principle was *equity or justice,* treating people fairly, in an even-handed and nondiscriminatory manner.

Consolidating the Three Principles

The work of the two commissions heavily influenced the subsequent direction of bioethics as a new field of scholarship and practice. The three principles became a standard organizing framework of bioethical discussions. Dilemmas in bioethics were explained in terms of a conflict between the basic principles, and solutions lay in properly balancing the competing values. Of course, different individuals and different cultures attach somewhat different weights to the competing concerns, and this is one reason why it is difficult to achieve consensus on most issues in bioethics.

The "Three Principles Approach" to bioethics was raised to a new level of philosophical sophistication and scholarship with the publication in 1979 of *The Principles of Biomedical Ethics* by Tom Beauchamp and James Childress. To the three principles of Beneficence, Autonomy, and Justice they added a fourth: Nonmaleficence, or the idea that one should do no harm. Although the principle has clear roots in Hippocratic texts, it could be argued that it is included in the principle of beneficence broadly understood. Acting in ways that benefit the patient entails refraining from harm, unless the harm is necessary to achieve a greater good. Since "nonmaleficence" seems expendable and has led to some confusion (Beauchamp and Childress 2001), it will be dropped it in the discussion that follows. (One frequently sees "nonmalfeasance" listed as the fourth principle, but malfeasance is a different concept, implying misconduct by a public official.)

Advantages and Limitations

The Three Principles approach has been extraordinarily useful in the development of bioethics as a discipline. It provided a common set of organizing categories accessible to scholars and practitioners from many disciplines and healthcare professions. Furthermore, it encouraged scholars from philosophy and religion to step back from their deep theoretical commitments and discuss important issues within a more neutral conceptual framework. After all, the pressing issues of bioethics, especially clinical ethics, need to be resolved. Decisions must be made, and they have lasting consequences. Endless theoretical disputes are a tempting luxury that should be avoided in an area of such practical importance.

Nevertheless, it is important to emphasize the limits of the dominant approach to bioethics. First, the virtue of the approach, that it facilitates discussion among individuals from various backgrounds, tends to limit the depth to which analysis is taken. Both accessibility of concepts and depth of analysis are valuable in a practical discipline, but there is an inherent tension between them. It is important to realize that the principles are only a convenient way to begin to organize our thoughts and to convey them to one another. They neither dictate nor limit any line of thought, but only point to certain general features of a case that should be relevant to an ethical understanding of the situation. Respecting autonomy does not mean just asking what the patient wants and assessing their capacity to decide. It may lead us to question the role of family dynamics and even deep social structures that influence this person's choices. Recent advances in genetics and neuroscience suggest the potential for radical alteration of human nature and motivation. Decisions about these technologies will raise anew, and in a more urgent fashion, perennial questions about human nature, justice, and the good society, taking us far into the traditional domains of social and political philosophy. We must be sure our analytical tools do not limit the depth of our discussions or circumscribe the questions we are disposed to ask.

Personhood and Moral Standing

Although the three traditional principles are undoubtedly central to bioethical analysis, they do not capture all of the critical concerns. Personhood, for example, is an equally important concept for understanding many issues, especially those surrounding reproduction. In decisions about abortion, for example, it is important to consider the potential benefits and harms to the woman both from continuing and from terminating the pregnancy, as suggested by the principle of beneficence. It is necessary to reflect on the right of a woman to make her own autonomous choices about reproduction and about the rightful limits of social control and coercion of individuals. We should also reflect on the justice of social arrangements that put a disproportionate burden for child rearing on women. But our analysis is not complete until we also ask about the *moral standing* of the developing human life. At what stage in development does it have rights of its own that we must respect? None of the three principles captures this crucial element of moral standing.

Moral standing is a central issue in all of the new technologies of assisted reproduction that will be refined and expanded in the twenty-first Century. Pitched political battles over cloning and stem cell research center around the moral status of the developing human life. Stem cell research suggests potential for treatment of previously untreatable diseases, and embryonic stem cells seem to be the most likely to be beneficial. But embryonic stem cells can only be obtained from a pre-embryo at the blastocyst stage, and the blastocyst cannot survive the extraction of the stem cells. If the blastocyst is a person with full moral standing, then it would be murder or an unacceptable human sacrifice to end its further development.

Moral standing is central to a number of other issues that will be hotly debated in the coming decades. Research beginning at the initial cleavage of the zygote could tell us much about what goes wrong in the process of human development and might enable prevention of early childhood diseases and developmental disorders. Genetic testing of pre-embryos (pre-implantation genetic diagnosis) will become more sophisticated and will lead to more selective abortions. The underlying ethical question will be the moral status of the developing human life, or the degree of protection that is morally required at each stage of development. Those who attribute full moral status from conception will reject any practices that compromise the life or interests of embryonic human life. Those who think that moral status increases as development proceeds will be increasingly challenged to justify interventions undertaken at different stages of development.

Personhood and Personal Identity

At the other end of life, patients suffering from progressive dementia such as Alzheimer's Disease slowly lose the ability to interact with their environment. At a certain point they can no longer recognize family or friends and may be unable to swallow food or fluids. If personhood and moral standing are understood in developmental terms, then we need to ask whether moral standing diminishes or even vanishes, as the distinctly human qualities of cognition and purposeful action are lost. In a sense, the profoundly demented individual is not the same person as before, having lost all former goals and purposes and having a distinctively different set of interests from the previous self. This has led some thinkers to assert that the demented individual is a different person from the earlier self who may have completed an advance directive refusing life-prolonging treatment. If the patient is a different person, then the decisions of the previous self are no longer binding, and we should consider treating the patient according to our conception of his or her best interests. Should respect for autonomy diminish as patients lose the capacity to evaluate their current interests, or does it represent a stronger and more durable value?

Decisions about the moral status of severely demented individuals will become more pressing as the incidence of dementia increases. The Baby Boom generation will begin to retire between 2010 and 2015, and by 2030 most will be in their 80s. An estimated 4–5 million people currently suffer from Alzheimer's Disease. Unless a cure or a more effective treatment is found, the number is projected to rise to about

7 million in 2030 and about 14 million in 2050. (There are no hard data on the prevalence of AD, but these figures represent common estimates. For one representative study, see Brookmeyer et al. 1998.) In addition to questions about the moral standing, best interests, and autonomy of demented patients, there will also be concerns about the cost of care. Treatment of end-stage dementia is intensive and expensive. Non-demented but frail elderly citizens will need increasing levels of health care, putting pressure on public funding and raising questions about the justice of spending large amounts on patients who are not cognitively capable of appreciating the benefits. Indeed, spending on health care for a very elderly population will likely stress the national budget and siphon money from other social needs, such as education and programs to reduce social and economic disparities, thus threatening the common good.

The Common Good

Another concept that has received limited attention under the dominant approach has been the common good, or the welfare of the community. Bioethics as developed in the United States has been focused on the interests and rights of the individual. The principle of justice broadens the scope of concerns, but it is usually understood to require a fair distribution of goods. The impact of a decision or policy on the overall, long-term interests of the community is often ignored. Bioethics has been focused primarily on the acute care setting, where the immediate needs and interests of specific individuals demand recognition. When we turn to issues in public health, however, the interests of the larger community become prominent. And as we evaluate developing technologies that can alter our genetic inheritance and control our mental states, we will need to consider carefully the impact on the entire human community, both present and future.

Issues in Genetic Medicine

It is clear that issues in genetic medicine will arouse intense ethical debate through the coming decades. We have had only a glimpse of the potential predictive power of genetic knowledge, but there is no doubt that its scope and precision will continue to increase. Genetic therapies have so far proven elusive. Nevertheless, as the experience with cloning tells us, we should be prepared for a breakthrough at any time. Although we cannot anticipate all of the ethical problems that will be raised, we are already familiar with a number of salient concerns. These center around the uses of genetic knowledge and the consequences of genetic interventions.

Genetic Knowledge

There is great potential for popular misunderstanding of the current predictive power of genetic knowledge and of the social implications of genetic discoveries. Sensationalist reporting of the latest discovery of "the X-gene" can lead to a naïve genetic determinism that exaggerates dangers and downplays the critical role of environmental influences. Moreover, there is at present little power to counter the influence of genetic predispositions or to "correct" genetic mutations. We should therefore exercise restraint in our discussions of genetic discoveries and seek to educate patients and the public about the limits of genetic testing. Beneficence and autonomy both require that genetic testing be conducted only when all of these implications are understood and consent is given. It will be especially challenging to ensure that genetic counseling is available to those undergoing genetic testing, so that they will understand all of the implications of their results.

Of course genetic knowledge carries implications for others besides the client being tested, and it will be necessary to balance their interests against the confidentiality owed to the individual client. Genetic counselors and other healthcare professionals must think in terms of families and not just individual patients, thus enlarging the traditional focus on the best interests and autonomy of the individual patient. It will be particularly difficult to balance these sometimes competing interests as the range of genetic knowledge continues to expand.

While we may need to share genetic knowledge about a patient with those whose health is also implicated, it will be increasingly important to safeguard genetic knowledge from third parties that might use it in inappropriate ways, such as denying medical insurance coverage. Insurance companies will argue that justice and fairness require that they have access to some genetic information; otherwise the affected individual can take advantage of confidential knowledge concerning the likelihood of serious illness or early death and load up on medical or life insurance. These are not new issues, but they will become even more difficult to manage because of the scope and complexity of genetic information. The whole system of risk rating that underlies private insurance coverage in the United States will be greatly stressed, and it may be undermined if access to genetic information is inequitably allowed.

Technology now on the horizon will allow the increasing use of genetic information in reproductive decisions. *In vitro* fertilization allows a wide range of genetic testing on pre-embryos. One of the cells of an 8-cell zygote can be removed from a laboratory animal and used for pre-implantation genetic diagnosis (PGD), and the remaining seven cells will develop normally. As this technique is perfected for use in human reproduction and as genetic knowledge advances, there will be a wider range of conditions for which termination of the developing life will be sought. The moral status of embryonic life will continue to be an issue along with the rights of prospective parents to exercise control over the genetic inheritance of their offspring. Disability groups will protest with increasing poignancy that PGD implies that their condition is a problem to be eliminated, thus discounting the value of their lives and further marginalizing them socially. It is even possible that, out of concern for the common good of society, there could be countervailing pressure on families with a history of genetic illness to take measures to avoid passing on their illnesses, including perhaps involuntary testing and termination, sterilization, or exclusion from medical coverage. PGD could become an extremely divisive issue, implicating the deeply held values of reproductive liberty, non-discrimination, social justice, and the common good.

Genetic Intervention

Although the ability to treat diseases through genetic intervention is currently quite limited, it would be a mistake to assume that the barriers to successful genetic therapies are insurmountable. Of course the development of genetic medicine will require research with human participants, with all of the attending ethical issues of balancing risks and benefits, assuring informed consent, and spreading the risks and benefits of research, but it seems inevitable that genetic interventions will be developed. There will be much discussion, however, about possible ethical limits to manipulation of our genes. For one thing, we will need to decide whether to prohibit germ cell modifications that would be passed on to successive generations. Germ-line alterations raise questions about the right to alter the genetic inheritance of future individuals without their consent (which of course cannot be obtained). In addition, there would be fear of the unknown consequences of permanent alterations to the human gene pool, reflecting a concern for the common good that includes future generations.

Therapy and Enhancement

Genetic manipulation could presumably be used to accomplish a wide range of purposes. The general public seems prepared to accept a strategy of altering regular somatic cells (as opposed to germ cells) in an attempt to cure, treat, or prevent serious illnesses. Genetic therapies are seen as a new, and potentially more efficient, means to accomplish these commonly accepted goals of medicine. There is resistance, however, to interventions that seek to enhance desirable traits such as strength and mental agility. Whereas therapy lies within the legitimate domain of medicine, enhancement is seen by some to lie outside its proper bounds.

While it strikes most people as intuitively sensible, the distinction between therapy and enhancement will not bear a great deal of weight. First, it is conceptually indistinct. Would enhancing the immune system be a proper use of genetic technology? What about slowing the rate of human aging? Where do we draw the line between acceptable treatment for short stature and unacceptable enhancement of height? Second, where the distinction seems clear, we do not accept it in the rest of medicine. Cosmetic surgery is only one example of accepted medical practice aimed at enhancement rather than the treatment of disease.

Interventions aimed at enhancement can raise issues of fairness, however, by conferring an advantage in competing for important goods. If some individuals had access to significant genetic enhancement of intelligence, memory, endurance, and longevity, for example, they would clearly have an advantage over others who did not. In societies that value equality of opportunity, such an advantage would be considered *prima facie* unjust. Such advantages could lead to extreme inequalities at the international level, as individuals in wealthier societies would be able to obtain enhancements not affordable in less affluent nations. Current global inequalities would be magnified as the citizens of wealthy countries became progressively more capable of amassing wealth and power through enhanced abilities and longer lives.

Conclusion

The three principles of beneficence, autonomy, and justice will certainly remain at the center of bioethical discussion in the twenty-first century. No matter how technologically sophisticated and powerful they become, medicine and nursing will continue to focus on the needs of the individual patient. With increasingly complex technologies, however, it may become more difficult for beneficent professionals to determine the best interests of their patients, and correspondingly more difficult for patients to exercise their autonomy by making intelligent and well-informed choices about their own interests. Since genetic knowledge has implications for family members, patient confidentiality will be a more nuanced issue. Moreover, developing technologies always raise the problem of fair access, since in the beginning at least, they tend to be quite expensive. Issues of justice arose dramatically in bioethical discussions with the development of kidney dialysis and life support half a century ago, and they will continue to surround the introduction of every new technology.

Genetic and reproductive technologies will keep issues of personhood and moral standing front and center. As genetic modification becomes possible on a practical scale, questions could be raised about personal identity: How much modification is possible before we have a new person? It is even conceivable that three factors could combine to raise questions about our identity as humans. Genetic modification could enhance abilities that would be augmented by bionic and cybernetic technology, including implanted computer chips, to produce individuals with super-human powers. It may be that such a (highly speculative) "posthuman future" would require novel ethical concepts. But so far there seems to be nothing about genetic medicine itself that indicates such a need.

References

Beauchamp, T. L., and J. F. Childress. 2001. *Principles of Biomedical Ethics,* 5th ed. New York: Oxford University Press.

———. 1979. Principles of Biomedical Ethics. New York: Oxford University Press.

Brookmeyer, R., S. Gray, and C. Kawas. 1998. Projections of Alzheimer's disease in the United States and the public health impact of delaying disease onset. *American Journal of Public Health* 88 (9): 1337–1342.

Katz, R. V., B. L. Green, N. R. Kressin, C. Claurdio, M. Q. Wang, and S. L. Russell. 2007. Willingness of minorities to participate in biomedical research studies: Confirmatory findings from the Tuskegee Legacy Project Questionnaire. *Journal of the National Medical Association* 99 (9): 1052–1060.

President's Council on Bioethics. 2008. *Former bioethics commissions.* http://www.bioethics.gov/reports/past_commissions/index.html (accessed October 7, 2008).

CHAPTER 5

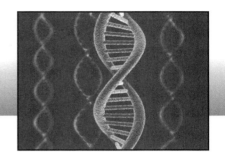

Redefining the Conventions of Informed Consent: Challenges in the Genomic Era

Robbie J. Dugas, DNS, RN, CFNP, CANP
Melinda Granger Oberleitner, DNSc, RN, APRN, CNS

Introduction

Ethical issues involving informed consent and genetic testing are becoming increasingly complex in light of the evolution and availability of genetic testing for specific disease entities. New questions regarding informed consent are being raised by professional, public, and private entities. A critical component of the nurse's role, regardless of practice setting, is often active participation in the informed consent process, specifically in the area of genetic testing (AACN 1998; Collins and Jenkins, 1997; Grady 1999; ISONG and ANA 1998; Scanlon and Fibison 1995; Touchette, Holtzman, Davis, and Feetham 1997). Knowledge of ethical issues associated with genetic testing is essential to nurses as they counsel clients (in this section, the term client will refer to participants in health care) who come in with questions that may engender ethical dilemmas in the clinical setting.

There are ethical questions that address the rights of the individual and family members as well as the roles of the community and the state in regard to genetic testing and research. This chapter addresses ethical issues surrounding informed consent and will present questions and unresolved issues related to how genetic technologies affect informed consent. Future implications for the individual, family, and society are discussed.

Evolution of Informed Consent Legal Doctrine

Historical meanings and definitions of informed consent and methods for obtaining informed consent are being challenged in the genomic era, with more questions being raised than ever before. Preserving the rights of both the individual and the family, as well as maintaining the ethical and legal obligations of the community and state, remain paramount in the genomic era. Client autonomy and decision-making related to informed consent have taken on new meanings with the mapping of the human genome. The genetic revolution will have an impact on how individuals, families, and communities handle health issues, and society at large will change as new discoveries become commonplace in healthcare settings. The importance of the client's understanding and the presentation of genetic information are critical in preserving the rights of all parties involved in informed consent.

Traditionally, the doctrine of informed consent has been predicated on the physician–patient relationship in decisions about diagnostic testing and medical or surgical treatment. In the United States a series of landmark legal decisions beginning in 1914 established the right of a competent individual to be the sole decision maker about "what shall be done with his/her own body" (Luce 2003; *Schloendorff v. Society of New York Hospitals* 1914). In *Salgo v. Leland Stanford Junior University Board of Trustees* (1957), the California appellate court established that informed consent must include the nature of the medical procedure, its purpose, the attendant risks, and the various alternatives to this procedure. In 1972, in another landmark case, *Canterbury v. Spence*, the court established the *reasonable person* standard of disclosure which states:

> the scope of the practitioner's communication to the patient must be measured by the patient's need, and that need is the information material to the decision...all risk potentially affecting the decision must be unmasked. We agree that risk is thus material when a reasonable person, in what the practitioner knows or should know to be the patient's position, would be likely to attach significance to the risk in deciding whether or not to forgo the proposed therapy.

Informed consent for research involving human subjects was formalized in the Nuremberg Code, which included the concepts of personal autonomy, freedom from coercion, freedom to withdraw, and full disclosure of information. In 1979, reacting to specific examples of subject abuse in the interest of research, the U.S. National Commission for Protection of Human Subjects of Biomedical and Behavioral Research issued the Belmont Report. These two documents are the ethical and legal foundations for the conduct of biomedical research with human subjects (Pelias 2001). The requirement for protection of research subjects through the informed consent process described in the report has been codified into federal policy (45 CFR, Part 46 (1983, 1991) and applies to all federally funded research (Hamvas, Madden, Nogee, et al. 2004).

Current review of federal regulations governing biomedical research with human subjects reveals that the intent and language of the regulations as currently written are not readily adaptable to genetic research, leaving insufficient protection in the current informed consent process. Pelias (2001) recommends that genetics research and family history recordings should be the focus of new provisions that could be added to current regulations or issued as independent guidelines specific to research in genetics. The new guidelines or provisions should provide more stringent safeguards for:

- the confidentiality of family history information,
- acknowledgement of the right of human subjects to exercise autonomy and self-determination as new information is received from research in genetics, and
- strong protection for subjects in decisions regarding the use of their tissue samples in research at any time in the future (Pelias 2001).

Organizations such as the American Society of Clinical Oncology (ASCO) strongly recommend that research on biological samples that are not anonymous from the time of collection (for example, tissue from biopsies and other surgical procedures) be considered human subjects research. Research involving these tissues should be guided by federal regulations, including informed consent provisions. Stewardship of specimens beginning with initial collection may be problematic, particularly in large research studies (ASCO 2003). Therefore the possibility of utilization of these biological samples for future genetic research should be considered. The prospect of future research on tissue samples should be explicitly stated in the informed consent, thereby allowing the individual to refuse consent.

The Health Insurance Portability and Accountability Act (HIPAA) of 1996 was prompted largely by concerns about unregulated access to a client's genetic information that might lead to discrimination in access to employment or insurance (Burke 2002; NIH 1997). However, HIPAA does not fully define genetic information and it does not prohibit the use of genetic information obtained from sources other than genetic testing, for example, family history. HIPAA protects against potential discrimination by health insurance providers for those people who are covered by group or employment-based health insurance. It does not extend the same protection to people who are covered by individual insurance policies or to people who lack access to COBRA (Consolidated Omnibus Budget Reconciliation Act) coverage after terminating employment-based insurance coverage (ASCO 2003).

In an attempt to safeguard individual autonomy, 41 states have enacted legal protection for genetic discrimination (Hamvas, Madden, Nogee, et al. 2004). Now, with the coming of a new genetic age, we must ask if informed consent standards mandated by current case law are sufficient to provide appropriate protections. We are especially concerned about the lack of legal protection of genetic information under individual insurance policies and protection for people who lack access to COBRA. It is likely that these laws will need to change in order to secure the rights of the individual.

Federal legislation, such as the Rehabilitation Act of 1973 and the Americans with Disabilities Act of 1990, prevents discrimination on the basis of handicap or disability. However, neither act includes provisions related to genetic discrimination. State legislation varies; some states protect against loss of insurance coverage and benefits, and insurance rate discrimination for individuals undergoing genetic testing. However, additional legislation is needed to limit medical testing by employers and to ensure that the information collected or tests performed are job-related exclusively. In the absence of legislation, we should require that all genetic testing and counseling be conducted so as to protect the identity of the person receiving services, similar to the way HIV (human immunodeficiency virus) testing is currently conducted in the United States (Bove, Fry, and MacDonald 1997). And what are the implications for family members as genetic information becomes available? If genetic testing could be done in a protected manner, would this eliminate the need for informed consent, thereby preventing genetic discrimination?

Client Autonomy and Informed Consent

The advent of the genetic age has created an expanded notion of the genetic identity of an individual or "client autonomy" with regard to genetic information (Goldworth 1999). Client autonomy is the ability to govern oneself and make deliberate choices about one's own future. The principle of client autonomy is understood as a decisional privacy, or the right of an individual to make one's own decisions, without duress or coercion, about possible options to pursue. A person should have the right to make choices regarding one's self, based on one's own values and beliefs, and to choose and act freely concerning what is done with one's body without controlling interventions of others (Goldworth 1999; Grady 1999).

In the past, client autonomy in medical decisions has changed from complete dependence on the advice of the physician to a more client-centered, non-directive approach. Client autonomy in informed consent primarily revolves around the client, or the client and the guardian or representative. Guidelines for preserving a client's autonomy in informed consent have previously meant providing adequate information in the appropriate cultural and educational context. In instances of genetic-related testing or treatment, this would ensure free, unpressured decisions. According to Grady (1999), discussion of privacy, implications for family members, impact on future choices, possible discrimination, and psychological reactions should all be part of the informed consent process.

The primary goal of genetic counseling is to promote client autonomy. This is accomplished by helping individuals understand their options in selecting an appropriate course of action in view of their family values and the risks. Preserving the process of decision-making by individuals and family members and safeguarding freely given informed consent for genetic counseling, testing, and therapeutics are two of the most important nursing responsibilities related to genetic services (Monsen 2000).

Some state and federal healthcare regulations have restricted client autonomy and the process of informed consent regarding genetic information. Genetic screening for phenylketonuria (PKU) has been an integral part of medical practice since the inception of newborn screening in the 1960s, when it was considered a milestone in the detection of genetic disorders (Pass, Lane, Fernhoff, et al. 2000). Screening for preventable conditions like PKU that can be ameliorated by early detection, and treatment is mandated by law in all but two states.

In some regions, little consideration was directed toward the question of obtaining parental informed consent prior to screening newborns for PKU. Personal autonomy and privacy were breached because informed consent was not obtained from the parents of newborns (Pelias and Markward 2001). Debate over mandatory screening weighed the negative aspects of invasion of parental autonomy and privacy against the positive benefits of screening. In fact, its inception preceded the promulgation of federal regulations related to informed consent by several years (Andrews, Fullarton, Holtzman, and Motulsky 1994). As new screening procedures for genetic mutations become more streamlined and cost-effective, we can expect to see these become a common practice in the twenty-first century. We may see the day when federal or state regulations outweigh the rights of individuals, informed consent is eliminated, and screening becomes mandatory. If this occurs, will parents have the right to refuse consent for screening and detection of genetic and other disease entities (Pelias and Markward 2001)? Can we expect individuals to willingly give up some of their privacy for the greater health and economic good of society?

The Use of Genetic Information

Institutionally governed and legally defined requirements for the consent process in healthcare settings, which have previously preserved the individual's autonomy and protected the rights of research subjects, are now being disrupted. Today institutions are struggling to devise informed consent language that describes the risks and benefits of participation in genetic research, primarily to protect the institution's interests and not those of the participant. The availability of individual DNA samples in institutions (from saved tissue perhaps stored for years) will probably lead to the rapid acquisition of new knowledge concerning genotype-phenotype correlation. Moreover, as new technology increases our capacity to identify an individual's genetic composition, consents that permit future genetic testing could be utilized for an unlimited number of possibilities that would not be specified at the time of tissue collection (Wilcox, Taylor, and Sharp 1999; Paasche-Orlow, Taylor, and Brancati 2003).

The issue is no longer an individual's privacy but how genetic information will be utilized and in what context. The misuse of information is the greatest concern of the public and of many nurses (Terry and Terry 2001; Cassells, Jenkins, Lea, et al. 2003). If appropriate institutional oversight and policies were available to strengthen the consent process, would this allay some concerns? The central ethical issue is the state of client autonomy. The central ethical question is what the individual is willing to give up for the collective good. Should we create an environment where public policy favors the greater good of society over the genetic rights of the individual? Will the possible health and economic benefits from genetic information so far outweigh the attendant risks that such testing and treatment technologies will become commonplace with minimal regard for autonomy in consent and decision making?

Client rights, particularly those related to self-determination, are being challenged in this new genomic era. In many countries, new laws have established a legally effective informed consent, giving the patient or research participant the ethical right to self-determination and to dictate what is done with one's own body. In the process of genetic testing, information about one's disposition to disease or the lack thereof can have profound psychological, relational, social, and physical ramifications. If consenting to genetic testing involves the involuntary surrender of DNA material for genetic research, one wonders about misuse of the resulting information. Unauthorized access to such information could lead to discrimination by health insurance companies and employers, or discovery by family members. Thus an individual would lose all rights to privacy and confidentiality of personal health information. The risks and benefits of the informed consent process have been modified by the nature of information gained through genetic testing. Legislation must specifically prohibit the misuse of genetic information. Otherwise, members of society will continue to fear genetic testing (Giarelli and Jacobs 2000).

Family Members and Informed Consent

In the pre-genomic era, family linkage or kinship was defined as those who were connected by "blood" and as those who were regarded as family or kin (Richard 1996; Finkler 1991; Miller 2005). Today, with the findings of human genome research , the healthcare system can define family and kinship relations by genetic testing, which can clearly show patterns of inherited disease. This clarification of family and kinship relationships raises the ethical question whether informed consent should still involve only the client or include the family or the extended family, all of whom may have a stake in the genetic information obtained.

Genes are heritable and their health effects may appear over several generations. The American Society of Human Genetics (ASHG) suggests that information is not private if family members know it (ASHG 2000). Knowing that a person is genetically disposed toward a specific disease is a direct indicator that close members of that person's family may also be disposed. With the invention of new reproductive technologies, the concepts of paternity, maternity, and siblingship are taking on new meaning, and a new language is being developed to reflect this change (Yoxen 1986; Carsten 2000). New identities are being created based upon detailed genetic profiles, and thus there is renewed interest in the meaning of family and kinship (Dolgin 1997; Franklin 1997; Strathern 1992, 1995).

Since genetic testing reveals not just the genetic makeup of the individual but information about other family members, there are questions of confidentiality and privacy as well as rights with regard to informed consent and genetic testing. When individuals sign a consent form for genetic services, the information revealed may affect the lives and decisions of family members. We are confronted with questions about the right to give consent and to privacy and confidentially of such information on the part of others in a family. Does the individual have a right to information about his or her own genotype and what it conveys? Should this genetic information belong to the family as well?

According to the ASHG (2000) Social Issues Subcommittee on Familial Disclosure, client–professional confidentiality may be broken when there is sufficient evidence that there is a substantial amount of genetic risk to others. The professional may have a "duty to warn" if there is potential harm to relatives that are serious, imminent, and likely, and if treatment or prevention of disease is available. The principles of nonmaleficence and of beneficence, as reflected in *Tarasoff v. Regents of the University of California*, (1976), support the moral obligation of practitioners to non-patient members of the community when serious harm can be prevented. Conversely, in those instances in which a genetic test reveals, for example, a biological marker for increased cancer risk in a family, current case law is underdeveloped and is not uniform regarding a physician's "duty to warn" family members not under that physician's care. Duty varies from state to state. Does a warning to relatives in the scenario presented above compromise their autonomy? What if relatives desire not to know genetic risks within the family (ASCO 2003)?

Client autonomy related to informed consent could mean exposing genetic information about multiple members of a family without their awareness or approval. Indeed, the revelation of family history information without the prior approval of all family members could be viewed as problematical. Will family members' values and choices be violated and unprotected? Privacy and confidentiality may also be disrupted. Consider the following scenario:

> Mrs. B. takes her four-year-old son to the pediatrician to have genetic testing performed for Huntington disease. Mrs. B. is very persistent with the practitioner in having this test done. Even though genetic testing is primarily unnecessary at this time, she states, "I want the genetic test done so I can help to plan my child's future medical care now." Mrs. B. signs the informed consent, independent of her husband's approval, and proceeds to have the genetic test performed. She informs the practitioner that she is aware that her husband has a positive family history of Huntington disease and that his grandfather died of respiratory failure related to the disease. She also informs the practitioner that she is unaware if her husband has the gene for Huntington disease; he has previously discussed genetic testing with her and made the decision not to get tested. Mrs. B. tells the practitioner that her husband is very religious and has stated, "If I do have the disease then it is God's will and I will know soon enough."

> Mrs. B. is informed that the genetic test on her son has returned "positive" for Huntington disease. She reiterates to the practitioner that she does not intend to inform her husband of the child's positive test results because of his previous remarks to her. Now the practitioner must decide the disposition of the results. Should the practitioner inform Mr. B. of the genetic test results since this is his child too? What about

the child's rights of consent? Usually genetic testing is done when the child reaches a level of understanding and can make a reasonable choice about genetic testing. Has the mother's assent violated the child's consent rights? What about the paternal consent for a child to have genetic testing? Is the father's approval overlooked and disregarded? What about the non-disclosure of information to the father? Is this an ethical violation?

Not all questions posed here will have viable answers available because the promulgation of federal laws and regulations governing genetic discoveries always lags behind them. We do know we are confronted with questions about the right to give consent and to privacy and confidentiality of such information on the part of others in a family. Consent must be fully and freely given. In the above scenario, the child is obviously too young to consent to genetic testing. Infants and very young children are universally regarded as incompetent in matters of consent for testing or treatment. Testing of infants and young children generally depends on the consent of the parents. The mother, in this situation, is the sole decision-maker in the genetic testing process. She assumes the father would reject genetic testing for their minor child, so he is excluded from the decision. Where there is disagreement between the wishes of parties involved, the genetic professional may suggest testing be postponed until all parties involved can reach agreement. They should be offered the support, referrals, and education needed to make an informed decision. Professional guidance should also be made available to assist individuals, such as the father in this case, who may have difficulty coping with the results of genetic testing (Rieger and Pentz 1999).

Valid Informed Consent: Recommendations for the Genomic Age

Genetic testing should be carried out within the bounds of voluntariness, informed consent, and confidentiality (ISONG 1998). Valid informed consent in genetic testing requires that individuals receive complete, impartial, and truthful information regarding the testing from providers who have the most current knowledge and skills related to genetic testing. Clients must receive sufficient, and correct, information to understand the impact that genetic testing may have on their lives.

The individual must have the capacity to consent. The general approach to obtaining informed consent is to regard persons who have reached legal majority as competent to consent for themselves and legal guardians as competent to consent for minors or incapacitated persons. Requests for genetic tests by competent adults generally meet with little or no objection. The protocol most widely used and advocated is that the professional provide pre-test counseling regarding both the positive and negative aspects of learning the results of tests. Generally, the professional should honor the decision of the adult client because the adult is presumed to have full capacity to make his or her own decisions and to give valid informed consent unless there is legal or medical evidence to indicate otherwise.

Requests for genetic testing of older children and adolescents are more problematic because minors are considered to be legally incompetent and testing is often requested by their parents. However, many professionals recommend that consideration be given to the maturity and the personal views of the minor, even though they are presumed not to be legally competent to give consent or to obtain treatment for some medical problems. Indeed, there is a growing practice of seeking assent of some young persons prior to beginning medical treatment even if they are not legally able to provide a valid consent. What happens when parents want a minor to be tested for a genetic disorder and the minor does not agree or does not wish to know the results of the test? In a situation where there is disagreement between the wishes of the parents and the wishes of the minor, the genetic professional may suggest testing be postponed until all parties can agree.

Testing of infants and young children generally depends on the consent of their parents. Infants and very young children are universally regarded as incompetent in issues of consent for testing or treatment. However, there are exceptions to parental consent in cases of state-mandated screenings. For the most part, these exceptions are legally and ethically justified by the benefits gained by society as a whole (Pelias 1998). Should there be exceptions to parental consent for genetic testing? Are all parents aware that in some situations testing of their offspring is mandatory and they cannot opt out?

Consent must be given fully and freely, without coercion. Clients must feel they have the right to accept or reject genetic testing or related clinical therapies. The client must know they will not suffer any negative effects from healthcare providers or insurers. Consent is not considered valid without the voluntariness of the individual (Scanlon and Fibison 1995; Bove, Fry, and MacDonald 1997).

Summary and Conclusions

Ensuring confidentiality of genetic information, nondiscriminatory treatment of persons who are affected with or are carriers of genetic disorders, and attempting to get valid informed consent from every person undergoing genetic testing are fraught with potential unresolved ethical, legal, and societal dilemmas (Bove, Fry, and MacDonald 1997). The challenge to nursing will be to educate patients and family members about genetic testing, their involvement in research endeavors, and all the uncertainties that will accompany informed consent in the evolving age of genomic health.

Genetic concerns, as a component of professional nursing practice, are daily becoming more common. Nurses involved in genetic counseling are often confronted with ethical issues at every phase of education and counseling. The challenge for nurses is to facilitate an environment of confidentiality and privacy in which valid informed consent can be obtained while meeting the needs of the patient, of families, of healthcare practitioners, and of society at large (Cassells, Jenkins, Lea, et al. 2003).

References

American Association of Colleges of Nursing (AACN). 1998. *The essentials of baccalaureate education for professional nursing practice*. Washington, DC: AACN.

American Society of Clinical Oncology (ASCO). 2003. *ASCO policy statement update: Genetic testing for cancer susceptibility*. Alexandria, VA: ASCO.

American Society of Human Genetics (ASHG). 2000. *Should family members about whom you collect only medical history information for your research be considered "human subjects"?* (Policy Paper). Bethesda, MD: ASHG.

Andrews, L., J. Fullarton, N. Holtzman, and A. Motulsky, eds. 1994. *Assessing genetic risk: Implications for health and social policy*. Washington, DC: National Academy Press.

Bove, C.M., S. T. Fry, and D. J. MacDonald. 1997. Presymptomatic and predisposition genetic testing: Ethical and social considerations. *Seminars in Oncology Nursing* 13 (2): 135–140.

Burke, W. 2002. Genetic testing. *New England Journal of Medicine* 347: 1867–1875.

Canterbury v. Spence, 464 F 26, 787 (US App: DC, 1972).

Carsten, J. 2000. Introduction: Cultures and relatedness. In *Cultures of relatedness*, ed. J. Carsten, 1–37. Cambridge: Cambridge University Press.

Cassells, J.M., J. Jenkins, D. H. Lea, K. Calzone, and E. Johnson. 2003. An ethical framework for addressing global genetic issues in clinical practice. *Oncology Nursing Forum* 30 (3): 383–390.

Collins, F., and J. Jenkins. 1997. Implications of the human genome project for the nursing profession. In *The genetics revolution: Implications for nursing*, ed. F. R. Lashley, 9–14. Washington DC: American Academy of Nursing.

Dolgin, J. 1997. *Defining the family: Law, technology, and reproduction in an uneasy age*. New York: New York University Press.

Finkler, K. 1991. *Physicians at work, patients in pain*. Boulder: Westview Press.

Franklin, S. (1997). Making representations: The parliamentary debate on the Human Fertiliza-tion and Embryology Act. In *Technologies of procreation: Kinship in the age of assisted conception,* eds. J. Edwards, S. Franklin, E. Hirsch, F. Price and M. Strathern, 96–131. Manchester: Manchester University Press.

Giarelli, E., and L. A. Jacobs. 2000. Issues related to the use of genetic material and information. *Oncology Nursing Forum* 27: 459–467.

Goldworth, A. 1999. Informed consent in the genetic age. *Cambridge Quarterly of Healthcare Ethics* 8: 393–400.

Grady, C. 1999. Ethics and genetic testing. *Advances in Internal Medicine* 44: 389–411.

Hamvas, A., K. Madden, L. Nogee, M. Trusgnich, D Wegner, H. Heins, and F. S. Cole. 2004. Informed consent for genetic research. *Archives of Pediatric and Adolescent Medicine* 158: 551–555.

International Society of Nurses in Genetics (ISONG) and American Nurses Association (ANA). 1998. *Statement on the scope and standards of genetics clinical nursing practice.* Washington, DC: American Nurses Publishing

Luce, J. M. 2003. Is the concept of informed consent applicable to clinical research involving critically ill patients? *Critical Care Medicine* 31 (Supplement): S153–S160.

Miller, B. D. 2005. *Cultural Anthropology.* 3rd ed. New York: Pearson Education.

Monsen, R. B. 2000. An international agenda for ethics in nursing and genetics. *Journal of Pediatric Nursing* 15: 212–216.

National Institutes of Health (NIH). 1997. *Genetic testing for cystic fibrosis.* http://consensus.nih.gov/1997/1997GeneticTestCysticFibrosis106html.htm (accessed September 12, 2008).

Paasche-Orlow, M. K., H. A. Taylor, and F. L. Brancati. 2003. Readability standards for informed consent forms as compared with actual readability. *New England Journal of Medicine* 348: 721–726.

Pass, K. A., P. A. Lane, P. M. Fernhoff, C. F. Hinton, S. R. Panny, J. S. Parks, et al. 2000. U.S. newborn screening system guidelines II: Follow-up of children, diagnosis, management, and evaluation. Statement of the Council of Regional Networks for Genetic Services (CORN). *The Journal of Pediatrics* 137 (4 Supplement): S1–S46.

Pelias, M. Z. 1998. Legal and ethical issues in genetic testing and informed consent. In *Genetic Counseling in the Dawn of the 21st Century,* eds. C. S. Bartsocas and P. Beighton, 10–17. Athens, Greece: HTA Medical Publications.

———. 2001. Federal regulations and the future of research in human and medical genetics. The *Journal of Continuing Education in the Health Professions* 21: 238–246.

Pelias, M. K., and N. J. Markward. 2001. The human genome in the public view: Genetics, geneticists, and eugenics. *St. Thomas Law Review* 13 (4): 827–849.

Richard, M. 1996. Families, kinship, and genetics. In *The Troubled Helix,* eds. T. Marteau and M. Richards, 249–273. Cambridge: Cambridge University Press.

Rieger, P. T., and R. D. Pentz. 1999. Genetic testing and informed consent. *Seminars in Oncology Nursing* 15: 104–115.

Salgo v. Leland Stanford Jr. University Board of Trustees, 317 p2d 170 (Cal. App., 1957).

Scanlon, C., and W. Fibison. 1995. *Managing genetic information: Implications for nursing practice.* Washington, DC: American Nurses Association.

Schloendorff v. Society of New York Hospitals, 105 NE 92 (NY 1914).

Strathern, M. 1992. *After nature: English kinship in the late twentieth century.* Cambridge: Cambridge University Press.

Strathern, M. 1995. Displacing knowledge: Technology and the consequences for kinship. In *Conceiving the New World Order,* eds. F. Ginsburgh and R. Rapp, 346–364. Berkeley: University of California Press.

Tarasoff v. Regents of the University of California, California Supreme Court; July 1, 1976. 131 California Reporter 14.

Terry, S. F., and P. F. Terry. 2001. A consumer perspective on informed consent and third-party issues. *The Journal of Continuing Education in the Health Professions* 21: 256–264.

Touchette, N., N. Holtzman, J. Davis, and S. Feetham. 1997. *Toward the 21st century: Incorporating genetics into primary health care.* New York: Cold Spring Harbor Laboratory Press.

Wilcox, A. J., J. A. Taylor, and R. R. Sharp. 1999. Genetic determinism and the over-protection of human subjects. *Nature Genetics* 21: 362.

Yoxen, E. 1986. *Unnatural selection? Coming to terms with the new genetics.* London: Heinemann.

CHAPTER 6

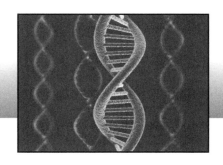

Genetic Inheritance, Identity, and the Proper Role of Nursing

Sharon J. Olsen, PhD(c), MS, RN, AOCN

...illness, health, disability, and difference are all connected to a person's identity, [the] sense of who [one] is. A person's identity is not formed in isolation. It is always formed against a certain background, a culture and a history, in dialogue with other human beings. My self-description is connected to your description of me, and our descriptions of one another are connected to the descriptions of others. Thus what counts as an illness or a disability—or on the other hand, as normal biological variation—will itself depend on its cultural historical location.

(Elliott 1999, 48)

In 1865, Gregor Mendel uncovered a simple and revolutionary truth: the unique identity of a garden pea is faithfully transmitted, generation after generation, to its descendants (Mendel [1865] 1965). James Watson and Francis Crick (1953) deciphered the form of this identity, deoxyribonucleic acid (DNA), and launched a new era of molecular studies in the life sciences. Just 50 years later, scientists with the Human Genome Project (International Human Genome Sequencing Consortium 2004) decoded, published, and downloaded onto a single CD-ROM the "building blocks" of life in the form of a string of nucleotides known to code for human characteristics, our anatomy and physiology—our biologic identity, our genotype—constituted by our ancestors and expressed in each of us as unique and human. The term genomics evolved to describe the product of the combinations of many genes and the environment working together to result in our physical characteristics, our phenotype. In the not-too-distant future, a person's unique genetic identity is projected to be accessible for perhaps as little as $1000 and a small blood sample (Robertson 2003).

In tandem with the genetic revolution, perhaps not intentionally but evident nevertheless, health and disease have been increasingly geneticized. It is now possible to identify certain disease-predisposing gene mutations and to thereby label healthy individuals as *at risk* (Kenen 1996; italics my own). This at-risk health status introduces an element of uncertainty about one's likelihood of developing disease, which results in a particular type of personal, familial, and social vulnerability. If, as Elliott suggests, personal identities are constructed from internalized perceptions of how others describe us, and you and I in turn describe ourselves as others have described us, then healthcare providers must consider the moral and ethical implications of their use and application of at-risk language. This will be an ever-increasing concern as molecular geneticists, scientists, and clinicians correlate newly discovered gene mutations with disease, the healthcare market develops corresponding predisposition testing technology, and increasing numbers of at-risk individuals are identified.

The moral questions I explore in this chapter address a number of related concerns that I have attempted to bring into line with my conceptualization of nursing's unique role in the genomic revolution. Do healthcare providers alter clients' perceptions of their personal identity by imposing at-risk status? Does at-risk status have implications for how clients create their own identities or how others view them (e.g., as an at-risk individual or a member of an at-risk group)? Do healthcare providers do an injustice in their likely unconscious but nevertheless regular reinforcement of at-risk status during periodic patient encounters across the spectrum of lifelong surveillance? What are the ethical obligations of nurses toward their patients and families in this context and what are our obligations as strategic members of a rapidly evolving and genetic technology-driven healthcare community? In essence, what concerns us here is that healthcare providers have unquestioningly appropriated and ascribed at-risk terminology without considering its impact as an identity label for individuals, families, and groups.

Elliott suggests that the way one frames an ethical question determines the ethical response one articulates. The position taken here is that identity is central to how one views oneself and, as such, is an important determinant of health and health-seeking behavior (Hunt, Davidson, Emslie, and Ford 2000). This position is framed by evolving genetic terminology, contemporary understanding of the concepts of identity, mutation, inheritance and vulnerability, the nature of the genetic counseling experience, and the geneticization of health and disease. As scientists and healthcare professionals increasingly carve out greater numbers of individuals and groups with a predisposition for specific genetic diseases, new threats to personal identity may be introduced.

Nurses, the largest group of healthcare providers, have only recently begun to articulate moral stances in the evolving world of genetic health care. The subject of this paper is of legitimate concern for nursing, in that as a discipline and a profession, nursing has a central aim and social mandate of health. Nursing's focus is the person and the family; and its method is a relational ethic of caring that is informed by science that takes context and experience into account, and legitimizes subjective data (Donaldson and Crowley 2004; Sarter 2004). If nurses are to effectively promote and facilitate health, they must understand how patients and families interpret, internalize, and ascribe genetic risk for disease, and work with them to maintain or improve health status.

Evolving Genetic Terminology

As genetic mutations are mapped to diseases and diseases are recognized to occur more frequently in certain families or groups, the language surrounding these processes has quickly adapted. *Genetic disease* and *at-risk* health status are two diagnostic terms that have evolved to describe healthy individuals and groups predisposed to certain diseases.

Genetic Disease

The term *genetic disease* came about as molecular biologists recognized that increasing numbers of medical diagnoses had a genetic basis. The term is not simply another type of diagnosis, it inherently implies relationships. By its nature, it identifies a problem in one person but at the same time labels biologically related relatives (Armstrong, Michie, and Marteau 1998). It implies a certain lack of health and carries with it an innate uncertainty about and lack of control over one's future health. Further, it carries a social vulnerability in medical, employment, and other public contexts. Finally, the term is value-laden, reflecting our understanding and lived experiences of a disease based on information garnered from a very personal social context impregnated by the media and experiences of friends and family members with the disease.

At-Risk Health Status

Kenen (1996), a sociologist and anthropologist, has explored the concept of at-risk health status in depth. She notes that the term evolved from public health in the 1970s in response to efforts to medicalize such normal processes as pregnancy and childbirth (e.g., high-risk pregnancy). Once an at-risk health status was diagnosed, "patients" (in this case, healthy pregnant women) were expected to conform to "specific behavior patterns and norms" (1545), including prescriptions for prevention. Ultimately, the prescribed behaviors became standardized, then institutionalized, and at last they became social norms promoted by healthcare practitioners as well as society.

Kenen describes the at-risk diagnosis as a "gift of knowing" offered under the auspices of a belief that knowledge is intrinsically good and enables patients to make more informed decisions. But she also acknowledges a number of downsides: an at-risk diagnosis may merely affirm risk and offer no cure, it may label a patient so that society sets specific expectations for one's behavior (e.g., informing other at-risk relatives, avoiding disease causing factors), or it may foster self-blame, stigmatize, or set up the expectation that one is obliged to undertake certain disease-prevention behaviors. In addition, by the nature of risk-based diagnoses (diagnoses based on extrapolating population risk to individuals), disease certainty is ambiguous and uncertain. As such, it can set up individuals for the perception that they have a chronic illness. This seems especially important in adult onset conditions wherein disease expression is not anticipated until later in life (if at all), leaving patients constantly on alert for symptoms.

Though Kenen's article was written just as the genetics of common inherited adult-onset disorders was being introduced into clinical practice, she did accurately predict many of the public, medical, and institutional responses that we have seen develop over the past decade. Take for example the case of inherited breast and ovarian cancer. Once the offending gene mutations were identified in the mid 1990s, a cascade of discoveries in patient care followed. Predictive gene tests were identified, the diagnostic genetic technology was patented, and high-risk cancer genetics clinics proliferated. Insurance reimbursement for genetic counseling and gene testing was solicited and won. Practice standards for gene testing and lifelong prevention and surveillance behaviors (including regular check-ups, screening tests, and prophylactic operations) were published. In the 1990s, national high-risk cancer genetics registries evolved to facilitate further basic and behavioral research (Anton-Culver, Ziogas, Bowen, et al. 2003). Today, primary care providers recommend standardized practice guidelines for long-term surveillance, and at-risk status for inherited breast and ovarian cancer is treated as a chronic illness.

An important problem associated with treating healthy individuals as if they have a chronic illness is that busy providers may concentrate solely on issues relevant to the genetic disease (e.g., updating pedigrees and prescribing and tracking disease surveillance in the form of more frequent clinical breast exams, pelvic exams, mammograms, ultrasounds)—in essence looking for disease. As evidence for this genetic disease/chronic disease focus, a recent analysis of 23 studies on the screening behaviors of women with an inherited risk for breast or ovarian cancers found no evidence for medical attention to or concern for prevention or screening behaviors related to other chronic adult conditions such as cardiovascular disease, diabetes, or osteoporosis (Olsen, unpublished dissertation).

Of further concern are studies of physician practices that suggest patients with chronic diseases tend to receive limited or no counseling or direction regarding health promotion, disease prevention, or screening (Rost, Nutting, Smith, et al. 2000; Redelmeier, Tan, and Booth 1998; Chernoff, Sherman, et al. 1999; Klinkman 1997). Other data suggest that widespread media coverage of topics related to breast cancer (compared with limited attention to cardiovascular disease) has sensitized women to the extent that they may place undue emphasis on breast cancer risk. By the same token, they may ignore health risks associated with other more common complex disorders such as cardiovascular disease, the number one cause of mortality in women (Blanchard, Erblich, Montgomery, and Bovbjerg 2002; Legato, Padus, and Slaughter 1997; Mosca et al. 2000; Erblich, Bovbjerg, Norman, et al. 2000).

Identity

Identity, as Carl Elliott puts it, is at once the self-actualization of our embodied interpretation of unconscious but externally expressed biologic variation, our life choices and experiences, and the interpretation of our public and private social exchanges. Indeed, it is our self-image: private, but in the same moment public. It is historically grounded in our ancestry as well as future-directed in our descendents.

Schechtman (1996) asserts that identity is bound up in our sense of self. It is that which we consider important to who we are and the personal properties we identify with. These might include sister of a breast cancer survivor, artist, liberal Democrat, trustworthy, Christian, and so on. Schechtman feels that much of our unique identity is bound up in our history, our relationships with others, how we are treated by others, and the experiences we have encountered or perhaps weathered. All of these experiences and properties merge to form our personal sense of self or our identity. It is that which makes each of us qualitatively different from any other individual, and it evolves with time and experiences.

Mutation and Identity

As molecular geneticists focused on sequencing the human genome, medical geneticists have continued to search for distinctive genes associated with disease. What has emerged is a picture of disease as mutation-driven, variable in expression (e.g., the manifestation of physical traits, pathophysiology), and dependent on the uniqueness of the individual's place in a specific social and physical environment. Mutations, in evolutionary terms, are inevitable and necessary for the survival of a species. In everyday existence, mutations occur randomly. They may be repaired via the normative action of other genes or they may go unrepaired. Unrepaired genes may never lead to disease, can singularly and directly cause disease, or may require additional action in combination with other genes, environmental exposures, or life experiences to trigger disease. Additionally, mutations can be inherited and result in the perpetuation of the same disease, disorder, or syndrome among new family members. Mutations may also lie silent (unexpressed) for generations.

As our scientific understanding of the inheritance of disease-causing mutations evolved, behavioral scientists intensified their efforts to understand disease patterns in families. Today, using family history and pedigree construction, medical geneticists and clinicians identify family members who may be carriers of, or at risk for, selected genetic diseases or disorders. A vast system of molecular genetic technology and genomic health care has rapidly evolved to support this new diagnostic capability, including specialized genetic counseling clinics, a vast array of gene tests, a cadre of specially trained genetic professionals, and standardized care management protocols and guidelines. Today, analysis of peripheral blood or tissue can pinpoint the aberrant gene and, once identified, the offending mutation can, assuming informed consent, be tested in family members (note, previously healthy individuals can now be ascribed at-risk status). If mutation-positive, carriers are prescribed recommendations for disease prevention, where they exist. It is noteworthy that providers have also come to label healthy individuals and family members with a known gene mutation as *patients*, effectively modifying the family member's condition of health as well as their status in the family. Thus disease risk is geneticized, medicalized, and institutionalized, and healthy individuals come to be "patients" who are ascribed an "at-risk" health status or diagnosis.

Genetic Inheritance and Vulnerability

As interpretive and relational beings, individuals and families have historically under-stood inheritance in terms of a family tendency to display similar physical features, character, personality, mannerisms, personal habits, health, and proneness to illness (Walter, Emery, Braithwaite, and Marteau 2004). On a day-to-day basis, most peo-ple do not normally reflect on themselves as genetic beings. However, public polls suggest that our everyday assessment of genetic inheritance is tied to patterns of social bonding (Richards 1997). We are the products of our parents and grandpar-ents, and ultimately we are biologically, psychologically, and sociologically tied to society as human beings, genomes being differentiated one from another by only 0.1%. Kant is credited with believing that "personal identity depends on the exis-tence of objects in space outside of the ego" (Pellegrino and Thomasma 1981, 109). Hence relationships, culture, experience, and our biology will bind our identity. Per-sonal experiences of a relative's illness, including suffering, and the number of rela-tives with the genetic disease, perceptions of the contribution of various personal and lifestyle characteristics, even age and gender considerations concerning the fre-quency of the disease in society at large, all contribute to the salience of genetic dis-ease for the individual.

Elliott (1999) affirms that identity is "always formed against a certain background, a culture and a history, in dialogue with other human beings." A recent meta-analy-sis offers some insight into how family members construct their perception of risk for genetic disease (Walter, Emery, Braithwaite, and Marteau 2004). The authors found that personal experience of a relative's illness, witnessing suffering or a long disease trajectory, and the relative emotional closeness of an affected relative were all important mediators of risk perception. Mental models of health, disease causation, and inheritance were found to be actively created and often contrasted with prevail-ing scientific knowledge. For some, genes were no more important than other shared environmental or behavioral factors. Bad luck, chance, and fate contributed prominently to these causation models. However, a sense of personal vulnerability was constructed as individuals regularly reassessed their causation models based on disease-related deaths and new diagnoses in biological relatives. For some, a personal perception of risk encouraged action. Family members, too, experienced some degree of vulnerability and uncertainty about their personal risk for genetic disease. The authors suggested that it was likely that coping and behavior change strategies were also colored by beliefs about how diseases occurred within and across family experiences as well as relationships outside of the family. Clearly a host of factors are engaged as individual family members or the collective family selectively integrate personally salient features of a disease that runs in the family.

Elliott cautions that although identity is relatively constant, it is subject to transformation—precisely because "our inner selves do not exist separate from our outer selves" (1999, 32). Our identity, the public as well as the private, is central to our understanding of health and to how we respond to disease or the threat of disease. Nurses encounter disease-induced identity transformations regularly. For example, it is not uncommon for cancer survivors to relate how the cancer experience "changed" them. How it altered their once "taken for granted" body image, their perceptions of the way life should be lived, of what is really important in life, and how it altered religious or spiritual beliefs. Many cancer survivors lose trust in the familiar symptoms of their own body; aches and pains once ignored are met with uncertainty, fear, and preoccupation. What was familiar is no longer so. Shaha's practice-derived theory concerning the Omnipresence of Cancer (Shaha and Cox 2003) suggests colorectal cancer patients learn to "co-exist" with their diagnosis as they begin "life after the cancer diagnosis" (Shaha, Cox, Hall, et al. 2006, 37–38). Such a transformation cannot help but have implications for one's perception of "self."

Genetic Counseling

The genetic counseling appointment marks an encounter between lay understandings of genetics on the one hand and the scientific framework of modern human genetics on the other (Armstrong, Michie, and Marteau 1998). Genetic counseling sessions involve the coming together of two agendas and can entail up to two hours of discussion. On the counselor's side, there is the transmission of expert knowledge about the patient's familial genetic problem and the crafting of individualized recommendations based on the specifics of the patient's personal and family medical history. On the other, the patient (possibly including some family members) seeks information and solutions for what has been socially and medically described as a problem: a genetic diagnosis. A power imbalance between the patient and the professional is inevitable, but the genetic counselor's traditional mode of non-directive counseling is medicine's way of limiting its consequences. Non-directive counseling supports a high level of patient autonomy in decision making. Extensive and complex genetic information is shared in the name of informed choice, and emotional support is offered. In the end, patients are the final arbiters of their own decisions about gene testing and the adoption of prevention and lifelong surveillance recommendations.

Despite the fact that a number of scholarly publications offer step-by-step guidelines for the counseling process, little is really known about the nature of this information giving and counseling process. Armstrong, Michie, and Marteau (1998) performed a rigorous qualitative analysis of 30 genetic counseling sessions across six different counselors. What they found was a highly structured and ritualized process. In the first part of the session, maps of inheritance and illness were formalized and a significant amount of complex genetic information was imparted. In the second phase "the possibilities for evading from the web [pedigree] that had been created" were explored. Ultimately "the patient was drawn into the matrix as a 'self' constituted by genetic linkages…genetic status was nonnegotiable…There was never discussion of 'who you are' as this was pre-given by the density of the genetic map: identity was located in genetic make-up" (1657).

In this study, Dr. Armstrong and his colleagues explored the influence of genetic counseling on identity transformation. They suggested that a "new identity" was not given but that a "revealed identity" emerged. That is, the patient's identity was revealed by the genetic links in the family pedigree. Accordingly, the genetic counselor revealed who the patient "had always been"—a concealed identity was revealed. The authors concluded by suggesting that "the patient might leave the consultation with varying degrees of revealed identity that have implications for the future, but…are also likely to involved a reassessment of self in the past" (1658).

Koch and Svendsen (2005) have described another approach to genetic counseling. They claim that "preventing genetic disorders is considered a common good" (829). They suggest that in a democratic society, all family members are entitled to the genetic knowledge produced in genetic counseling and each member is responsible for their own health. In their essay, the authors suggest that:

> …acquiring knowledge about genetic risks and embarking on preventive action is the "right" way of relating to oneself [ala taking personal responsibility for health], the family [saving lives of relatives] and eventually society [maintaining a healthy population]. The prime technique used is to appeal to people's sense of responsibility towards the family and articulates an ethics of rights and entitlements of relatives. As such this social technology promotes "the healthy life" as well as "the healthy family." (831)

Though such an approach appears socially responsible and oriented to the greater good, the down side is that knowledge is only empowering when it is beneficial. This approach does not take into account that some patients may be unwilling or unable to exercise the authority and responsibility that they would be given. Additionally, given the variable nature of gene expression for disease there is an inherent degree of uncertainty that cannot be "democratically" eliminated from this mode of "social technology." Though the goal is to save lives, responsibility for developing or preventing disease seems to lie with the patient. This logic is consistent with Kenen's suggestion that the "individual is supposed to try to avoid becoming ill" (1996, 1548). Kenen suggested that in the "at-risk health role" individuals were "not entitled to relinquish [their] obligations" toward health. Instead doctors expected them to fulfill their "at-risk health role" by "going for diagnostic tests and/or changing behaviors" (1549). Providers using this approach might be cautioned: Is this inadvertent but subtle abuse of power appropriate?

Genetic counseling is a consultation service, not unlike referring a patient with heart problems to a cardiologist where the patient is examined, family history is taken as part of the health history, expert information and recommendations are offered and discussed, and a follow-up letter is forwarded back to the referring provider. However, genetic counseling is qualitatively different from the typical "referral." Information taken, as well as given, has the potential to alter patient perceptions of themselves and their biological relatives, as well as how society views them. Skirton and Eiser (2003) suggest that because both clients and counselors bring to the process of genetic counseling their own knowledge, values, and beliefs, it is critical to take time to understand the client's previous knowledge and psychosocial experiences surrounding the condition and to assist them to integrate past and present understandings and perceptions. Meilander (1991) reminds us that "our identity has been secured through bodily ties—in nature, with those from whom we are descended; in history, with those whose lives have intertwined with ours" (44). Providers cannot divorce the person and their identity from the body. Nor can we equate identity with genetic make up. Precisely because genetic status is not negotiable there must be an opportunity to discuss "who you are."

Good and Right Genomic Nursing Practice

Rothman (2003) speaks of an increasing number of strangers at the bedside in patient care. In genetic health care, there is no bedside; traditional providers, physicians and nurses, are conspicuously absent. Genetic counselors and medical geneticists are the dominate providers in this arena primarily because of their command of complex genetic information.

Though interest and numbers are growing, nurses have been reticent to venture into this area as training in genetics has not been, nor is it currently, a routine part of formal nursing education. This must change. Today, we know that all disease has a genetic component and about 10% of disease has an inherited predisposition. In absolute numbers this means a significant number of individuals and families are at risk for or will be diagnosed with a genetic disease.

Nurses account for the largest group of healthcare professionals; 2.9 million plus (USDHS 2006). They practice in an ever-widening array of settings and geographic locations. While medical geneticists and genetic counselors are relatively few in number given the rapidly growing demand for genetic and genomic health care, it is critical that all nurses gain skill and flexibility in the core competencies of genetic and genomic nursing (Jenkins, Calzone, Lea, and Prows 2006). This will enable them to reinforce the message of the genetic counselor and work closely with individuals and families to overcome uncertainties and maximize health across healthcare settings. In this way, nurses take up their moral and professional responsibility to promote personal, familial, and communal coping strategies that make possible the successful internalization of evolving and complex genetic information and sustain critical lifelong health promotion and disease prevention and surveillance behaviors.

It is certain that genetic and molecular scientists will continue to actively search for disease-causing mutations. Once these are found, gene tests will be developed (today over 900 gene tests are available), and not only families with inherited predispositions for these diseases, but also clinicians will seek evidence-based strategies for preventing the relevant genetic disease. In today's healthcare system, individuals and families are encouraged to take increasing responsibility for their health and medical information. The moral nature of nursing, rooted in goals of health and healing, emphasizes the quality of the inter-human relationship over the particular choice that comes out of that relationship (Pellegrino and Thomasma 1981). Nurses are well prepared to support and advocate for those who may be unwilling or unable to exercise authority and responsibility for their own health or, to maximize the self-assessment and coping skills necessary to master the day-to-day uncertainty that can come with lifelong disease surveillance.

But, perhaps more importantly, nurses need genomic competency because there is a critical lack of attention to the "subjective vulnerability" of the at-risk individual (Bergum 2002). In genetic counseling sessions, patients may be at once incriminated by their pedigree and responsible for passing on a genetic disease. The patient's commonly held sense of self may be threatened. Nurses can facilitate more than just a cognitive understanding of the molecular biology of a genetic disease. They have the moral responsibility to take an active role as collaborators in the genetic healthcare team, to extend the scope and reach of the genetic experts. Beyond the genetic counseling consultation, at-risk individuals and their families will return to their everyday existence and usual sources of health care. Recent research confirms that they will reassess their sense of health and disease, their sense of self and family, and their understanding of their sense of place in society (Kenen, Ardern-Jones, and Eeles 2003). Kenen and colleagues' research suggests that perceived risk becomes "chronic risk" whereby a "biographical disruption of identity" becomes "pervasive and chronic, though at times intermittent" (321). Such a finding suggests that it is necessary to periodically assess the psychological, social, and spiritual coping resources that individuals and families use to promote a healthy sense of self. This will be especially salient across the normal occurrences of family life events that lead individuals and family members to reassess their sense of vulnerability: child-bearing decisions, disease-related deaths, and new diagnoses among biological relatives.

The nature of the caring relationship in nursing is to assist individuals to heal themselves (Bergum 2002; Thomasma 1999). Pellegrino and Thomasma (1981) suggest that in health "we see ourselves identified with our bodies, facing the world and acting on it in essential unity. In illness the body is interposed between us and reality...the body stands opposite to the self; instead of serving us, we must serve it" (203–208). This is likely also true for the at-risk individual. For those confronted with the at-risk health status, provider attention to the genetic disease must not supersede attention to the more holistic focus on overall health and wellness. With undue attention to the molecular, a healthy body may no longer feel healthy—it has a *genetic disease*, it is vulnerable and untrustworthy. This newly discovered vulnerability can extend to family members because it is frequently the "patient's" responsibility to share genetic information with biological relatives, to alert family members of their possible risk status, to expose never before considered feelings about passing on an inherited predisposition, and to possibly stigmatize with a disease.

Further, at-risk individuals and family members are prescribed responsibility for following stepped up and lifelong screening regimens and presented with options for prophylactic surgery or chemoprevention. All these experiences have the potential to overwhelm and will likely take time to integrate. Reassessment of one's health status and more importantly one's identity cannot be accomplished during the genetic counseling session. Further, issues and concerns may take time to present themselves. Because nurses offer skills that can readily assist patients to successfully transition through periods of vulnerability, they can help individuals and families integrate these new genetic life experiences and get on with their lives with a sense of wholeness and health.

Support during times of vulnerability requires the nurse and the patient to enter into a healing relationship. Right and good healing occurs as an interaction that is committed to engaging with the patient and family as they journey through this vulnerable period (Bergum 2002). Together the nurse and the patient target problems the patient has with their genetic disease, with family, or with disruptions in their social and work structure—all in relation to their values. The nurse by the very act of entering into this relationship declares publicly that they have "special knowledge and skills, that can heal, or help, and that [they] will do so in the patient's interest, not [their] own" (Pellegrino and Thomasma 1981, 209).

Reflections on the Initial Moral Questions

In this final section, I return to the questions set out at the beginning of this chapter. Do healthcare providers alter clients' perceptions of their identity by imposing at-risk status? Perhaps first, it is necessary to establish that healthcare providers do impose at-risk status. Definitions of "impose" include to require, to compel, and to force upon. Generally, genetic experts and medical providers establish diagnoses via family history and genetic testing. Family history or a positive genetic test suggest a diagnosis and, because the individual does not have disease, at-risk health status is ascribed by default. Further, adherence to lifelong surveillance will necessitate regular visits to healthcare providers for follow up tests and examinations wherein "patients" will likely repeatedly hear the words "because you are at risk for ___." Taken together, I would suggest that genetic, medical, and nurse providers likely do impose an at-risk health status. A diagnosis is required and a genetic disease is imposed but, because "disease" per se is not present, providers are compelled to ascribe at-risk health status. If, as Elliot (1999) says "my self-description [my identity] is connected to your description of me…," then an imposed diagnosis or at-risk health status would have implications for identity. In fact, the work of Kenen, Ardern-Jones, and Eeles (2003) provides evidence that identity is in fact transformed in a small sample of healthy women with an inherited predisposition for breast or ovarian cancer.

Does at-risk status have implications for how clients create their own identity or how others view them (e.g., as an individual or member of an at-risk group)? Kenen,

Ardern-Jones, and Eeles (2003) describe women who "went back and forth in their minds between being aware of the changes in their self identity due to their increased risk of developing cancer and trying to bracket off the at-risk status and getting on with their lives" (321). If healthy patients and families see themselves "identified with [their] bodies, facing the world and acting on it in essential unity" (Pellegrino and Thomasma, 1981), then the salience of new information that suggests the body is perhaps now less trustworthy and perhaps more vulnerable should be examined. "First, do no harm," a central ethical precept of both medicine and nursing, demands nothing less. Further, because "our identity has been secured through bodily ties...with those from whom we are descended" (Meilander 1991), and at-risk health status inherently implies familial involvement, it is clear that providers effectively extend the reach of one individual's diagnosis to an entire family. As such, the salience of new genetic information for family members must not be overlooked, nor should the reciprocal implications for intra-familial relationships.

Finally, what are the particular ethical obligations of nurses toward their patients and families in the context of genetic health? Much of this has been described above, but the role of the nurse in genetic health care is only beginning to be explored. It is critical that all nurses develop a baseline understanding of genetics and its role in disease prevention, development, and treatment. Such knowledge is central to our understanding of what nurses can and must do to ensure that patients and families can build on their strengths and become autonomous, maximally functioning, healthy, integrated beings. As strategic members of a rapidly evolving, genetic technology-driven healthcare community, nurses must collaborate with genetic experts if we are to 1) understand how patients and families interpret and internalize genetic information and how genetic information influences patient and family identity, decision making, and health behavior, and 2) develop interventions that maximize successful adaptation. Identity is not formed in isolation.

References

Anton-Culver H., A. Ziogas, D. Bowen, D. Finkelstein, C. Griffin, J. Hanson, C. Isaacs, C. Kasten-Sportes, G. Mineau, P. Nadkarni et al. 2003. The cancer genetics network: Recruitment results and pilot studies. *Community Genetics* 6: 171–177.

Armstrong, D., S. Michie, and T. Marteau. 1998. Revealed identity: A study of the process of genetic counseling. *Social Science and Medicine* 47 (11): 1653–1658.

Bergum, V. 2002. Beyond the rights: The ethical challenge. *Phenomenology + Pedagogy* 10: 53–74.

Blanchard, D., J. Erblich, G. H. Montgomery, and D. H. Bovbjerg. 2002. Read all about it: The over-representation of breast cancer in popular magazines. *Preventive Medicine* 35: 343–348.

Chernof, B.A., S. E. Sherman, A. B. Lanto, M. L. Lee, E. M. Yano, and L. V. Rubenstein. 1999. Health habit counseling amidst competing demands: Effects of patient health habits and visit characteristics. *Medical Care* 37 (8): 738–747.

Donaldson, S. K., and D. M. Crowley. 2004. The discipline of nursing. In *Perspectives on Nursing Theory,* eds. Pamela Reed, Nelma Shearer and Leslie Nicoll. 4th Edition. Philadelphia: Lippincott Williams and Watkins.

Elliott, C. 1999. *Bioethics, culture and identity: A philosophical disease*. London: Routledge.

Erblich J., D. H. Bovbjerg, C. Norman, H. B. Valdimarsdottir, and G. H. Montgomery. 2000. It won't happen to me: Lower perception of heart disease risk among women with family histories of breast cancer. *Preventive Medicine* 31: 714–721.

Hunt, K., C. Davidson, C. Emslie, and G. Ford. 2000. Are perceptions of a family history of heart disease related to health-related attitudes and behavior? *Health Education Research Theory and Practice* 15 (2): 131–143.

International Human Genome Sequencing Consortium (IHGSC). (2004). *International Human Genome Sequencing Consortium describes finished human genome sequence.* http://www.genome.gov/12513430 (accessed October 7, 2008).

Jenkins, J., K. Calzone, D. H. Lea, and C. Prows. 2006. *Essential core competencies and curricula guidelines for genetics and genomics.* Silver Spring, MD: American Nurses Association.

Kenen, R. H. 1996. The at-risk health status and technology: A diagnostic invitation and the "gift" of knowing. *Social Science and Medicine* 42 (11): 1545–1553.

Kenen, R., A. Ardern-Jones, and R. Eeles. 2003. Living with chronic risk: Healthy women with a family history of breast/ovarian cancer. *Health, Risk and Society* 5 (3): 315–331.

Klinkman, M. S. 1997. Competing demands in psychosocial care: A model for the identification and treatment of depressive disorders in primary care. *General Hospital Psychiatry* 19: 98–111.

Koch, L. and M. N. Svendsen. 2005. Providing solutions—defining problems: the imperative of disease prevention in genetic counseling. *Social Science and Medicine* 60 (4): 823–832.

Legato, M. J., E. Padus, and E. Slaughter. 1997. Women's perceptions of their general health, with special reference to their risk of coronary artery disease: Results of a national telephone survey. *Journal of Women's Health* 6 (2): 189–198.

Meilaender, G. C. 1995. *Body, soul, and bioethics.* Notre Dame, IN: University of Notre Dame Press.

Mendel, G. 1865/1966. Experiments on plant hybrids. In *The Origin of Genetics: A Mendel Sourcebook,* eds. C. Stern and E. R. Sherwood, 1–48. San Francisco: Freeman.

Olsen, S. 2008. *Prevalence and predictors of cancer and cardiovascular disease prevention behaviors among healthy women with an inherited predisposition for breast and ovarian cancer.* The Catholic University of America. December 2008. Unpublished dissertation.

Pellegrino, E. D., and D. C. Thomasma. 1981. *What is medicine?: A philosophical basis of medical practice.* New York: Oxford University Press.

Redelmeier, D. A., S. H. Tan, and G. L. Booth. 1998. The treatment of unrelated disorders in patients with chronic medical diseases. *The New England Journal of Medicine* 338: 1516–1520.

Richards, M. P. M. 1997. It runs in the family: Lay knowledge about inheritance. In *Culture, Kinship and Genes,* ed. A. Clark, 175–194. Basingstoke: Macmillan Press.

Robertson, J. A. 2003. The $1000 genome: Ethical and legal issues in whole genome sequencing of individuals. *The American Journal of Bioethics* 3 (3): W35–W42.

Rost, K., P. Nutting, J. Smith, J. C. Coyne, L. Cooper-Patrick, and L. Rubenstein. 2000. The role of competing demands in the treatment provided primary care patients with major depression. *Archives of Family Medicine* 9: 150–154.

Rothman, D. 2003. *Strangers at the bedside: A history of how law and bioethics transformed medical decision making.* New York: Aldine de Gruyter.

Sarter, B. 2004. Philosophical sources of nursing theory. In *Perspectives on Nursing Theory,* eds. Pamela Reed, Nelma Shearer, and Leslie Nicoll. 4th ed. Philadelphia: Lippincott Williams and Watkins.

Schechtman, M. 1996. *The constitution of selves.* Ithaca, NY: Cornell University Press.

Shaha, M. and C. Cox. 2003. The omnipresence of cancer. *European Journal of Oncology Nursing,* 7 (3): 191–196.

Shaha, M., C. Cox, A.Hall, A. Porrett, and J. Brown. 2006. The omnipresence of cancer: Its implications for colorectal cancer. *Cancer Nursing Practice* 5 (4): 35–39.

Skirton H., and C. Eiser. 2003. Discovering and addressing the client's lay construct of genetic disease: An important aspect of genetic healthcare? *Research and Theory in Nursing Practice* 17 (4): 339–352.

Thomasma, D. C. 1999. Toward a new medical ethics: Implications for ethics in nursing. In *Interpretive Phenomenology: Embodiment, Caring, and Ethics in Health and Illness,* ed. by Patricia Benner. Thousand Oaks, CA: Sage Publications.

U.S. Department of Health and Human Services (USDHS) Health Resources and Services Administration Bureau of Health Professions. 2006. *The registered nurse population: Findings from the March 2004 National Sample Survey of Registered Nurses.* Bethesda, MD: USDHS.

Walter, F.M., J. Emery, D. Braithwaite, and T. M. Marteau. 2004. Lay understanding of familial risk of common chronic diseases: A systematic review and synthesis of qualitative research. *Annals of Family Medicine* 2 (6): 583–594.

Watson, J. and F. Crick. 1953. Molecular structure of nucleic acids: A structure for deoxyribonucleic acid. *Nature* 171: 737–738.

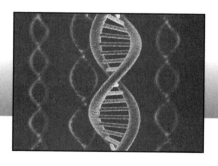

CHAPTER 7

Danger and Genomic Technologies

Rita Black Monsen, DSN, MPH, RN, FAAN

Introduction

New and emerging approaches to maintenance of health and management of illness challenge healthcare professionals, including nurses, to continually update their knowledge and skills. Genetic technologies and the geneticization of health care proliferate at a rapid pace across the world. Societies and community leaders are often reluctant to develop policies and regulations in the face of these changes and may rely on the advice of experts in medical technology to chart their courses of action. Frequently, individuals and families who might benefit or be harmed by such new developments are called upon to testify about their experiences and recommendations. Law and policy makers are also influenced by the economic and political potentials that accompany these ventures. Moreover, there is a need for continued monitoring and adjustment of protections as applications of technology expand. I believe that there are three dangers associated with genetic technologies and genomic healthcare approaches as they are delivered to patients, families, and communities, indeed society as a whole. These are danger of discrimination associated with genetic testing and discovery of inherited risk for illness; danger of commercial exploitation of individuals, families, and communities as genetic technologies proliferate in agriculture, health care, and athletics; and danger associated with inadequate preparation of healthcare professionals to utilize gene-based diagnostics and therapeutics appropriately for the improvement of health and quality of life of entire societies.

Danger of Discrimination

The Coalition for Genetic Fairness, an organization that joins healthcare professionals, consumers, and representatives of the biotechnology and pharmaceutical industries, is calling for a national law protecting individuals from discrimination in employment and insurance coverage based upon genetic make-up (CGF 2006). Protection against misuse or limitation of genetic information (Haga and Willard 2005), including how information is used to determine risk classification for health insurance and employment, varies widely between states. Indeed, testimony by various groups before a federal advisory board revealed that people were fearful of genetic testing because of the potential for discrimination. Such a law has received overwhelming support from elected leaders in the federal government (Greely 2005), and would augment existing state legislation as well as the Americans with Disabilities Act of 1990. Combating fears of discrimination in the community is important, according to Francis Collins, Director of the National Human Genome Research Institute, because reluctance to participate in testing and trials for gene-based diagnostics and therapeutics is likely to slow progress toward efficacious management of illness (CGF 2006).

One important example of discrimination by an employer is the case of the Burlington Northern Santa Fe Railway Company (Haga and Willard 2005) where 36 employees were threatened with denial of payment for injury claims because the railway asserted that genetic information it had collected relieved it of responsibility for work-related disability. The Equal Opportunity Commission settled with Burlington for $2.2 million in a 2001 suit that demonstrated misuse of genetic information based on routine testing for genetic defects without employee knowledge and consent (Schafer 2001).

In contrast, IBM recently announced its commitment to hiring practices and decisions for health insurance coverage not based upon genetic information. This precedent by a company with over 300,000 employees may shape corporate employment policies (Haga and Willard 2005). If not, we face the liklihood that public fears of unfair practices and discrimination based on genetic information will curtail research that could deliver safe, cost-effective genomic health care to those in need in the future.

Danger of Commercialization

The biotech industry provides advancing technologies for the production of consumer goods, industrial equipment and products, and new pathways for research and development. This is one of the fastest growing sectors of the United States and world economies despite enormous front-end investments required for the discovery and development of successful products. In the area of agriculture, the Department of Energy Office of Science, Office of Biological and Environmental Research reports that in 2003 about 167 million acres in 18 countries were sown with transgenic crops (plants or animals that have DNA from different organisms, also known as genetically engineered), principally insecticide- and herbicide-resistant corn, soybeans, canola, and cotton (Human Genome Project Information 2004).

Agriculture in the United States accounts for 63% of the world's transgenic crops. Cultivation of these plants is leveling out, but on the increase in developing countries. Genetically engineered crops have entered the food supply in the United States and several areas of the world with very little substantiation of their safety for human consumption (National Academy of Sciences 2004), thus raising questions about potential health effects. Human Genome Project Information (2004), an organization sponsored by the Department of Energy Office of Science and Office of Biological and Environmental Research, notes that considerable controversy and debate surround genetically engineered foods, with unanswered questions about safety, labeling, consumer knowledge of associated risks, environmental protection, and reduction of hunger around the world.

The National Academy of Sciences (2004) issued a landmark report on the safety of genetically engineered foods, which noted that genetic engineering was associated with "unintentionally introduced changes in the composition of foods" (ix). Conventional breeding methods do result in potentially hazardous foods, evidenced by the fact that "most crops produce allergens, toxins, or antinutritional substances" (3), but using genetic engineering technology that is not adequately tested for safety may also contaminate the nation's food supply. The report urges thorough safety testing before introduction to the market, monitoring and tracking to detect changes in population health associated with genetically engineered foods, and ongoing development of analytic technologies that use informatics, epidemiological methods, and dietary surveys of food consumption patterns across the United States that will ensure food safety.

Further dangers of commercialization reside in exploitation of human curiosity and, perhaps, desires to capitalize on peoples' wishes to enhance their health. The direct marketing of genetic tests to the public can generate considerable profits without the expense of health assessments and appropriate counseling by nurses and other professionals, as seen in the offerings of one biotech company, Sciona (http://www.sciona.com/; accessed October 7, 2008). This is a privately owned organization that provides the results of analysis of as many as 19 genes related to bone and cardiovascular health with a mailed-in specimen of buccal mucosa (taken with a swab of the inner cheek). The report is returned to the consumer with "a complete snapshot of their overall risk profile and recommendations for achieving optimal health without a specific disease focus." The company offers kits that determine insulin resistance, antioxidant and detoxification factors, and "inflammation health" and makes recommendations for diet and lifestyle to promote health. Indeed, the company believes that "people are capable of interpreting fairly complex information when it relates to their own well-being" and does offer the statement that "when the implications of the information are likely to impact on medical interventions, the service will only be provided through a qualified practitioner."

The danger that I discern in claims such as these is based on volumes of research and many years of collective clinical experience in the community of genetics healthcare professionals. Professionals who provide genetic counseling take great care to place genetic testing in the context of thorough examination of individual and family health histories, family pedigrees, supportive counseling when disclosing the results of genetic testing, and careful follow-up of patients and families to prevent misinterpretation of genetic information and needless anguish among relatives and offspring. Direct marketing of genetic tests like these and other tests that estimate risks for specific cancers has the potential to seriously harm patients and families when they are offered without adequate support and counseling.

Finally, genetic testing and or gene-based therapeutics to give humans extreme characteristics and abilities may be detrimental to health and well-being. These measures may enhance strength, endurance, appearance, or other features, but they may entail exploitation of the person and family with possible negative side effects later in life. One such measure is the genetic testing of athletes to find characteristics that could lend themselves to treatments that might enhance performance. This technology is not widespread now, but may encourage "gene doping" or procedures to improve strength and endurance in sports (Genetics and Public Policy Center 2005). Professional athletes and the many industries surrounding professional and amateur sports may risk impaired health or illness by introducing genetic material that supposedly would lead to success, fame, and lucrative incomes. While gene-based therapeutics is an area of great potential, there are risks of unanticipated effects such as the introduction of genetic material that may or may not yield the desired result. What kind of informed consent would be necessary for such modifications? What are the risks for unexpected effects immediately and long-term? Once genetic material is introduced, how could it be removed if the individual no longer wanted such modifications? These questions have no satisfactory answers, and our ability to offer solid protections with gene-based therapeutics may be limited for some time to come.

Danger of Inadequate Preparation of Healthcare Professionals

Perhaps one of the greatest dangers to patients, families, communities, and society lies in the inadequate preparation of clinicians in healthcare settings where genetic concerns and questions arise. Freedman, Wideroff, Olson, and colleagues (2003) surveyed American family physicians and found that these providers felt unprepared to respond to patient questions about emerging genetic information and testing. These findings have been supported by several surveys of nurses, nursing faculty, and other providers that began over 20 years ago. Still, we recognize that knowledgeable health professionals are essential (Feetham, Thomson, and Hinshaw 2005).

In 1996, the National Coalition for Health Professional Education in Genetics (NCHPEG) gathered representatives from the professional organizations serving the U.S. healthcare field, consumer groups, and the biotech and pharmaceutical industries to promote education in genetics and thereby improve the health of our population. Today, NCHPEG comprises 140 organizations and operates a website that connects these groups and others with educational programming, competencies for professional practice dealing with genetics and genomic technologies, and resources for curriculum development and assessment of genetic knowledge.

Without adequate preparation to respond to the concerns of patients and their families, nurses and other providers cannot meet their obligations for truth-telling, for preserving the autonomy of those they serve, and for providing the necessary counseling that safeguards informed consent and supportive care. Without sensitivity to the cultural and spiritual commitments of families and population groups, healthcare professionals risk providing services and conducting research that are irrelevant, and perhaps damaging and oppressive. Nurses' professional responsibilities to stay informed and seek correct information about genetics and genomics in health care are paramount if we value our careers in nursing.

References

Coalition for Genetic Fairness (CGF). 2006. Home page. http://www.geneticfairness.org (accessed September 12, 2008).

Feetham, S., E. J. Thomson, and A. S. Hinshaw. 2005. Nursing leadership in genomics for health and society. *Journal of Nursing Scholarship* 37: 102–110.

Freedman, A. N., L. Wideroff, L. Olson, W. Davis, C. Klabunde, K. P. Srinath, B. B. Reeve, R. T. Croyle, and R. Ballard-Barbash. 2003. U.S. Physicians' attitudes toward genetic testing for cancer susceptibility. *American Journal of Medical Genetics* 120: 63–71.

Genetics and Public Policy Center. 2005. *Gene Doping: Human Genetic Technologies and the Future of Sports.* Genetics Perspectives on Policy Seminars sponsored by Johns Hopkins University and the Pew Charitable Trusts. October 11, 2005. Johns Hopkins University, Washington, DC.

Greely, H. T. 2005. Banning genetic discrimination. *New England Journal of Medicine* 353: 865–867.

Haga, S. B., and H. F. Willard. 2005. Act now to prevent genetic discrimination. *The Washington Post,* December 20, 2005. http://www.washingtonpost.com/wp-dyn/content/article/2005/12/27/AR2005122700889.html (accessed October 7, 2008).

Human Genome Project Information. 2004. *What are genetically modified (GM) foods?* http://www.ornl.gov/sci/techresources/Human_Genome/elsi/gmfood.shtml (accessed October 7, 2008).

National Academy of Sciences. 2004. *Safety of genetically engineered foods: Approaches to assessing unintended health effects.* Washington, DC: The National Academies Press.

National Coalition for Health Professional Education in Genetics (NCHPEG). 2008. www.nchpeg.org (accessed October 7, 2008).

Schafer, S. 2001. Railroad agrees to stop gene-testing workers. *The Washington Post,* April 19, 2001. http://www.washingtonpost.com/ac2/wp-dyn/A34877-2001Apr18?language=printer (accessed October 7, 2008).

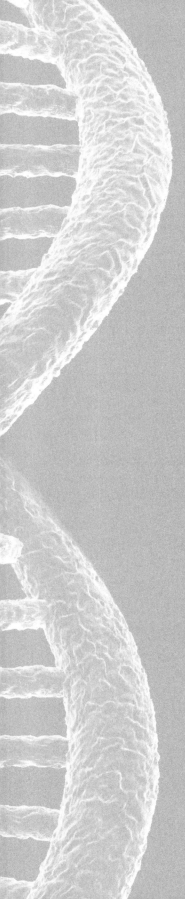

PART 2

Religious and Cultural Perspectives of Communities and Societies

We present here papers from some of the major cultural communities in the world. Culture encompasses the beliefs, mores, and behaviors of groups of peoples and guides their decision-making the face of changes in health and family life. Genomic technologies, which bring new knowledge about the inheritance of risk for illness, can lead patients and families to consider the possibilities of testing and treatment that may never have been available in their past experience. For many communities, the guidance of culture and the advice of elders and religious leaders provides helpful avenues for action. In some instances, people seek information about prior decisions in similar circumstances. But in the case of genetics and genomics, there may be no precedents upon which to draw. People may seek advice from those outside of their cultural groups, and may be supported and consoled as they learn about the dilemmas that others have coped with.

These chapters are included to provide a glimpse into the thinking and decision making patterns seen in several religious and cultural traditions, some not directly discussing genomic technologies. They may be helpful as we collaborate with peoples from diverse cultural and religious communities to inform them about their options with regard to genetic and genomic health.

PART 2 ❧ CONTENTS

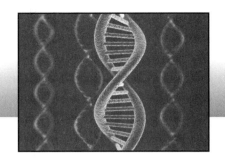

CHAPTER 8

Hinduism and Sikhism: Genetic Counseling Aspects

Elizabeth A. Gettig, MS, CGC
Triptish Bhatia, PhD

A case study: Years ago one of the authors [EG] provided prenatal diagnosis and genetic counseling to a couple living in the United States who had immigrated from Bangalore, India. Both members of the couple were 35 years of age and engineering professionals. An amniocentesis was performed which revealed a diagnosis of Trisomy 18. They elected termination of the pregnancy and cremation of the remains of the baby by the hospital. Several weeks later the couple re-contacted the center asking if ash from the cremation or any other material was available, as they wished to conduct a ceremony to commemorate the life of the baby at their Hindu temple. Due to mid-trimester development, little or no ash was available to the couple. The counselor did ask to speak to their priest to gather more information about the ceremony and determine if any alternatives could be found. After a very thoughtful discussion with the priest, the genetic counselor mentioned that the laboratory did have slides which had cells from the baby. There were extra slides available. The priest was asked if the slides could be used in the ceremony. The counselor delivered three slides to the priest who crushed them with a mortar and pestle to create a fine sand similar to ash. This material was used in the ceremony, which brought great comfort to the couple.

The case above illustrates how working with clergy in a culturally sensitive manner can provide support and comfort to families. Only by mutual exchange could a satisfactory resolution be made. To communicate effectively with other cultures, genetic care providers must pursue cultural competency. We review issues of Hinduism and Sikhism (in India and the United States) and offer aspects of the religion and culture that may assist in communication. Although there are significant differences between the Hindu and Sikh cultures and vast diversity within them, there are shared traditions: a belief in rebirth, a concept of karma (in which experiences in one life influence experiences in future lives), collective decision making, an emphasis on the value of purity, and a holistic view of the person that affirms the importance of family, culture, environment and the spiritual dimension of experience. When offering genetic testing and counseling it is important to keep the tenets of these religions in mind. The growing number of south Asians in the United States and the increase in genetic services in India demonstrate the need for trans-cultural understanding. Many who immigrate from India continue with traditional religious practices. Some practices may be westernized a bit but the roots remain in India. Therefore we address traditional Indian values in this chapter.

Genetic testing programs and genetic training programs have emerged worldwide (Table 1). These services and programs reflect varying approaches to the patient and to the student in training. As India develops more genetic resources we have sought to contrast our current similarities and differences in serving families with genetic conditions. In the Hindu and Sikh traditions, there is no great distinction between culture and religion, and medical decisions are grounded in both religious beliefs and cultural values. We focus on Sikhs and Hindus in this paper, but recognize the vast number of cultures and languages in India and among those who have emigrated to the United States and other parts of the world.

Cultural self-awareness is the key because it enables healthcare providers to recognize that as cultural beings, they may hold attitudes and beliefs that can detrimentally influence their perceptions of and interactions with individuals who are ethnically, culturally, and racially different from themselves. A threefold approach of developing awareness and knowledge of one's own culture, developing awareness of the client's culture, and learning specific skills to minimize the impact of one's own biases and prejudices toward the multicultural interaction aids in developing ethno-cultural self awareness (Sue and Sue 1999).

TABLE 8–1
Global Genetic Counseling Training Programs

Country	Program
Australia	Charles Sturt University
	Griffith University
	University of Melbourne
	University of Newcastle
Canada	McGill University
	University of British Columbia
	University of Toronto
China	Peking University Center of Medical Genetics
Cuba	National Center for Medical Genetics
France	University of Marseille
Israel	Haddasah Hebrew University
Japan	Chiba University
	Kawasaki University
	Kinki University
	Kitasato University
	Kyoto University
	Ochanamizu University
	Shinsu University
Netherlands	University of Groningen
Norway	University of Bergen
Saudi Arabia	King Faisal Hospital and Research Center
South Africa	University of Cape Town
	University of Witwatersand
Spain	University of Barcelona
	University of Pompeu Fabra
Sweden	Uppsala University

ᵔ CONTINUED

TABLE 8-1
Continued

Country	Program
Taiwan	National Taiwan University
United Kingdom	Cardiff University University of Manchester
United States	Arcadia University (Beaver College prior to July 16, 2001), Glenside, PA University of Arkansas (Online Consortium with Nebraska, Kansas, Oklahoma) Boston University School of Medicine, Boston, MA Brandeis University, Waltham, MA California State University, Northridge, CA Case Western Reserve University, Cleveland, OH Howard University, Washington, DC Indiana University Medical Center, Indianapolis, IN Johns Hopkins University/National Center for Human Genome Research, Bethesda, MD Medical College of Virginia, Virginia Commonwealth University, Richmond, VA Mt. Sinai School of Medicine, New York, NY Northwestern University Medical School, Chicago, IL Sarah Lawrence College, Bronxville, NY University of Arizona Health Science Center, Tucson, AZ University of California, Irvine, Orange, CA University of Cincinnati College of Medicine/Children's Hospital Medical Center, Cincinnati, OH University of Colorado Health Science Center, Denver, CO University of Maryland School of Medicine, Baltimore, MD University of Michigan, Ann Arbor, MI University of Minnesota, Minneapolis, MN

↪ CONTINUED

TABLE 8–1
Continued

Country	Program
	University of North Carolina, Greensboro, NC
	University of Oklahoma Medical Center, Oklahoma City, OK
	University of Pittsburgh, PA
	University of South Carolina, Columbia, SC
	University of Texas Medical School, Houston, TX
	University of Utah Health Sciences Center, Salt Lake City, Utah
	University of Wisconsin, Madison, WI
	Wayne State University, Detroit, MI
United States Academics Programs (Nursing) in Genetics	Columbia University
	University of Iowa
	University of California, San Francisco
	University of Pittsburg (PA)
	University of Washington

Sources: ABGC 2008; ICGP 2006.

General Facts: India and the United States

To undertake our task of contrasting India and the United States some basic facts are needed. India is one of the oldest civilizations on the planet, dating back over 5,000 years. The United States has a relatively short history. India's first major civilization flourished for a thousand years beginning around 2500 BCE. By the nineteenth century, Britain had assumed political control of virtually all Indian lands. Nonviolent resistance to British colonialism led by Mohandas Gandhi brought independence in 1947. The subcontinent was divided into the secular state of India and the smaller Muslim state of Pakistan. A third war between the two countries in 1971 resulted in East Pakistan becoming the separate nation of Bangladesh. Despite impressive gains in economic investment and output, India faces pressing problems such as the ongoing dispute with Pakistan over Kashmir, massive overpopulation, environmental degradation, extensive poverty, and ethnic and religious strife (CIA 2006).

India has over a billion citizens, a third of whom are less than 15 years of age, compared to a total population of less than 300 million in the United States with 20% of the U.S. population less than 15 years of age. (Indian Ministry of Home Affairs 2001). The land mass of India is slightly more than one-third the size of the United States. The growing Indian population is straining its natural resources. The life expectancy is 64 years, contrasted to about 78 years in the United States. The population growth rate in India is 1.4% and .92% in the United States. The infant morality rate in India is 5.6% with the rate in the United States being 0.65 % (CIA 2006).

India has a diverse set of spoken languages among different groups of people. At least 30 different languages and around 2,000 dialects have been identified. The Constitution of India has stipulated Hindi and English to be the two official languages of communication for the national government. Additionally, it contains a list of 22 scheduled languages. (Wikipedia n.d.).

Internationally literacy is defined as those who can read and write after age 15. Using this definition the Indian literacy rate is 59.5% (70.2% males; 48.3% females) compared to the U.S. rate of 97% (equal between the sexes). There are 147 million people in the U.S. workforce and 482 million in the Indian workforce.

The leading causes of death are shown in Table 8–2 and are contrasted with the United States and the World Health Organization (WHO) (NCHS 2005; Infoplease 2002; WHO 2000). Being a developing country, India is still fighting with its overload of infectious diseases. HIV/AIDS in India is at a critical stage. Diarrheal diseases such as cholera and dysentery caused by poor sanitation and unsafe water claim thousands of lives annually in addition to loss of life from tuberculosis and malaria. Relevancy of genetic health conditions compared to those infectious in nature has not emerged as a pressing health issue. The priorities are different as vast numbers of people still live in poverty, at least 25% of the population. This does not mean that genetic diseases are not present in India, but genetics takes a different place in terms of importance in health care (Verma 2000). There is scarcity of genetic awareness among the public and health provider community with the possible exception of beta-thalassemia and other hemoglobinopathy programs (Figure 8–1). The general public may not know about these diseases and therefore are unable to recognize and understand their symptoms and origin, though they observe the familial nature of conditions. The public may feel helpless and may not seek help to understand these conditions. They are referred by their family physicians for genetic testing and special services that may be quite limited (Verma 2005).

TABLE 8–2
Leading Causes of Death—India, World, United States

India (1998)	World (2002)	United States (2001)
Heart Disease	Heart Disease	Heart Disease
Pneumonia	Stroke	Cancer
Diarrhea	Pneumonia	Stroke
Perinatal	HIV/AIDS	COPD
Stroke	COPD	Injury
Tuberculosis	Diarrhea	Diabetes
Traffic Accidents	Tuberculosis	Pneumonia/Influenza
Measles	Malaria	Alzheimer's Disease
HIV/AIDS	Cancer trachea/bronchus/lung	Kidney Disease
Tetanus	Traffic Accidents	Septicemia

Source: National Center for Health Statistics 2005

Relevant Ethnocultural Groups

Cultural differences are important factors in communicating health-related information and health beliefs. There are culture-related myths, behaviors, and beliefs that influence the way people listen to genetic counselor or health professional. This, in turn, influences decision making. Understanding cultural factors is important in designing culture-specific strategies for genetic counseling.

Though famine is not present in India, each day brings a quest to forage for food for many in the population. Begging in cities is commonplace but often is an organized gang activity. In general, people in India don't seem to complain about illness as much as Americans. At a public hospital, it may take hours to be seen by a physician, but the crowds patiently and calmly wait their turn. The physician–patient

FIGURE 8–1
Beta-thalassemia

Beta-THALASSEMIA (b-thal) is a genetic disorder of red cells caused by the reduction or absence of *b*-globin-chain production, which occurs because of mutations in the *b*-globin gene. It is inherited in an autosomal recessive manner. The impact on child health and families is distressing. For example, a study of 200 families with thalassemic children in Mumbai showed that treatment costs made up 20–30% of family income (Sangani , 1990). This financial burden is due in part to the fact that diagnostic and treatment services are often available only through private practices and only to the minority that can afford them.

The *b*-thalassemias have extremely diverse clinical phenotypes. At the severe end of the spectrum, many homozygous or compound heterozygous patients present with severe anemia requiring regular blood transfusion to sustain life, whereas at the mild end the heterozygous state is characterized by mild hypochromic, microcytic anemia with elevated HbA2 levels (Weatherall 2001). Certain communities of India, like Sindhis, Gujratis, Punjabis, and Bengalis, are more commonly affected with *b*-thalassemia, the incidence varying from 1% to 17%. To minimize the tremendous health burden imposed by the disease, it is desirable to have genetic counseling and prenatal diagnosis facilities available in the country. The success of pre-natal diagnosis and genetic counseling depends on the knowledge of the spectrum of b-thal mutations in the population (Agarwal et al., 2000). The heterogeneous nature of *b*-thal is well known, with more than 200 different mutations reported to date. Apart from such a vast molecular variability, each ethnic population has its own cluster of specific mutations (Weatherall and Clegg 2001). In Asian Indians, five common and ten less common mutations, with a variable number of rare mutations, are defined (Varawalla et al. 1991). Therefore, to successfully implement programs aimed at reducing the incidence of thalassemia, and to make them more cost effective, knowledge about the mutation spectrum and hence specific genetic testing for the disease is important.

exchange is often unidirectional with little comment and certainly few questions from the patient, a stark contrast to the expectations and practice of medicine in the United States.

India is a relationship-based culture. This means it takes time to establish trust and one should not hurry. Friendship and kinship are often more important than expertise, but titles and diplomas are prized. In the United States an attitude of "seize the opportunity" is commonplace, while in India there is a tendency to believe what goes around comes around so that opportunities will come again later. Humility is seen as a virtue, as is showing deference to elders. Humor is found throughout the Indian culture. As a group the Indians share the U.S. tendency for risk taking.

India is a spiritual nation. It is noted as the birthplace of Hinduism, and around 500 BCE two other religions developed in India, namely, Buddhism and Jainism. Hinduism is one of the ancient religions of the world. It is supposed to have developed about 5000 years ago. Hinduism differs from Christianity and other Western religions in that it does not have a single founder, a specific theological system, a single system of morality, or a central religious organization. It consists of a multitude of different religious groups which have emerged since 1500 BC. Today, only about 0.5% of Indians are Jains and about 0.7% are Buddhist. In ancient times Jainism and Buddhism were very popular in India. India is also the home to one of the largest Muslim populations (Indian Ministry of Home Affairs 2001). These three ancient religions, Hinduism, Buddhism, and Jainism, are seen as the molders of the India philosophy. In this chapter, we focus on Hinduism and Sikhism, which were established in northern India approximately 500 years ago by Guru Nanak. Although Hindu and Sikh cultural and religious traditions have profound differences, they both traditionally take a duty-based rather than rights-

TABLE 8–3
Religions of India

Religion	Percent of Population
Hinduism	81
Islam	13
Christianity	2
Sikhism	2
Buddhism	1
Jainism	About 0.5
Zoroastrianism	About 0.01
Judaism	About 0.0005

Source: Indian Ministry of Home Affairs 2001.

based approach to decision making. Table 3 illustrates current religious affiliations of the Indian population.

Hinduism

The dominant religion in India today is Hinduism. About 80% of Indians are Hindus. Hinduism is not really a religion but a way of life. Regarding health issues, spiritual well-being comes from leading a dedicated life based on non-violence, love, good conduct, and selfless service, and ultimately from experiencing the Truth within. The approach to spiritual well-being varies according to individual temperament. The Truth may be realized through devotion to a particular aspect of God, self-analysis, austerities, selfless service, or meditation. Hinduism ascribes to the theory of Karma (the law of cause and effect). Each individual creates their own destiny by thoughts, words, and deeds. (Klostermaier 1998).

It must be noted that these religious beliefs are not universal among all Hindu Indians. In the healthcare setting, it is helpful to have a basic understanding of the individual patient's chosen religion and how that person practices and lives out that faith. Illness, accident, and injury result from the karma one creates and are seen as a means of purification.

Sikhism

Sikhism is the fifth largest religion, with approximately 20 million Sikhs worldwide. The word "Sikh" means disciple or follower. Sikhs who have undergone the Khalsa baptism ceremony adhere to the Khalsa Code of Conduct, which defines social practices, ethical rules of conduct, acceptance of the teachings of the gurus, and wearing of five physical articles of faith (or five Ks) as follows:

- Kes (also referred to as Kesh, kais, kesa): Uncut hair, including body and facial hair. Hair on the head is worn in a topknot. Not all Sikhs, particularly in Western countries, adhere to this practice.
- Kangha: A comb carried as a symbol of hygiene, to keep the hair neat and to hold the topknot in place. Bald Sikhs also wear a kangha.
- Kara: A steel or iron bangle worn on the right wrist as a sign of loyalty to the guru, as a reminder to the wearer to restrain their actions, and to remember God at all times.

- Kirpan: A sword, often a short one, approximately four inches in length or a smaller steel replica. The kirpan is typically worn underneath the clothing and symbolizes defense for all that is just.
- Kachha: Knee-length pants tied with a drawstring, generally worn as an undergarment, symbolizing sexual restraint.

Men who are members of the Khalsa must wear a turban. However, the turban is not one of the five Ks. Women are not required to wear a turban, but may do so if desired. A scarf instead of a turban is acceptable for women. The turban is a means of keeping the hair neat and tidy. It consists of a lengthy piece of cloth and is generally tied as an inverted V over the forehead. The color and shape of the turban, and the manner in which it is tied, can indicate a Sikh's age, geographical origin, and political preference. A keski, or small under-turban about one-fourth the size of the outer turban, may be worn only when not in public.

The goal of Sikhs is to build a close, loving relationship with God. Sikhs believe in a single God, who is referred to by different names depicting the virtues like Kartar (creator), Nirankar (formless), or Akal Purakh (immortal entity). But the most common name used is Waheguru, meaning "God is wonderful." This concept is similar to Islam, whose followers believe in a single God who has 99 names. Some Sikhs believe that their religion is a re-purification of Hinduism; they view Sikhism as part of the Hindu religious tradition. Many Sikhs disagree; they believe that their religion is a direct revelation from God—a religion that was not derived from either Hinduism or Islam.

Health Beliefs: Karma and Rebirth

Because Indians see their health as interwoven with other life and spiritual elements, it is not uncommon for an illness to be thought of as an opportunity to be taught a lesson in life. This philosophy opens the door for more holistic forms of medicine. Herbal medicines, sometimes referred to as Ayurveda, an ancient holistic system of medicine, may be practiced.

The Indian system of medicine is known as Ayurveda, which means "knowledge of life." Indian medicine mixes religion with secular medicine, and involves observation of the patient as well as the patient's natural environment. A large percentage of people in India rely on herbal remedies as the principal means of preventing and curing illnesses. In the Ayurveda system, the body is composed of three primary forces, termed dosha. The state of equilibrium between the dosha is perceived as a state of health; the state of imbalance is disease. By examination the Ayurveda physician finds out the position of the three dosha (Tridosha). Once the aggravated or unbalanced dosha is known, it is brought into balance by using different kinds of therapies.

The notion of karma and a belief in rebirth is important for many Hindu and Sikh patients as they make decisions surrounding birth and death. Karma is a law of behavior and consequences in which actions in past live(s) affects the circumstances in which one is born and lives in this life. Thus a patient may feel that their illness is caused by karma (even though they may completely understand biological causes of illness). Hence, an illness may be seen as a result of actions in this life or a past life. In many Hindu and Sikh households there is an attachment to traditional medicines (e.g., Ayurveda and Siddha), which may be used together with modern medicine (Azariah, Azariah, and Macer 1998).

Throughout a pregnancy, it is believed that the developing child is vulnerable to evil spirits. It is therefore the tradition of many Hindu families to perform rituals to protect the mother and the unborn baby. In south India, during the fifth month of pregnancy, some of the ceremonies preformed include Valakappu, Puchutal, and Saddha. These vary according to different regions in India, but they are each performed in the woman's house. During the eighth month of pregnancy, another ritual, called Simantam, takes place in the husband's house. Many Indian women additionally protect themselves from evil spirits by wearing a type of amulet called a valai or valayal, which means, "to surround." It is believed to create an invisible barrier that keeps the pregnant woman safe from the influence of evil spirits.

For Hindus, noting the exact time of a baby's birth is important for the child's horoscope. Traditionally a baby is born in the home of the wife's parents with a midwife present, but not the husband. In a Western hospital, the Hindu husband may be present at the birth. Generally, breast feeding by Indian women is practiced and encouraged. It is usually continued anywhere from six months to three years. It is common for breast milk to be supplemented with cow's milk and diluted with sugar water. The recuperation time for the mother and baby usually lasts for 40 days after birth. During that time, the mother is encouraged to remain at home, where she is to obtain adequate rest and is offered special food along with regular meals. Males are not circumcised. Traditionally, the child is named in a celebration on the 10th day after birth. In the West, the child is sometimes named at birth.

Supported by their belief in karma, most Hindus do not approve of abortion, with no exceptions for rape or deformities. Termination by abortion sends the soul back into the karmic cycle of rebirth. However, birth control, natural or artificial, is approved and practiced. In an American hospital, a Hindu woman would most likely not request special care. She would want her husband's advice on any medical decisions. Hindu tradition does not approve of mercy killing, assisted suicide, or suicide. Prolonging life artificially is up to the individual. However, letting nature take its course is common in Hindu tradition. The making of a living will or advance directive (such as for the donation of organs) is up to the individual (Coward and Sidhu 2000).

Sikhs believe in samsara (the repetitive cycle of birth, life, and death), karma (the accumulated sum of one's good and bad deeds), and reincarnation (rebirth following death). These beliefs are similar to Hinduism. The goal of human life is to break the cycle of births and deaths and to merge with God. There is great emphasis placed on daily devotion to the remembrance of God. Sikhs have rejected the caste system of the Hindu religion. They believe that everyone has equal status in the eyes of God. This is a very important principle that permeates all Sikh beliefs, behaviors, and rituals.

For Sikhs, health beliefs include recognition that all humans suffer. Suffering stems from two sources—failure to appreciate God's creation and failure to control the mind. Alcoholic beverages, narcotics, and tobacco are avoided by most. The five Ks are worn at all times, even during hospitalization, illness at home, or when washing. The healthcare provider should consult the patient or family before removing any of these items.

Children are considered a gift from God. The father will wish to whisper the Mul Mantra (Guru Nanak's first poetical statement) into the newborn's ear as soon as possible following birth. The mother may be secluded for a period of 13 to 40 days following delivery. This is considered a period of impurity. Birth control is acceptable. Artificial insemination is permitted if the sperm is from the husband. Elective pregnancy termination is generally unacceptable. Children's hair will be left uncut. Boys may undergo a ceremony of turban-tying in the gurdwara at 10 to 12 years of age. From this point forward, the turban should be treated with the same care and symbolism as with adults. Teenage boys will not shave.

Sikhs, like Hindus, may have a large extended family, which includes all members of the Sikh community. Elders are valued and cared for by the family. Men and women have equal status. However, women are expected to cover their legs. Women may wear loose trousers called salvars and a shirt that reaches to the knees. It is advisable to provide same-sex caregivers, including physicians, particularly for women. Again, family members are likely to stay with a relative who is hospitalized. Health providers should allow family participation in care as much as possible. During hospitalization, family members may bring karah parshad (a special food that has been blessed) to the ill relative. If at all possible, the hospitalized person should be allowed to have a small piece of this food, even if on a restricted diet.

Collective Decision Making: Hindu and Sikh

Extended families are common and provide family members with social support and financial security. Because of the value placed on independence and privacy in Indian culture and the desire to save face, family issues, including healthcare decisions, are frequently discussed within the immediate family before seeking outside help. Hindu and Sikh families are traditionally close-knit in India or wherever they have immigrated. A Hindu or Sikh hospital patient would want relatives to visit and close family members to help in the making of any medical decisions, such as whether or not to operate. In public hospitals in India, a family member is usually present at all times. If the patient is connected with a Hindu temple or ashram in the United States, the patient may request the Hindu priest or guru to visit.

If the patient is older than the visiting relative, the visitor would be expected to stand unless invited to sit by the patient. Respect for one's elders is engraved in Hindu culture, along with warm, affectionate family ties. In a hospital setting, personal devotions may consist of prayer, meditation, and the reading of scripture. A small picture or statue of a deity may be used in prayer. A mantram (a sound vibration representing an aspect of the Divine) may be recited on a mala (prayer beads strung together, similar to a rosary). Facing north or east is preferred, but not required. Relationships between siblings tend to be close. Many times brothers live together for both financial and familial reasons. After marriage, if families live apart, siblings and their families continue to meet throughout the year for religious holidays and special occasions, as well as vacations.

End-of-Life Issues

As in most cultures, a Hindu in America would prefer to die at home. However, if unavoidable, dying in a hospital would be acceptable. The dying patient may wish to be alone, with relatives, or with their priest or guru (if possible). In the chapel of the funeral home, a Hindu priest, if available, would do the last rites. It is believed that the soul will reincarnate again and again until its karma is exhausted. Giving in to mourning for the dead is said to make it more difficult for the soul of the deceased to leave the earthly plane. The ideal is to remember the deceased with happy thoughts, as the soul will receive those thoughts. Of course, given human nature, mourning for the dead is natural, but excessive mourning is not recommended.

For Sikhs, cultural practices surrounding death include reading scriptures and singing hymns during the last hours of a Sikh's life. Hope, rather than sadness, should characterize the death of a Sikh. Expressions of grief for one who has lived a happy and long life are limited or not seen at all. It is believed that crying will inter-fere with a peaceful departure of the dying person. Expressions of grief may be more liberal if a person dies early in life or from some unnatural cause. The family will likely wish to prepare the relative's body following death. This involves washing and dressing the deceased by wrapping in a white shroud, leaving the five Ks in place. The head will be wrapped in a turban. If no family is available, the head of the deceased should be kept covered. All hair should be left untrimmed. The face should be cleaned and the eyes and mouth closed. Sikhs are generally cremated within 24 hours of death if possible. Stillborns and neonates may be buried. Autopsy is accept-able, but generally not desirable unless required by law.

Purity, Modesty, and Marriage

Arranged marriages are still common, but the process has changed, especially among more cosmopolitan Indians. The two to be wed have time to become acquainted (even date) before making a decision to marry. The decision of whether to date is made fairly quickly to prevent a relationship that will not culminate in marriage. It is felt that a close relationship should only be shared with one individual. The fear of a close relationship is tied to the concept of premarital sex tainting the women and robbing her of purity, which jeopardizes her potential for finding a suitable spouse. Modesty is highly valued among Indians and patients are decidedly more comfortable and secure with same-sex care providers.

In Indian society, the roles of men and women are distinct. Women manage the home by keeping all financial, family, and social issues in order. Women are more passive in the Indian culture and men typically are the breadwinners and managers of matters requiring interaction with individuals in the community, e.g., health care. This type of behavior implies that men have a dominant and authoritative role because they are the primary point of contact with society. However, these roles are beginning to change among educated Indians in the larger cities of India and among immigrants in progressive or permissive societies such as the United States. For Hindus and Sikhs, modesty is highly valued and leaving the body covered as much as possible is recommended. Eye contact may be avoided between children and adults, men and women.

Male Offspring Preference

There is a general bias in favor of males over females in Hindu and Sikh culture. The roots of this bias are twofold. In Hinduism, for example, the eldest son is required to light his father's funeral pyre and to perform yearly rituals for the well-being of the father in the next life. The eldest son is also the head of the extended family and has the responsibility to protect and provide for the women in the family; this includes a moral obligation to ensure that sexual mores are preserved. Sons at marriage receive a dowry with their wife, which adds to the family wealth. Daughters, in taking a dowry with them at marriage, do the reverse. The responsibility of eldest sons to provide for and protect the women in their extended families means that there is often a strong male dominance in matters of consent (Coward 1993).

Informed Consent

Researchers and investigators have argued that getting fully informed written consent may not be possible in developing countries, where illiteracy is widespread (Schrag 2001; Hansson 1998). Gender dynamics, the family unit, financial constraints, and religion influence the researcher–participant relationship as well as the decision-making process In India, getting fully informed written consent from subjects may not be easy, given the large number of languages and dialects spoken, migration of people from one state to another, etc. These difficulties have led to many investigators resorting to partial consent, at times only verbally (Mudur 1997). But with more strict ethical guidelines and collaborative research projects, obtaining consent where those seeking help are appropriately informed about the issues and options for care is becoming mandatory.

Privacy and Confidentiality

There is no word for "rights" in traditional Hindu and Sikh languages. Lack of privacy is pervasive in India. The culture is collectivist and individual space is not a recognized concept, let alone seen from a U.S. perspective as positive and important. People in India like to be in groups and may even feel sorry for the Westerner if they are on their own.

In spite of the stigma associated with many genetic diseases, confidentiality is not a big issue in India. The whole family and sometimes extended family come together for counseling sessions and discuss the situation among them. Family is a valued emotional and financial support for these persons as a public support system is not very well developed in India. Families are definitely concerned about information going beyond family as it may affect marriage alliances. A genetic disease in families may discourage good marriage proposals.

India provides state-supported healthcare systems throughout the country and diminishes concerns regarding job or insurance discrimination. Currently, the fee for genetic testing or counseling is born by the families themselves, as the healthcare system is either a state facility or a private provider, neither of which allows payment from the state. The public healthcare system is free for the general public, but hospitals are not well equipped and few genetic tests are available. Moreover, in rural areas there are no proper healthcare resources available and in the case of genetic testing, clients go to private doctors and private hospitals. There are not many health insurance companies in India and providers are limited to a few major cities. Persons with genetic diseases are not discriminated against if they have government jobs. They continue in their jobs after a genetic diagnosis.

Support Groups

Support groups are a source of information and help for persons with genetic illnesses. However, such organizations are not yet well organized in India.

Genetic Information Providers

In India doctors are considered very respected and trusted professionals, and most of the time they are providing genetic information. Their patients are dependent on them and expect their advice. Most patients find themselves less equipped to make decisions, especially medical decisions. Their external locus of control demands others to make decisions for them and in this case it is the providers of genetic information. Hence they expect the doctors to be directive, in contrast to the U.S. tradition of nondirectiveness. In India, medical advice is taken by and large with full faith.

Conclusion

In short, Hindus and Sikhs have value-based cultures. They are more religious minded. Decisions in life-related issues are governed and influenced by powerful others, be it family or healthcare providers. In contrast to U.S. culture, genetic awareness is more limited and hereditary conditions or traits are accepted as God's wish, with the family as the primary caregiver to those affected. No public support system is available for genetic testing and the burden is on the society and family exclusively. Genetic counseling with Hindu and Sikh families requires that genetic counseling be group-oriented and that it involve the heads of families or recognized authorities in the society.

Acknowledgement

The authors wish to thank specific members of the *Indo-U.S. Project on Schizophrenia Genetics* (University of Pittsburgh, Pittsburgh, PA and Dr Ram Manohar Lohia Hospital, New Delhi, India), our Pittsburgh colleagues Vishwajit Nimgaonkar, MD, PhD, Monisha Tarneja, MPH, and our Delhi colleagues, Smita N. Deshpande, MD, DPM, N. N. Mishra, PhD, Smita Saxena, MS, MPhil. and Harikrishnan Alingal, MS, MPhil. Thank you for sharing your expertise with us.

References

Agarwal, S., M. Pradhan, U. R. Gupta, S. Sarwai and S. S. Agarwal. 2000. Geographic and ethnic distribution of b-thalassemia mutations in Uttar Pradesh, India. *Hemoglobin* 24: 89–97.

American Board of Genetic Counseling (ABGC). 2008. *Accredited Programs.* 2008. http://www.abgc.net/english/View.asp?x=1440 (accessed October 9, 2008).

Azariah, J., H. Azariah, D. R. J. Macer. (eds). 1998. *Bioethics in India (Proceedings of International Bioethics Workshop in Madras: Biomanagement of Biogeo-resources).* Christchurch, NZ: Eubios Ethics Institute/University of Madras.

Central Intelligence Agency (CIA). 2006. *The World Factbook: India.* https://www.cia.gov/library/publications/the-world-factbook/geos/in.html (accessed September 18, 2008).

Coward, H. 1993. *World religions and reproductive technologies.* vol. 2. Ottawa: Royal Commission of New Reproductive Technologies, Research Studies.

Coward, H., and T. Sidhu. 2000. Bioethics for clinicians: 19. Hinduism and Sikhism. Canadian *Medical Association Journal* 163 (9): 1167–1170.

International Genetic Counseling Programs (IGCP). 2006. *Genetic counseling education: Connecting the global community.* http://igce.med.sc.edu/internationaldirectors.asp (accessed October 9, 2008).

Hansson, M. O. 1998. Balancing the quality of consent. *Journal of Medical Ethics* 24: 182–187.

Indian Ministry of Home Affairs. 2001. *Census of India.* http://www.censusindia.gov.in/ (accessed October 9, 2008).

Infoplease. 2002. *Top 20 Causes of mortality throughout the world.* http://www.infoplease.com/ipa/A0779147.html (accessed September 18, 2008).

Klostermaier, Klaus. 1998. *A concise encyclopedia of Hinduism.* Oxford: Oneworld.

Mudur, G. 1997. Indian study of women with cervical lesions called unethical. *British Medical Journal* 314 (7087): 1065.

National Center for Health Statistics. 2005. *Deaths—leading causes.* http://www.cdc.gov/nchs/fastats/lcod.htm (accessed October 9, 2008).

Sangani B., P. K. Sukumaran, C. Mahadik, H. Yagnik, S. Telang, F. Vas, R. A. Oberroi, B. Modell, and S. M. Merchant. 1990. Thalassemia in Bombay: The role of medical genetics in developing countries. Bulletin of the World Health Organization 68 (1): 75–81.

Schrag, B. 2001. *Commentary: Crossing cultural barriers—Informed consent in developing countries.* http://www.onlineethics.org/CMS/research/rescases/gradres/gradresv5/cultural/culturalc1.aspx (accessed September 18, 2008).

Sue, D. W., and D. Sue. 1999. *Counseling the culturally different: Theory and practice.* New York: J. Wiley & Sons.

Varawalla, N.Y., J. M. Old, R. Sarkar, R. Venkatesan and D. J. Weatherall. 1991. The spectrum of b-thalassemia mutations on the Indian subcontinent: the basis for prenatal diagnosis. *British Journal of Haematology* 78: 242–247.

Verma, I. C. 2000. Burden of genetic disorders in India. *Indian Journal of Pediatrics* 67 (1): 893–898.

Verma, I. C. 2005. *Clinical Diagnosis and Genetic Counseling–Sir Ganga Ram Hospital.* http://www.sgrh.com/dept/gene/gene.htm#Clinical%20Diagnosis (accessed October 9, 2008).

Weatherall, D. J. 2001. Phenotype and genotype relationships in monogenic disease: Lessons from the thalassemias. *Nature Reviews Genetics* 2: 245–255.

Weatherall, D. J., and J. B. Clegg. 2001. Inherited hemoglobin disorders: An increasing global health problem. *Bulletin of the World Health Organization* 79: 704–712.

Wikipedia. n.d. Official languages of India. http://en.wikipedia.org/wiki/Official_languages_of_India (accessed September 18, 2008).

World Health Organization (WHO). 2000. *Women's Health in Southeast Asia,* vol. 1. New Delhi: World Health Organization.

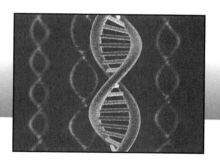

CHAPTER 9

"Every Generation...": A Jewish Approach to Questions of Genetic Research, Testing and Screening, and Gene Therapy

Rabbi Michael L. Feshbach

The sun sets over rolling meadows as I drive by, through the far reaches of Rockville and towards our home in North Potomac, Maryland, casting shadows over the white fences and the wandering cattle. The farmland helps defy the definition of our area as "strictly" suburban. But we know, with a hint of sadness and a sense of inevitability, that the clock is ticking on the cows and the farm. The land is owned by an elderly woman, the last of generations of family farmers, but has been pre-sold on the occasion of her death. Our future neighbors will be gleaming new office buildings, still more space in the sprawling complex that makes up the bio-tech "boomtown" so visible all around us. The farm will someday give way to additional administrative wings and research labs of endeavors like the Human Genome Project.

In the meantime, fights break out at school board hearings all around the country over teaching science in light of passionate personal commitments to the surface and superficial readings of the first two chapters of the book of Genesis. Many people in this country seem to believe in a literal Adam and Eve, and oppose the idea of the evolution of the species.

And yet, and yet… There is another way, a spiritual approach that takes religious tradition *seriously,* but not *literally.* I have always believed that Adam and Eve were not the actual first, but the quintessential prototypes of all human beings, that the story, in fact, is a powerful tale of what happened not so much *before* our time, but *within* our lives. For this first couple was given one rule, and one restriction: do not eat of the fruit of the tree of knowledge. (The "fruit," by the way, was an "apple" only in Christian interpretation. In Judaism it was either a fig—after all, didn't they wrap themselves in fig leaves?—or an "etrog," a cousin of the lemon. Early Christian interpretation used an apple because that fruit had connotations of sexuality in the Roman world, and Christian interpretation has seen this story as being about sex. Jewish tradition does not interpret it in this way.) One might be advised not to reach out, not to know what you have not known, not to go where you have not gone before. Stay put, and stay safe; remain in the Garden.

But to reach out for new knowledge is what *makes us* who we are. The human story, then, *begins* with the eating of the fruit. It is what takes Adam and Eve from naïve innocence into the world of adult human experience. More than that: this may be a story of divine disappointment that we could not stay "close" in our original created state, but it is also a story of human growth. For me, at least, this is not about a sin that taints all future generations, but the next step in the human path.

For we are going to reach out for new knowledge. We are going to reach for the stars, and split the atom. We are going to poke and prod into the stuff and substance of the world around us, to climb mountains because they are there. It is who we are. The spiritual, the religious, the moral question is not will we seek new knowledge, not "what if," but, in the face of what we find, "what now?"

Rabbi David Saperstein, head of the Religious Action Center of Reform Judaism, has forcefully remarked (and I paraphrase his observation here) that every generation has felt itself at the cutting edge of history. The only difference is that "because of our recent sweeping changes in technology, they were wrong, and we are right."

In my own words: every generation has felt itself on the verge of a Brave New World, with unprecedented abilities and "everyday" realities that would seem miraculous to those who lived in centuries past. But today, in a world of the split atom and the double helix, of space exploration and environmental degradation, of mutated crops and newly stubborn famines, of heart implants and heartless poverty which denies access to even basic medical care to growing billions at the bottom rungs of the chain of human existence, today it is clear that we alone stand in a place where no one else has stood: able to shape or alter all life on this planet—or destroy it; able to tinker with the very fabric of human life—or dehumanize all our interactions with each other. They were wrong. And we are right: the decisions we make today will affect our human future forever. We are able to be saviors or monsters. The tragedy is that we are so torn as a society that different people will use each of these words to describe the very same act.

How clearly this is the case in what we face with the new frontiers of bioethics. Such questions have been in the headlines of late, from Terry Schiavo to *Million Dollar Baby*. But since the human experience of dealing with the unexpected and ambiguous, with love and loss, with aging and diminution of our abilities, of frustrating "grey" when we want "black and white," since this experience is universal, the more relevant question is why aren't these issues in the headlines *all* the time?

Of relevance, perhaps, to our discussion about genetic research and therapy, puzzling and problematic words of warning emerge from the Jewish tradition, in the midst of the over-hyped and under-read Ten Commandments. For there, in the midst of what Jewish tradition considers the Second Commandment, are the following words: "For I, the Eternal your God, am an impassioned God, visiting the iniquity of the ancestors onto the third and fourth generation of those that despise me, but performing loving kindness onto the thousandth generation of those who love me and keep my commandments." This is what Jewish tradition considers the Second Commandment (Catholics and Protestants actually count the "Ten" slightly differently: one more indication of the inappropriateness of governmental endorsement and display of a set of religious writings).

How is this related to genetics? It is a reminder, if ever one was needed in this postmodern world that emphasizes this truth again and again, that "we are who we were," that we are shaped in ways beyond conscious understanding by our parents and our past, that we inherit not only potential we did not earn, but also problems we do not deserve.

To begin to define a Jewish approach to this Brave New World of genetic testing and gene therapy we must distinguish between two modalities, two different ways of approaching Jewish texts. In our tradition there is both *halachah* and *aggadah*, "law" and "lore," distinct elements (unless said with a thick New York accent, in which case they almost blend together). The first is the realm of the Jewish legal tradition: what's a Jew to do? The second is the world of homiletics and legends, stories and tales from which underlying insights may often be teased out, but which were not originally meant to tell us what to do.

While the division is not as clear cut as this, as an oversimplification of the matter more traditionally observant Jews (Orthodox and some Conservative Jews) live in the world of Jewish law. For them, *halachah*, as interpreted by the interaction between ancient texts and modern practitioners, determines action. For more liberal Jews (Reform, Reconstructionist, and some Conservative Jews), *halachah* offers guidance, but *aggadah* may be a way of reading new situations into the tradition as well. The fact is that both "law" and "lore" are important sources of values, and often when faced with the delicate act of trying to figure out what an ancient tradition has to say about a very new situation, we will turn to both expressions of the Jewish spirit, and still not be sure of what "Judaism" has to say about any given topic.

The entire enterprise of using ancient sources to address modern ethical situations is fraught with peril: it is inevitable, if a tradition is to remain "relevant" to the modern world, yet it is problematic. One of the best treatments of this balancing act is found in an article from a decade ago by ethicist Louis Newman called "Woodchoppers and Respirators: The Problem of Interpretation in Contemporary Jewish Ethics" (1995).

Indeed, when approaching any topic of Jewish life it is useful to keep in mind the axiom that "where there are two Jews, there are three opinions." Judaism has no central hierarchical structure that determines doctrine, and even within similar streams or denominations of Judaism (Reform, Conservative, Reconstructionist, and Orthodox), opinion on a subject is a matter of building a bridge between the past and the present, and thus depends on argument, persuasion, communal consensus, and continual openness to new insights.

There are often surprising outcomes of these discussions. To cite just two examples: the normally more "liberal" Reform movement scholar Mark Washofsky (2000) argues strongly for using great caution in the removal of a feeding tube, and the normally more restrictive Conservative movement's Elliot Dorf argued for more open conditions for allowing it. An Orthodox rabbi named Azriel Rosenfeld argues for the possibility, in the future, of allowing genetic manipulation of offspring even for non-therapeutic purposes, such as to enhance certain desirable characteristics (intelligence and appearance); Conservative Rabbi David Golinkin views such techniques as permissible only for what we would commonly understand as medical purposes.

132

And as implied above, disagreements exist even between those in the same denomination. Rabbi Elliot Dorf often writes from the "liberal" end of the Conservative movement, and is challenged by others in his movement; Rabbi Mark Washofsky writes from the "traditional" end of Reform Judaism and encounters many more liberal voices amongst his colleagues.

All denominations of Judaism, however, are beginning to address questions relating to genetic testing and gene therapies with increasing frequency. A common thread to all branches of Judaism is the notion of *pikuach nefesh,* the "saving of a life." To save a life all the proscriptions of Jewish law may be set aside save three: you cannot commit murder, rape, or idolatry even to save your own life. But there is general agreement that anything else can be done—anything else—if it will save a human life.

The temptation, then, is to end the discussion before it begins. The Talmud or Jewish law codes could even have directly addressed questions they never actually dreamed of, such as an amniocentesis or mapping the human genome, prohibited all of it, and those prohibitions could be set aside if the benefit of doing so would be to save human life.

It should surprise no one by now to realize that the question is more complicated than that. For what is pikuach nefesh? How broad a brush do we use? Or how specific a threat are we talking about?

Autopsies, for example, are generally prohibited by Jewish law, as a kind of desecration of the body, which is supposed to be buried: intact, untampered with, in its natural state, *as soon as possible* after a death has occurred. An autopsy required by the state may be allowed by traditional authorities, under the principle of *dina d'malkhuta dina* ("the law of the land is the law," that is, the laws of the land we live in, in most cases, have the power of Jewish law as well), but even then the autopsy must be done *quickly.* But what about an autopsy that might be medically beneficial to others? A liberal reading of pikuach nefesh would allow the autopsy, for the chance that the information gleaned might someday save someone else. A more strict interpretation (followed, in this case, by most traditional authorities) would argue that if a specific autopsy of a particular person might be of *direct benefit* in saving the life of a *specific, known* other individual, then, and only then, might an autopsy be allowed.

So the principle of saving life is valuable to keep in mind, as a reason why some genetic testing might be permitted in Jewish tradition. But it is not a *carte blanche.* It cannot serve as a blanket protection to cover all cases.

What, then, does Jewish tradition have to say about key questions in the ever-changing, cutting-edge world of genetic research, testing and screening, and gene therapy? I will examine several partially overlapping areas under consideration: the amniocentesis procedure, Tay-Sachs screening of adults, Huntington disease, and breast cancer screening. This will begin to paint a general picture of how Jewish tradition treats these subjects, and how Jewish patients might turn to, base their decisions on—or perhaps rebel against—this background. It is an important part of Jewish tradition to give credit to one's sources and one's teachers: in the remarks that follow I base my comments extensively on the writings of Mark Washofsky (1995) (Reform), Elliot Dorff (Conservative), and Fred Rosner (Orthodox), whose respective works on Jewish bioethics have become important references in this field.

Prenatal testing to obtain genetic information about a fetus in utero is a rapidly evolving field. Even in the time since my youngest child was born in 2001, new options are available to obtain more information in less obtrusive ways. Observations that once required an amniocentesis can be made earlier now simply through enhanced sonogram technology and other tests. In this way the risk–benefit analysis and the age recommendation that I am familiar with (maternal age of 35 being the "tipping point" between the rate of risk of miscarriage and the rate of benefit of detecting genetic abnormalities) will undoubtedly change in the relatively near future. What will also shift as the technology changes, then, is the ethical consideration of whose "interests" are being served, and of who is the "patient" in question.

Having said that, however, I believe that one of the major issues behind prenatal testing remains the same no matter what method of testing is used to employ the information. It is the underlying question of what to do with the information. It is the debate about abortion.

As it plays out within Jewish circles, there is actually one aspect of this debate about which there is universal agreement. In the case of a threat to the life of the mother, abortion is *mandated*. It is not seen as a choice. It is not seen as an option. It is an *obligation*. All branches of Judaism are in agreement about this point (which rarely happens about anything).

The question, though, is *why?* How we answer this question will determine whether abortion is allowed by Jewish tradition in other situations. And here, as expected, there is heated disagreement. As a brief, oversimplified rendition of this argument: *If* abortion is allowed to save the mother because the fetus is considered a "pursuer," and abortion is allowed as a kind of "self-defense," then the fetus does seem to have the status of a person, and would not be allowed for other reasons. *If*, on the other hand, the fetus is considered "merely water" for the first period of development, or "like a limb" of the mother, then abortion may be allowed for other compelling reasons, although not, in the second case, for just *any* reason (since self-mutilation is not allowed; you cannot cut off your arm just because you want to).

In general, many Orthodox rabbis today believe that abortion should be limited to the extreme situation of danger to the life of the mother, and the non-Orthodox branches of Judaism (Reform, Conservative, Reconstructionist, along with *some* Orthodox authorities) allow for abortion in cases where the pregnancy poses a danger to the health of the mother as well, including in this consideration emotional and mental health.

These are not abstract issues. And the question of the cultural and religious environment in which a patient lives is directly relevant to medical decisions. My wife and I lived in Erie, Pennsylvania through our first two miscarriages, all of our first successful pregnancy and much of our second successful one. My wife was just 35 at the time of the birth of our first child, and we explored with our physicians and, having had two previous miscarriages, struggled with the question of whether to have an "amnio." Only a few places in Erie performed the procedure, and when we mentioned to people whom my wife worked with that we were thinking about getting it, they responded: "Why? What would you do with the information, anyway?" In a heavily anti-abortion environment, getting this information was seen as…almost superfluous.

But the fact is that there are certain outcomes that *would* have led us to terminate a pregnancy. And I can't say for sure how we would have reacted if the results had been problematic. Certainly in anticipation of some conditions we would have cried, and prepared. But in others… many—perhaps most—of those dealing with this question vis a vis Jewish tradition would not require a couple to bring a child to term who would die a horrible and painful death in the days soon after being born.

On the question of abortion, then, Judaism is not "pro-choice" per se, if by "pro-choice" one means "do whatever you want." But because the decision is seen to rest on a case-by-case basis, and depend on the particular medical circumstances *and* on the impact it would have on the *individual* family involved, Judaism can, I believe, fairly be described as being *politically* "pro-choice." This matter should be in the hands of the woman, the family, and the physician… and, for Jewish families, in consultation with Jewish religious tradition.

All of this is background to saying that prenatal genetic screening is generally allowed in Jewish tradition, without huge reservations in the non-Orthodox branches of Judaism, and with some hesitation by many Orthodox authorities. ("If the cure to these conditions becomes available in the future," an Orthodox argument might go, "then such screening would be rendered unnecessary." On the other hand, of course, if it were possible to correct such conditions *before birth,* the argument might tip the other way.)

What about, then, advance screening of adults for genetic conditions which they might pass on to their offspring? The condition that comes immediately to mind when discussing a Jewish approach to genetics is that of Tay-Sachs disease. According to the National Institute of Health, "Tay-Sachs is an inherited disorder caused by the absence of a vital enzyme, resulting in the destruction of the nervous system. It is always fatal; to date there is no cure."

A more detailed medical presentation of the condition describes Tay-Sachs as a fatal genetic lipid storage disorder in which harmful quantities of a fatty substance called *ganglioside* G_{M2} build up in tissues and nerve cells in the brain. The condition is caused by insufficient activity of an enzyme called *beta-hexosaminidase A* that catalyzes the biodegradation of acidic fatty materials known as *gangliosides.* Gangliosides are made and biodegraded rapidly in early life as the brain develops. Infants with Tay-Sachs disease appear to develop normally for the first few months of life. Then, as nerve cells become distended with fatty material, a relentless deterioration of mental and physical abilities occurs. The child becomes blind, deaf, and unable to swallow. Muscles begin to atrophy and paralysis sets in. Other neurological symptoms include dementia, seizures, and an increased startle reflex to noise. A much rarer form of the disorder occurs in patients in their 20s and early 30s and is characterized by an unsteady gait and progressive neurological deterioration. Persons with Tay-Sachs also have "cherry red" spots in their eyes (National Human Genome Research Institute n.d.).

The incidence of Tay-Sachs is particularly high among people of Eastern European Jewish descent. While there are both Jewish and non-Jewish carriers of the recessive TSD gene, 85% of its victims are Jews. Approximately one in 25 Jews is a TSD carrier. In the non-Jewish community the rate is one in 250. A carrier couple (that is, a couple in which *both* parents are carriers) is "at risk" and has a one in four chance with each pregnancy of producing a Tay-Sachs baby; the chance for an unaffected child is three in four. There are tests available which can determine whether adults are "carriers" of Tay-Sachs. Genetic counseling in general (as well as a specific recommendation that adults be screened for Tay-Sachs, preferably before the wedding but definitely before a pregnancy) is now a routine part of the pre-marital counseling offered by many rabbis. My own pre-wedding packet contains detailed information about Tay-Sachs (and can be seen at www.templeshalom.net/documents/marriage-packet.pdf).

Death from Tay-Sachs is painful, prolonged, horrible, and, at this time, inevitable. What possible objection could there be to doing everything in our power, from advance screening to prenatal testing, to eradicate the disease?

The objection, raised in certain circles of the Orthodox world, relates to the question of the impact of the information on the individuals found to be carriers, or on couples who are already engaged. There is a fear of a stigma attached to a person found to be a carrier, so that the person would be seen as "damaged goods," and thus less likely to find a mate. There are concerns about the stress that the information will cause to the carrier as well, and great fear about the chance that an already engaged couple would break their engagement upon learning that they are both carriers. The context to these concerns is the strongly pro-natal position of Jewish tradition: marriage is viewed as the ideal adult state, and having children is considered a *commandment*. (Interestingly, in an odd twist that is an early nod to issues relating to women's role and rights, the commandment to bring children into the world falls on *men*, rather than women—a recognition that child-bearing can be dangerous and for some women life-threatening, and one cannot be commanded to do something that might endanger one's life. An early illustration of *sensitivity* to women, however, was subsequently implication of this realization—for if a couple cannot have children, in some ultra-Orthodox circles the man is expected, indeed perhaps even pressured, to divorce his wife and try again with another woman. No matter the first couple's feelings for one another.) *Not having children* because of a statistical possibility that they might have Tay-Sachs disease is not, therefore, generally seen as an option in the Orthodox world.

The concerns expressed above, however, can be dealt with. In 1973 an organization called the Association of Orthodox Jewish Scientists issued a paper which called for "voluntary screening of young adults of an age in which marriage has become a serious consideration but before definite marital commitments have been made." Earlier screening would potentially lead to unnecessary additional stress, and screening of an engaged couple might lead to the dissolution of the relationship. The common practice in non-Orthodox Jewish circles, however, is to recommend such screening to an engaged couple and, as mentioned above, it is an issue usually raised as part of rabbinic pre-marital counseling. Most (but not all) Orthodox authorities would prohibit an abortion of a fetus found to have Tay-Sachs disease (and some ban amniocentesis altogether); most—perhaps the vast majority—of non-Orthodox authorities would allow an abortion is this case.

Rabbi Elliot Dorf, in his recent and very readable work *Matters of Life and Death: A Jewish Approach to Modern Medical Ethics* (1998), treats two other areas of genetic testing of adults: Huntington disease and breast cancer screening. As described by the National Institutes of Health (National Human Genome Research Institute n.d.), Huntington disease "results from genetically programmed degeneration of brain cells, called neurons, in certain areas of the brain. This degeneration causes uncontrolled movements, loss of intellectual faculties, and emotional disturbance." It is passed from parent to child through a mutation in the normal gene. The gene is dominant, which means that each child of a parent with Huntington disease has a 50–50 chance of inheriting the gene. It leads to dementia, disability, and death.

A pre-symptomatic test is now available for those individuals at risk for carrying the gene. The moral and spiritual question basically is this: do you *really* want a crystal ball? Do you want to know? Since the age of onset of the disease varies greatly, is it better to know what is coming and prepare, or live your life as long as you can? And in this age of the Internet and NSA spying, who knows who will get the information? Rabbi Dorf raises the immediate implications: How will this affect insurance? Employment? Choices about whether to marry, to have children? And, crucially, does one who knows that one faces a deadly disease later in life have an obligation to disclose this information? To whom, and under what circumstances? The gene for Huntington disease, once detected, is a direct and dire indication that one will contract the disease. What about a case of genetic probability, rather than certainty?

I sat with a young couple in my study just as I was getting ready to finish writing this chapter. They are getting married in a few months, and we are going through my usual procedures and questions, reviewing the details of the processional, the role of photographers, and the intricacies of whatever personal issues of communication or couples counseling they may want before the wedding. We reach and quickly move through the discussion of Tay Sachs. And then the bride-to-be asks me a pointed question. There is a strong history of breast cancer in her family. There are tests available now to detect a gene mutation (BRCA) that is a factor in many cases of breast and ovarian cancer. Much publicity has been given recently to the finding that Ashkenazic Jewish women have an elevated risk, in comparison to the general population, of carrying this mutation. She leans forward on the couch. Should she be tested?

And in one moment all the issues we have been discussing here come to a head. With two people in front of me, I feel the awesome weight of it all: the blessing and the curse of new knowledge, the opportunities (early action?) and risks (insurance companies?), the delicate dance of what the woman—and her husband-to-be—would do with the information, the inherent uncertainty of the whole business, at least at this stage, as the presence of the mutation alone is not perfectly predictive of what will come.

With the weight of the issues comes the irony of the question coming to me. Every practitioner should know the limit of his or her craft. The irony of my writing this article, in this case, is clear to me: my wife's sister is a nurse-midwife earning a PhD in Health Care; her husband is a philosophy professor and one of the leading ethicists in the country. Either of them, I felt, would be more equipped to sit in my chair at that moment, or to address so many of the issues here.

I suspect I am not alone in a sense of momentary isolation when facing questions of bioethics. These issues arise in similar settings, but with the unique stories and individual circumstances that come out of the human experience.

And so we remember that healing, whether the physical kind practiced by nurses and physicians or the spiritual and emotional kind practiced by caregivers and counselors and clergy, is an art as much as it is a science. What do we know about our bodies? What are the mysteries science has yet to solve, the secrets yet to spill?

Soon the whole of the genome will be laid out before us. And reaching out for new knowledge, for more information, is what we do as human beings. But I am reminded of Jeff Goldblum's character in *Jurassic Park,* who noted that we have spent so much time asking if we could do a thing that we have forgotten to ask whether it should be done. Or more to the point here: we have spent so much time asking about information that we do not always dwell on application. We come back to the line between "what if" and "what now."

Our bodies and our minds and life itself are a gift from the One who creates and shapes the world. All I know for sure is that we will—and we should—keep on reaching out. We should move forward into this new world, using our minds to understand our bodies. But may we carry on in a spirit of awe, and reverence, and love, with some humility left in the face of the miracle of life, for some room still for amazement at the fact...that we are here at all.

References

Dorff, Elliot. 1998. *Matters of life and death: A Jewish approach to modern medical ethics.* Philadelphia: Jewish Publication Society.

National Human Genome Research Institute. n.d. *Learning about Huntington's disease.* http://www.genome.gov/10001215 (accessed October 9, 2008).

National Human Genome Research Institute. n.d. *Learning about Tay-Sachs disease.* http://www.genome.gov/10001220 (accessed October 9, 2008).

Newman, Louis E. 1995. Woodchoppers and respirators: The problem of interpretation in contemporary Jewish ethics. In *Contemporary Jewish Ethics and Morality: A Reader,* eds. Elliot N. Dorff and Louis E. Newman. New York: Oxford University Press.

Rosner, Fred. 1991. *Modern medicine and Jewish ethics: 2nd Revised and Augmented Edition.* Jersey City, NJ: Ktav Publishing House.

Washofsky, Mark. 1995. Abortion and the Halakhic conversation. In *The Fetus and Fertility in Jewish Law: Essays and Responsa,* eds. Walter Jacob and Moshe Zemer. Pittsburgh: Rodef Shalom Press.

Washofsky, Mark. 2000. *Jewish living: A guide to contemporary reform practice.* New York: UAHC Press.

CHAPTER 10

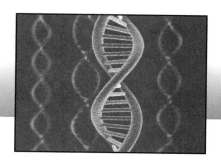

The Catholic Church Views on Genetic Testing: Indications for Genetic Counselors

Rebecca B. Donohue, MSN, FNP-BC, AOCN, APNG

Catholic Views on Genetic Services and Testing

Cultural diversity can present many challenges when a provider is planning a genetic counseling session. This diversity can be a result of religious as well as gender, racial, ethnic, and other backgrounds. Patients and their families expect to be treated with respect regardless of the personal religious beliefs of the healthcare professional. Some suggestions made by the counselor may violate the patients' religious beliefs and make them less receptive to counseling. A basic understanding of the Catholic Church's views on genetic testing may help avoid this dilemma.

In presenting these views, one must account for the structural differences between Catholicism and the rest of the world's religions. Catholicism is unique in that it recognizes the pope as the single central teaching authority. Technically, this can be regarded as a hierarchical-magisterial structure. Such is not the case for the most of the world's denominations, where human authority is more diffusive (W. Curtis Mallet, personal communication).

Moral principles are developed from revelation and reason with the authoritative interpretation of those principles. Conscience is then necessary to apply those principles. The Roman Catholic Church has a tradition of bioethical reasoning expressed in scripture, the writings of the church leaders, contemporary Catholic theologians, and encyclical documents (Markwell and Brown, 2001). Papal encyclical documents that address contemporary issues involved with bioethics are used here to assist with defining the Catholic bioethical principles guiding genetic testing. These encyclical documents include Pope Paul VI's *Humane vitae* (1968), and Pope John Paul II's *Evangelium vitae* (1995) and *Veritatis splendor* (1993a). Prior to discussion of these principles it is important to point out that "dissent from official teaching exists in all religious affiliations. Healthcare professionals should be aware of the fact that not all persons adhere to every tenet officially proposed by a particular denomination."

A basic understanding of the principles that guide Catholic Church decisions may help the genetic counselor anticipate how the proposed interventions may be received by the individual of Catholic faith. The Catholic Church maintains the following viewpoint regarding genetic testing (W. Curtis Mallet, personal communication):

- Life begins at conception and ends at natural death.
- Intercourse is only moral within marriage.
- Direct abortion (i.e., destruction of the embryo or fetus) is unacceptable.
- Artificial contraception is unacceptable.
- Natural Family Planning and ecological breast feeding are laudable.
- The moral value of genetic testing will depend upon the circumstances and intention of the person(s) involved.
- Presymptomatic and confirmational diagnosis is generally acceptable.
- Informed consent is non-negotiable.
- Genetic testing is in itself morally neutral.

The purpose of this chapter is to assist in understanding views of the Catholic Church concerning bioethics and genetic testing through discussion of principles guiding these views. Catholic faith principles described here are built on the framework of moral principles presented by Beauchamp and Childress (2001, 13). A basic understanding of the Catholic principles regarding genetic testing may help determine the best strategies to provide genetic services and ensure a proper informed consent process when counseling persons of the Catholic faith. Although principles are general norms requiring judgment, they are not exact guides that inform us in decision making for each action or circumstance as more detailed rules do (14).

Principles of Catholic Decision Making

Principles guiding the Catholic Church decision making with regard to health, therapeutics, and predisposition testing (inherited genetic susceptibility to a disease that may or may not result in disease development) programs are founded on the basic principle of respect, or reverence, for the dignity of human life, from which other principles arise. The Catholic Church views life as a sacred gift from God that is to be protected and nurtured from the time of conception to death. Respect for personal dignity and support of human life can be maintained through prevention of disease and by seeking out more effective therapies for illnesses (Committee on the Home Missions 1996).

Respect

Respect for persons as seen by the Catholic Church can be further divided into four principles: autonomy, beneficence, nonmaleficence, and justice. In respect of an individual's autonomy physicians, genetics counselors, and the public should understand that responsible use of genetic testing includes providing informed consent (Schneider 2002). The Catholic Church believes in the informed consent process and that this process must uphold human dignity and sustain human life, while protecting privacy and confidentiality (Middleton and Biegert, 2005; Bayley 2005).

Autonomy

The meaning of autonomy in this context is that an individual cannot be coerced into testing; that they must act autonomously. Some may argue that a person cannot act autonomously within religious organizations that direct personal decisions; that individuals that do not act on their own and submit to the authority of a religious organization loose their autonomy. In response to this Beauchamp and Childress state, "individuals can exercise their autonomy in choosing to accept an institution, tradition, or community that they view as a legitimate source of direction" (2001, 60). Respect for a person's autonomy requires the healthcare provider to acknowledge their right to hold views and to make choices based on their personal values and beliefs. Although the decision to have genetic testing is autonomous, genetic testing often involves testing of not only the individual but also family members such as parents, siblings, and children. It is important to understand that it is a Catholic tradition to consider future generations as well as living individuals (Committee on the Home Missions 1996). In this regard the genetic counselor should anticipate that the Catholic individual may wish to have family members involved in the entire decision-making process rather than make genetic testing decisions alone.

Beneficence and Nonmaleficence

Beneficence is defined as maximizing benefits for the individual while minimizing risks. Within the Catholic theological documents this would be referred to as "doing good." The Catholic Church teaches that you cannot consider beneficence without also considering nonmaleficence. Nonmaleficence means to do no harm; Catholic teachings call this "avoiding evil." To do no harm refers not only to the body and to emotional well-being, but also to spiritual well-being. In No. 1750 of *Cathechism of the Catholic Church,* Pope John Paul II (1993b) tells us that determination of whether an action is good or bad depends upon the specific act, the situation, and the intentions of the person acting. Genetic testing performed as a result of sound medical practice which sets the stage for either an effective treatment or a cure of disease is not only approved by the Catholic Church but is considered a blessing (Committee on the Home Missions 1996). Pope John Paul II told the World Medical Association in 1983, "Therapeutic interventions directed towards promotion of the personal well-being of the individual by healing of various illnesses such as are involved with chromosomal defects would fall within the logic of the Christian moral tradition" (Congregation for the Doctrine of Faith 1987).

The Catholic Church's definition of beneficence includes not only the promotion of the welfare of the individual, but also the promotion of the welfare of others. In this respect Catholics will want to ensure that they are not seeking what is best for themselves while risking harm to others. At the same time they may feel a moral obligation to proceed with testing that could benefit others, including future generations, even if they may have no obvious personal benefit.

Justice

The principle of justice implies fairness. The Catholic Church believes that it is each individual's responsibility to work for his or her own welfare as well as that of others. Personal sacrifices may be required when necessary for the common good. According to Pope John Paul II in No. 1925 of *Catechism of the Catholic Church* (1993b), "the common good consists of three essential elements: respect for and promotion of the fundamental rights of the person; prosperity, or the development of the spiritual and temporal goods of society; the peace and security of the group and of its members." For Catholics, genetic testing may be seen as an obligation to consider testing for the betterment of the community, as long as there will be no harm caused, even if there is no apparent benefit for the individual. The principle of justice implies that genetic testing services must benefit not only those who are able to pay for them, but also contribute to enhancing the common good of all in society. In this regard measures must be taken to make the benefits of genetic testing services available to those who are at greatest risk and have the greatest need while protecting all against discrimination based on the test results.

Catholic Church Views on Specific Tests

Some of the genetic tests currently available include carrier screening, preimplantation genetic diagnosis, prenatal diagnostic testing, newborn screening, presymptomatic testing to estimate the risk of developing cancers, presymptomatic testing to predict adult-onset disorders, and confirmational diagnosis of an individual with health problems. In attempting to determine the views of the Catholic Church regarding these genetic tests, the principles aforementioned need to be considered. While considering each of these tests, the nurse should be mindful of the dominant beliefs in the Catholic Church: respect for personal dignity and support of human life.

Carrier Screening

Testing for carrier screening for a disease is accepted by the Catholic Church in certain circumstances. Acceptable reasons for carrier screening include the use of results prior to marriage to determine if marriage is suitable, or use to help a couple accept and prepare for a possible disease in their child. Because of the Catholic Church belief that "each and every marriage act must remain open to the transmission of life" (Pope Paul VI 1968), the use of carrier screening to help a married couple determine whether or not to practice birth control, other than natural family planning, is unacceptable.

Preimplantation Genetic Diagnosis

Preimplantation genetic diagnosis is a test that screens for genetic flaws among embryos used in in-vitro fertilization, a process performed outside of the womb. In that the Catholic Church views any sort of insemination other than what occurs from the fruit of the marriage as unacceptable, the Catholic Church does not consider this type of testing an acceptable option (Congregation for the Doctrine of Faith 1987).

Prenatal Diagnostic Testing

Prenatal diagnostic testing is acceptable for the Catholic Church if it allows earlier, more effective treatment, or will help with acceptance of untreatable disorders. Prenatal diagnosis of the embryo and of the fetus while still in the mother's womb that allows earlier more effective treatment is acceptable, as long as the life of both the embryo and the mother are protected and the risk minimized. Keeping in mind the belief of the Catholic Church that life begins at conception and ends at the time of natural death, and the importance of doing no harm, prenatal diagnosis with the option of abortion depending upon the results is strictly forbidden (Committee on the Home Missions 1996; Congregation for the Doctrine of Faith 1987).

Newborn Screening

Newborn screening such as for phenylketonuria, Tay-Sachs, or sickle cell anemia is acceptable to the Catholic Church. This acceptability can be seen in that newborn genetic screening can identify treatable genetic disorders in newborn infants, allowing early intervention that can eliminate or reduce symptoms that might otherwise cause a lifetime of disability.

Presymptomatic Testing

Presymptomatic testing to estimate the risk of developing cancer may provide information that will allow an individual to reduce their cancer risk. Genetic testing is acceptable if testing can assist in determining a person at risk for a disease, thus allowing preventive or early detection measures to be used to eliminate or reduce risks.

Presymptomatic testing to predict adult-onset disorders such as Huntington's disease and Alzheimer's disease is controversial in medicine. In cases such as these, where there is no cure or effective treatment, and in light of the Catholic Church's desire to maintain personal dignity, a judgment is needed as to what advantage would be gained from testing the asymptomatic person. A positive result in a healthy individual is a devastating revelation that may predict a long and debilitating terminal illness. This may result in emotional and financial devastation to the client and the family. If the person has not yet had children, the test provides very strong motivation for careful consideration of family planning. Careful analysis of the psychological issues would be needed.

146

Confirmational Diagnosis

Confirmational diagnosis in a symptomatic individual can aid the medical diagnosis. Therapeutic intervention can be enhanced and healing facilitated by obtaining the correct diagnosis. This makes confirmational diagnosis acceptable to the Catholic Church (Middleton and Biegert 2005).

Summary

The Catholic Church adheres to the ethical principles stemming from the principle of respect, including autonomy, beneficence, and justice. Dominant beliefs in the Catholic Church are respect for personal dignity and support of human life. The Catholic Church believes the informed consent process must uphold human dignity and sustain human life, from conception to death, while protecting privacy and confidentiality. The Catholic Church believes that it is the duty of individuals to care for future generations as well as themselves; therefore Catholics may wish to have family members involved in the entire decision-making process for genetic testing. Adhering to the Catholic faith, individuals would want to ensure that, while they are doing what is best for themselves, no harm will come to others. Catholics may feel a moral obligation to proceed with testing that could benefit present and future generations, despite a lack of personal benefit. When preparing for counseling of an individual of Catholic faith the genetic counselor must consider the goal of testing, associated risks, and the positive and negative effects, whether medical, psychological, or spiritual.

Because genetic testing is a relatively new technology it is not always possible to find a position statement published by the Catholic Church on individual genetic tests. Genetic testing is in itself considered morally neutral by the Catholic Church, with the moral value of genetic testing dependent on the circumstances and intentions of the person involved. Since medical technology is constantly evolving, the Church prefers to explain the moral principles that must be respected in each human act considering the action, circumstances, and intentions involved. A particular test or procedure may be perfectly acceptable in one instance and unacceptable in another. Some procedures are always unacceptable (e.g., direct abortion, artificial contraception, cloning, IVF, AIS, destruction of embryos). With regards to tests one must always ask "What is the goal of testing?" "What are the risks?" "What are the possible positive and negative effects—medical, psychological, spiritual?" A genetic counselor should recognize the inappropriateness of administering religious and moral advice or making value judgments of official religious teachings, and refer patients with questions of this nature to their own religious leaders (W. Curtis Mallet, personal communication).

References

Bayley, C. 2005. Cancer and genetic medicine: An ethical view. http://www.chausa.org/Pub/ MainNav/News/HP/Archive/2005/09SepOct/articles/Features/HP0509m.htm (accessed September 18, 2008).

Beauchamp, T. L., and J. F. Childress. eds. 2001. *Principles of biomedical ethics*. 5th ed. New York: Oxford University Press.

Committee on the Home Missions. 1996. *Critical decisions: Genetic testing and its implications.* http://www.nccbuscc.org/shv/testing.htm (accessed October 9, 2008).

Congregation for the Doctrine of Faith. 1987. *Instructions on respect for human life and its origin and on the dignity of procreation replies to certain questions of the day.* Rome: Libreria Editrice Vaticana.

Markwell, H. J., and B. F. Brown. 2001. Bioethics for clinicians: 27. Catholic bioethics. *Canadian Medical Association Journal* 165 (2): 189–192.

Middleton, C., and M. E. Biegert. 2005. Planning for the age of genetics. http://www.chausa. org/Pub/MainNav/News/HP/Archive/2005/01JanFeb/Articles/Features/HP0501M.ht m (accessed September 18, 2008).

Pope John Paul II. 1993a. *Veritatis splendor.* Rome: Libreria Editrice Vaticana.

———. 1993b. *Catechism of the Catholic Church.* Citta del Vaticano: Libreria Editrice Vaticana.

———. 1995. *Evangelium vitae.* Rome: Libreria Editrice Vaticana.

Pope Paul VI. 1968. *Humane vitae.* Rome: Libreria Editrice Vaticana.

Schneider, K. 2002. The ethical issues. In *Counseling About Cancer: Strategies for Genetic Counseling,* 2nd ed., 291–293. New York: Wiley-Liss.

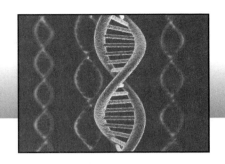

CHAPTER 11

Attitudes of Muslims Regarding the New Genetics: Testing, Treatment, and Technology

Noureddine Berka, PhD, D(ABHI)
Timikia Vaughn, MS
Verle Headings, MD, PhD
Barbara W. Harrison, MS, CGC
Robert F. Murray, Jr., MD, MS
Franklin R. Ampy, PhD
Imam Johari Abdul-Malik, MS

Allah has created you into peoples, tribes, and nations that you might know each other. Verily, the best among you are those who are most conscious of God [The Allah in Arabic].

Holy Qur'an

Introduction

Stephen R. Covey (1989), in *The 7 Habits of Highly Effective People*, advises the reader to "seek first to understand, then to be understood." This approach will serve practitioners well when caring for a patient from a background or faith that differs from their own. In this chapter we will attempt to give some sense of the perspective of the Muslim patient and the views of this community on life, death, health, disease, treatment, faith, and the roles of caregivers, family, and God in the healing process.

The Muslim Community in the United States

The Muslim (the name of the people who practice the religion of Islam) community in the United States is quite diverse, and over the past 30 years there has been a sharp increase in their diversity and number. About one-third of the estimated 6 million Muslims in the United States are U.S. citizens, another one-third are immigrants from South Asia (Pakistan, India, and Bangladesh), and the balance come from the Middle East, Africa (North and Sub-Saharan), Indonesia-Malaysia, China, Europe, and other parts of the world (Council on American Islamic Relations 2006). The Islamic community of faith, although from different national origins, shares a great deal with one another across racial and ethnic lines when faced with the realities of illness and death.

One out of six people on earth today are of the Islamic faith. The number of Christians and Muslims are about equal worldwide. Yet while Muslims total approximately 1.5 billion worldwide according to the estimates of adherents to the various religions of the world (Adherents.com 2005), Islam is the fastest growing religion or way of life in the United States and worldwide, and many authorities believe that Islam will soon become the second largest religion in America.

The Belief System

We hope to familiarize the reader with the basis on which the Muslim cosmology is based and to help explain the behaviors that nurses and other healthcare providers may observe during the course of a patient's care. In the field of health, we must realize that during a crisis, many people turn to their faith for guidance and support, while others may lose touch with their faith and cultural traditions. This is true among all people; Muslims are no exception and, also like others, may vacillate between all three modes in the course of an illness.

The core beliefs of the Muslim are based upon the scriptures of the Qur'an. The Qur'an is believed to be the book of revelation given to the prophet Muhammad (peace be upon him) from God delivered by the angel Gabriel. In the Islamic belief system all of the prophets—Adam, Noah, Abraham, David, Solomon, Moses, Jesus-Son of Mary-The Messiah and others—are all prophets of the One God (peace be upon them all). Muslims also guide their behavior and understandings from the authenticated traditions of the last prophet to humankind, Muhammad the son of Abdullah, born in 570 BCE in Mecca. His sayings and examples are collected in a separate set of texts referred to collectively as Hadith.

Muslims will refer to the Qur'an and the Hadith for clarification of almost every aspect of life, including matters of health, treatment, and standards of care. In order to address circumstances that did not exist in the time of the Prophet Muhammad (peace be upon him), Muslims will take their questions to the learned people who utilize Islamic paradigm-based reasoning to determine the appropriate course of action in the light of the Qur'an and the prophetic traditions. The priorities in Islam are: 1) one's children, 2) the needs of the many over the few, and 3) the greater good of society. The issue of autonomy is also central to the decision-making process, in that an individual Muslim still must choose what is the course of action that they feel best meets the objectives of God (Allah) for them. Each person, alone, is ultimately responsible before God for the choices made in life.

The core actions of the Islamic faith are as follows (for details on each, Table 11-1 on the next page):

- *Shahadah*—Testimony of Faith,
- *Salat*—Daily Prayers,
- *Zakat*—Alms Giving,
- *Ramadan*—The Month of Fasting
- *Hajj*—Pilgrimage to Mecca.

Six Beliefs

All Muslims, including so-called Sunni, Shiite, or other sub-divisions of the Islamic orthodoxy, hold these beliefs as essential and adhere to the practices they prescribe.

Allah

Muslims believe that there is only one God, who is the same God the One that Jews and Christians believe in. Thus, they could be considered uncompromisingly monotheist. They do not subscribe to the notion of the Trinity or the concept that God is incarnate.

Books

Muslims believe in the original books sent to the previous messengers of God, including Suhuf-Abraham, Psalms-David, Solomon, Torah-Moses, Jesus, and Muhammad (peace be upon him).

TABLE 11–1
The Core Actions of the Islamic Faith

Shahadah

Shadah means to bear witness before mankind that there is nothing worthy of worship except God and God alone, and to bear witness that Muhammad is the (last) prophet of Allah.

Salat

Salat means to pray five times a day at the times, in ritualistic purity, covering the parts of the body, in any clean space, facing the shortest distance to Mecca as prescribed by the prophet Muhammad, (praise be upon him). Muslim patients, their families, and other guests will often wish to pray in the hospital. This prayer requires bowing and prostration with one's face on the ground. Should the patient not be able to perform the full range of physical movements, they may lay or sit in their bed and perform the movements if only symbolically. These prayers occur after dawn, at noon, in the afternoon, after sunset, and after dusk; they need not be performed on the minute, but should be performed in the time range allowed. These may be made alone or by forming rows and praying together. Nurses should not be surprised if they enter a patient's room and find a small group of people on their knees with their faces on the floor using the sheets from the nearby vacant bed as a covering or prayer rug for the floor.

To the Muslim the whole world is a place of prayer. The belief that prayer changes things is something that Muslims hold in common with many faiths. Prior to performing the prayer there is a ritualistic washing or ablution. This ablution or *wudu* includes washing of the hands, rinsing of the mouth, rinsing of the nostrils, washing the face, forearms, wiping over the head and ears, and washing the feet. If a patient has a bandage, wiping off the bandage will suffice. Nurses may enter the patients' bathroom and find them or a guest with their foot in the sink as a way of acquiring the state of ritualistic purity for prayer. In most Muslim countries, there are special sinks built near the floor to make this process easier, especially for the sick.

Zakat

Zakat (alms giving) means to return part of one's excess wealth to the cause of society and the needy annually in order to purify the balance that remains with one. This sum is about 2.5% annually from the return on lawful investments or assets. Often the sick person or their family may give more in charity as a way to improve or to cure the condition. The principle that good deeds wash away bad deeds applies here as in other walks of life.

(continued)

TABLE 11–1
Continued

Ramadan

Ramadan means to fast during the ninth month in the lunar calendar (the month of Ramadan begins with the evidence of the crescent of the new moon). The fasting period starts at dawn, which may be more than an hour before sunrise, and continues until the sun drops below the horizon. During this period, the fasting person will abstain from all permissible (halal) food and drink (including water), as well as the feeding of one's passions, whether that be romance or road rage; neither lying with a passion nor arguing the truth is permitted during the hours of the fast. The rules of fasting are laid down in the second unit or surah of the Qur'an, "Oh you who believe, fasting is prescribed for you, as it was prescribed for those before you (Jews, Christians, others) that you might acquire a pious self-control due to God-consciousness." The Qur'an continues, "but any of you who are sick or on a journey the days missed should be made up from days later" (until one has completed the month worth of days, remembering that a lunar month may have 28, 29, or 30 days). Patients who must take medication are not required to fast, although many who are sick feel a sense of loss if they cannot observe the fast. Their priority before God Almighty is to care for the body that has been loaned to them and to maintain its health.

Hajj

The Hajj (pilgrimage) is a spiritual journey retracing the footsteps of the prophet Abraham, (peace be upon him), his wife Hajjar, and son Ishmail (peace be upon them). The period of Hajj occurs every year in the twelfth month, called Dhul-Hijjah. It is a time in which almost three million Muslim pilgrims from around the world come to Mecca. Pilgrims will leave their daily routines and acquire a state of simplicity, all equal before God. Muslims dress in a simple white garment made of two cloths for men or a plain dress for women. Pilgrims will gather in Mecca and on the ninth day of Dhul-Hijjah depart to the plains of Arafat outside of the city of Mecca to pray to the Almighty to receive forgiveness for all of their past sins. Upon completion of this journey, they return to their homes around the world as sinless as the day they were born.

Angels

Muslims believe in angels and see them as a special class of creatures who only do God's will (Qadr). Angels are made from light and can, on occasion, take the form of people. They are, by nature, good and cannot do evil. Angels are believed to be accompanying people wherever there is good and wherever God is praised. They have a host of functions including recording the deeds of people. There are many angels who have names mentioned either in the Qur'an or Hadith. The angel Gabriel has the duty of bringing revelation. The Angel of Death collects the souls of people at precisely the appointed time for the end of their lives, without fail or favor.

Messengers

Muslims believe that there are many prophets and messengers that have been sent to humankind. All prophets are equal before Allah. The Qur'an teaches that not all of the prophets are listed by name in the scriptures, yet the teachings clearly state that Muhammad (peace be upon him) is the last of the prophets. Most importantly, Muslims believe that the words of the prophet should be obeyed in our worldly affairs.

Qadr

God's foreknowledge and control over all affairs. Muslims believe that while people have limited free will, God is in control of everything that occurs and that everything is God's will (Qadr), and at the same time humankind is accountable for their intentions and deeds. Therefore, believers should try their best in every circumstance and then accept the outcome as God's will (Qadr). This may entail a powerful psychological toll in the battle with despair in terminal medical circumstances.

Day of Judgment and Life after Death: Heaven or Hell

The Muslim believes that the ultimate object of life is to worship God in all endeavors, hoping for the reward not necessarily in this life but in the "True" reality, the eternal life of the hereafter. For those of faith and good deeds, by God's mercy they will enter paradise to live there forever. For those who fail the tests of this life and reject faith, their reward will be damnation. Muslims believe that no true believer will be left in the hell-fire forever.

Disease

Disease and health are considered to be tests from the All-Merciful God in order for us to witness those people who will be truly faithful. Muslims accept germ theory and most scientifically proven models of material reality. Therefore, Muslims view medicine and its practitioners as people doing God's handiwork, yet believing that the ultimate healer is God alone.

The body of each human is considered to be a trust, a gift from God to be cared for until we return it to the True Owner. It is believed that the organs and limbs will testify either for us or against us on the Day of Judgment. The range of therapies available to the Muslim includes conventional treatment and medications, yet may also include aspects of prophetic or traditional medicine as well.

These practices include but are not limited to the reading or listening to the Qur'an as a treatment, prayer, the consumption of Zamzam water, honey, Black Seed oil, and other remedies. The patient is obliged to take the remedies that they believe will provide the best outcome for them, their family, and the society. Some of the faithful may learn for example that their cancer is inoperable and may decide to go to Mecca to pray and drink from the well of Zamzam. This approach, in the Islamic context, would not be rejecting therapy but choosing one therapy over another.

Medical Procedures

Modesty is a great consideration for the body of the Muslim whether alive or dead. It is desirable to have same-sex healthcare providers to protect the modesty of the patient and caregiver. This fact has given rise to a significant number of female physicians in the developing Muslim world, many of whom have migrated to the West for better training, practice opportunities, salaries, and state-of-the-art institutions to advance their careers medicine. This trend is also true in the nursing and allied health fields.

Medications should never be derived from a porcine source, nor should the medication contain alcohol except for medical necessity. Blood donation and transfusion is completely acceptable in Islam. Living donor organ transplantation is permissible only in cases in which there is a limited risk to the donor. The Muslim views the act of organ donation to be noble in the sight of God. Abortion or the willful termination of a pregnancy is only permissible under conditions determined with the help of a scholar in the Islamic faith or Imam to insure the proper Islamic ruling (fatwa) is taken. This method of decision-making may be seen as limiting a patient's autonomy; it also frees the individual of the moral burden if it is decided that termination of the pregnancy is an option. Other questions involving reproductive technologies and genetic applications in health care are likely to be discussed with a scholar in the Islamic faith or an imam to ensure that decisions are made in accordance with Islamic beliefs.

Other features of health care, including necessary physical contact and respect for personal space, are to be carried out to promote the health of the patient. If at all possible, members of the same gender should perform personal care for men and women, respectively. Muslims respect the knowledge and skills of nursing and medical personnel and expect that the wishes and lead of the patient will be followed.

Death and Dying

Muslims view death as part of the process of life and the journey to the hereafter in a way that perhaps many in the West only give lip service to. This by no means implies that grieving is not a part of the practice of Muslims. But the prophetic tradition informs us that, as the family begins gathering and grieving, they should not wail and mourn around the deceased out of respect for the feelings of the dead. Muslims believe that the soul remains aware and conscious although the body is not responding. There are no formal last rites, but some Muslim family members may wish to read from the Qur'an. Muslims wish to resolve personal issues with family members before death, but do not seek deathbed confessionals. Washing, scenting, and shrouding of the body is advocated. Muslims wish to have rapid burial, without embalming or coffins.

Autopsy examinations are generally only allowed if a strong case is made that such a procedure would help keep others from falling victim to the same disease. Thus organ donation remains a sensitive subject, but there exists support in the community of Muslim scholars to allow such procedures if done with respect for the remains of the dead. Medical research can be considered to be a charity by providing knowledge to future generations. The help of an Islamic clergy along with the family is an indispensable resource in this regard.

Muslims, Islam, Medicine, and Genetics

In healthcare settings it is generally useful to record cultural characteristics for the family, including ethnic background, religion, and occupation. In order to gain sensitivity and be of true assistance to the client, the counselor must become aware of various aspects of the dynamics involved in the couple's decisions. A couple's views and beliefs on reproductive issues are frequently shaped by their cultural and spiritual beliefs (Kimura 1990). Religious beliefs may provide answers to the search for meaning after an undesirable event, and it can be used to cope with the emotional trauma these events may cause. Understanding the process involved in making and coping with health-related decisions is vital to establishing rapport with a client in a healthcare decision-making session. Healthcare providers can assist patients who depend on their spirituality or religion by having some understanding of how, as a whole, individuals of a religion view various reproductive issues.

The number of individuals who follow a particular religion or spiritual teacher in the world is astounding. Yet, while Christianity has the estimated largest number of followers, Islam is a close second with an estimated 1.3 billion followers. According to the Council on American Islamic Relations, there are approximately 7 million people who are followers of the Islamic faith in the United States. In light of the growing number of practicing Muslims in the world population as well as the United States, efforts should be made to examine the opinions of these individuals regarding reproductive issues, including prenatal screening, congenital defects, termination of pregnancy, infertility, and assisted reproduction, that have a direct bearing on healthcare choices.

Islam's origins can be traced to the same land that bore Judaism and Christianity. The central tenet of Islam is the belief that "There is no deity save God, and Muhammad is the messenger of God" (Garrad and Sheikh 2001). The aim of this belief is for the Muslim to create peace in one's self, family, and society by actively submitting to and implementing God's will (Qadr) (Hedeyant and Pirzadeh 2001). Islam is comprised of a moral code, as well as a civil law, and this code serves as a foundation for all Muslims regarding any decision that they make in their lives. Although there is a central tenet to Islam, various cultures refine the tenets based on their sensitivities and inclinations. Notwithstanding, Imams and Islamic scholars are responsible for interpreting and conceptualizing religious teachings (Qur'an, Hadith, and the words of the scholars) for the wider Muslim community. The Imams are the Muslim leaders who give instruction and guidance to the local community (Garrad and Sheikh 2001). Among the Imams some are scholars of the religious texts and are often asked make a religious ruling (fatwa) on issues including medical concerns. At times these scholars are asked to answer questions that were never posed to the scholars of previous generations. Therefore these contemporary jurists will make ijtihad (paradigm-based Islamic reasoning) to issue a new understanding of the ancient texts.

The family structure of Islam is also outlined by the teachings of the Qur'an. The birth process, in the view of Muslims, is a sacred event in which certain rituals are preferably done after birth, but are not required. There are traditional understandings in Islam regarding conception, the termination of a life, and even preventive measures regarding contraception and birth control. While some forms of birth control are permissible in some cases the practice of abortion is permitted.

Several studies have examined the attitudes of individuals regarding reproductive issues, including prenatal testing, perception of risk, and consanguinity. A study was done in Saudi Arabia to determine the attitudes of Saudi families affected with hemoglobinopathies towards prenatal screening and abortion and the influence of a religious ruling called fatwa (Alkuraya and Kilani 2001). In this study, the authors noted that Islamic scholars have issued a fatwa that a pregnancy may be terminated prior to 120 days if the fetus is affected with a severe malformation and if the fetus life after being born would be a means of misery to both the child and the parents. Sheikh Mohamed Al-Hanooti of the Fiqh Council of North America is of the opinion that in the less than 120 days that abortion, in the cases of *zina* (sex outside of marriage), rape, incest, divorce, or uncertain marriage. Many imams agree that after 120 days, with a unanimous opinion of medical experts, termination of a pregnancy may be permissible to save the life of the mother or in cases of severe congenital malformations of the fetus.

In the study by Alkuraya and Kilani, 32 families with a family history of various hemoglobinopathies were interviewed to discuss their degree of suffering, prior genetic knowledge, attitudes toward prenatal diagnosis, and the factors that influenced that attitude. Learning about the relevant fatwa increased the number of people who would accept abortion in the study, but not the number of people who would actually undergo prenatal diagnosis. This was found to be true regardless of socioeconomic status or level of education. The study researchers concluded that the individuals might have rejected prenatal diagnosis because they believed it was aimed at an abortion. Despite their personal feelings, many participants in the study remained opposed to prenatal diagnosis and abortion.

A workshop was organized by the International Islamic Center for Population Studies and Research in Al-Azhar University in Cairo to discuss the issues surrounding infertility and assisted reproductive technologies (Serour and Dickens 2001). The workshop reviewed the issue of access to in-vitro fertilization services, pre-implantation genetic diagnosis, follicular maturation, and embryo implantation. The participants discussed the difficulties that have arisen in some Muslim communities because this technology is believed to conflict with some religious tenets and enacted Muslim law. Techniques that are used in standard in-vitro fertilization, such as ovum donation or sperm donation, are not acceptable because sperm donation is considered adulterous (Mor-Yosef and Schenker 1995).

It is stated that if the husband's infertility is beyond cure the infertility should be accepted or the wife justified if she seeks divorce. Pressure for divorce may frequently come from the family of the wife. One of the central ideas of Muslim identity is that the family structure should have an authentic lineage. Therefore, sperm donation is seen as fracturing the family genetic linkage. While sperm donation and ovum donation are not welcomed, pre-implantation genetic diagnosis has been considered to be a viable reproductive option (el-Hashemite 1997). The participants of the workshop organized by the International Islamic Center for Population Studies noted that in-vitro fertilization would provide an acceptable option for couples who cannot yet establish a pregnancy on their own, yet maintain their own genetic make up to create a child. The workshop recommended creating a committee for medical ethics that would monitor appropriate research that is respectful of the needs and interests of infertile couples.

The Attitudes of Muslims Toward Reproduction in the United States

The following study was conducted by one of the authors as a graduate student at Howard University to assess the attitudes of Muslims in the United States. The purpose of this study was to examine the attitudes of Muslims regarding reproductive issues by:

- Evaluating Muslim attitudes towards having a child born with birth defects that have a significant genetic component.
- Identifying the influences that are involved in the dynamics of the decision-making process in regards to reproductive issues.
- Examining Muslim beliefs about viable interventions in regards to reproductive issues.
- Identifying the coping strategies for Muslims when they deal with reproductive issues.
- Determining if the genetic counselor would be useful to someone who has increased probability of delivering a child with a significant genetic disorder.

Fifty Muslim men and women were recruited from the Washington, DC area. Muslims from these centers comprise individuals from diverse ethnic backgrounds and geographic areas, including the United States, Africa, the Middle East, and Asia. The questionnaire was distributed to participants a couple of hours after religious services. We obtained results from African American, African, Middle Eastern, and Indian Muslims. All written materials given to individuals were in English and an explanation of the study in the form of the preamble was given to each Muslim who indicated they would like to participate. To ensure confidentiality, no personal identifying information was obtained. Participants answered questions regarding the actions they would take if they were in one of the two scenarios. A description of genetic counseling was provided for those individuals not familiar with the profession.

Scenario 1 consisted of a situation in which a couple is informed by a genetic counselor that a soft marker for a moderate genetic condition was identified on ultrasound. The fetus was described as having a congenital heart defect; the suspected condition involved the child having certain facial features and moderate mental retardation. The couple was given the option to have amniocentesis, a prenatal genetic testing method. A description of the procedure was outlined as well as the risks associated with the procedure. The couple was informed that the risk of the procedure is 0.5% (1/200). The respondents were asked to judge the usefulness of the information the genetic counselor would provide in this scenario. They were also asked if they would take the information provided in this scenario into account in their decision-making process. They were asked questions regarding prenatal testing in this scenario and coping strategies they would utilize before and after making a decision. Scenario 2 was similar, but the fetus was more severely affected, possibly with a fatal condition.

The participants were asked about their beliefs regarding reproductive technologies in the event of infertility. The questionnaire also asked about consulting a religious leader for making important life decisions. Additional questions regarding reproductive issues were also included. We found that 62% of them were female; 86% had completed college or post-graduate studies; 82% of the participants surveyed were U.S. citizens and of those who were not, three quarters had been in the country less than ten years. Fourteen percent of the respondents identified themselves as African, indicating they were from the Sudan, Kenya, or Morocco; 52% were African American. 22% were from the Middle East, including Pakistan, Yemen, and Jordan; 12 were from Asia, including India, Singapore, and Cambodia. One third of the respondents reported that they did not have any children, 26% of the respondents had one or two children, and 42% of the respondents had three or more children.

When respondents were asked the frequency with which they sought a religious leader to help make important life decisions, 22% of them said rarely, 10% of them said occasionally, 34% said quite often, and 34% said very often. The following figures show the frequency of responses regarding prenatal testing by citizenship and utilization of reproductive technologies based on ancestry.

The first aim of the project was to evaluate Muslim attitudes towards having a child born with a medical condition that has a significant genetic component. We found that participants, regardless of age, education level, citizenship status, ancestry, number of children, or religious consultation, believed that the significance of a child with a birth defect was not due to imbalance or divine judgment against the parents, but rather other reasons. Participants wrote in their own beliefs about the relevance of a child with a significant genetic component. Many of these participants believed that having a child with birth defects was a test from God (Allah), as well as God's will (Qadr). Some participants also believed that this child was a blessing from God whether or not the child was born with a birth defect.

The second aim of the project was to examine the beliefs regarding viable interventions relative to reproductive issues. Viable interventions examined included prenatal genetic testing, termination of pregnancy, and the use of assisted reproductive technologies like in-vitro fertilization and pre-implantation genetic diagnosis for infertility. Of those who were not U.S. citizens, a third stated they would definitely pursue prenatal genetic testing, whereas only a few U.S. citizens (4.9%) would definitely have genetic testing. It is possible that those who are not citizens do not have these technologies available in their place of origin and would be more likely to take advantage of technologies if they were available. It is of interest that the distribution of the frequencies in scenario 2 where the child was more severely affected was not very different than in scenario 1. We speculated that the severity of the genetic condition would not change the likelihood of individuals deciding to have prenatal genetic testing in regardless of age, gender, education, citizenship status, ancestry, number of children, or religious consultation.

When respondents identified the reasons why they would not pursue testing in scenario 1, 51% of them indicated that knowing the diagnosis of the child prior to birth would not affect their feelings about the pregnancy in any way. The next most frequently cited reason (43%) was that they did not believe in termination if the child were to have the clinical features listed in scenario 1. In scenario 2 the most common reasons for not pursing genetic testing were the same as in scenario 1. This finding supports the conclusion that the attitudes of the Muslims involved in this study do not appear to be related to the severity of the genetic condition.

When asked why they would have prenatal genetic testing the most frequent response (66%) in scenario 1 was that knowing the diagnosis of the child would reduce anxiety, and for scenario 2 the most frequent response (53%) was that knowing the diagnosis would allow them to make financial and insurance preparations for their child. We concluded that even if prenatal diagnosis is a viable option, terminating the pregnancy for a genetic condition is almost never considered.

In addition to prenatal genetic testing and termination of pregnancy, we also examined the attitudes of Muslims towards assisted reproductive technologies in the event of infertility. Of individuals who identified themselves as African, 42% would probably not and 28% of them would definitely not use in-vitro fertilization; 45% of Middle Easterners said that they would use in-vitro fertilization if they were infertile, and only 9% would definitely not. For African Americans, 28% of them said that definitely would use in-vitro fertilization, 16% said they would definitely not. For those of Asian ancestry, the frequencies were both 33%. Each country in the Middle East and Africa has cultural differences, so we did not make larger-scale generalizations about this issue.

When respondents were asked to identify why they would not utilize IVF, the majority of them stated (66%) that they did not believe in having children outside of natural means. The second most frequent choice was that they preferred to adopt a child rather than conceive a child from artificial means. When the participants were asked what most bothered them about reproductive technologies, the most frequent response was that using these technologies was too much like playing God. We can speculate that they felt that the birth process is in fact considered sacred, and technology should not interfere in these matters. In addition, participants may have been hesitant to use them because of the method in which the sperm is often obtained in reproductive technologies. Some Muslims may believe that only the husband's genetic material should be used for conception.

The third aim of the project was to examine the influences on decisions regarding reproductive issues. In every demographic category examined, the majority of individuals (greater than 87%) stated they would seek consultation before deciding to undergo prenatal genetic testing. When asked to identify which individuals they would consult with, the three most frequent responses were spouse (88%), another family member (65%), or an imam or Muslim scholar (63%.) This finding sheds light on the fact that Muslims regard prenatal genetic testing as something that cannot be decided on at an initial genetic counseling session, preferring to first discuss their options with a variety of individuals in their social network before making a final decision about whether to pursue prenatal genetic testing.

The fourth aim of the study was to examine the coping strategies for Muslims when dealing with reproductive issues. When respondents were asked the methods of coping with continuing the pregnancy of a child affected with a moderate genetic condition, the three main coping outlets were talking with family members (64%), reading religious materials or texts (60%), and attending a support group for parents of children affected with a similar genetic condition. A majority (79%) of respondents reported that they would pray or meditate, 53% said they would read religious books, and 64% said they would attend a support group if they were to have a child severely affected with a genetic condition. The study revealed that those surveyed, regardless of the severity of the condition with which their child was affected, would turn to their religion through prayer, meditation, and reading of religious books to find comfort in coping with a child affected with a genetic disorder.

The last aim of the project was to determine the usefulness of the information a genetic counselor provided in scenario 1. A minority (31%) of U.S. citizens and a third of the respondents that did not identify themselves as U.S. citizens believed that the information provided by the genetic counselor would be useful. For many respondents genetic counseling is not easily accessible, and they may be appreciative of this information, even if they later decide against genetic testing.

This study sheds light on the fact that many Muslim followers may not pursue Western genetic tests such as amniocentesis, and if they did, termination would not be a common option for them. The perception of the Muslim in regards to having a child born with a birth defect is not seen as a burden, but rather as a test from God or God's will (Qadr). Care should be taken to remain non-directive when counseling individuals of the Islamic faith. We recommend that the genetic counselor explore the relevant options and cultural beliefs when assisting them in making reproductive choices.

References

Adherents.com. 2005. *Major religions of the world ranked by number of adherents.* http://adherents.com/Religions_By_Adherents.html (accessed October 9, 2008).

Alkuraya, F. S., and R. A. Kilani. 2001. Attitude of Saudi families affected with homoglobinopathies towards prenatal screening and abortion and the influence of religious ruling (Fatwa). *Prenatal Diagnosis* 21 (6): 448–451.

Council on American-Islamic Relations. 2006. *Western Muslim minorities: Integration and disenfranchisement.* http://www.cair.com/Portals/0/pdf/policy_bulletin_Integration_in_the_West.pdf (accessed September 18, 2008).

Covey, S. R. 1989. The *7 habits of highly effective people.* New York: Simon & Schuster.

el-Hashemite, N. 1997. The Islamic view in genetic preventive procedures. *Lancet* 350 (9072): 223.

Kimura, R. 1990. Religious aspects of human genetic information. In *Science, law and ethics,* Ciba Foundation Symposium. Chichester: Wiley.

Mor-Yosef, S., and J. G. Schenker. 1995. Sperm donation in Israel. Human Reproduction 10 (4): 965–967.

Serour, G. I., and B. M. Dickens. 2001. Assisted reproduction developments in the Islamic world. *International Journal of Gynaecology and Obstetrics* 74 (2): 187–193.

CHAPTER 12

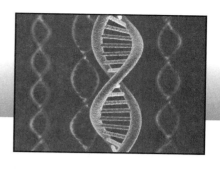

Genetics and Ethics from a Christian Perspective

Isaac M. T. Mwase, PhD, MDiv, MBA
Connie C. Price, PhD, MPS

Christian voices are being heard on most of the major issues in genetics. That is a good thing. It is important for all segments of humanity to have their perspectives considered as we make difficult choices about life, at the beginning and ending of life and in between. Christian voices have always commanded attention in discussions about the nature of persons; these need to be heard particularly now in a world characterized by biotechnological innovation. When we consider what ought to guide decisions by Christians about the use of various biotech innovations, among the topics we have to address are the following: creation and evolution, the nature of persons, beginning- and end-of-life issues, and health and health care. These topics provide a framework for exploring Christian perspectives on genetics and ethics.

Creation and Evolution

Views about the origins of the universe, life, and of human life play a crucial role in Christian perspectives on genetics and ethics. It matters to Christians whether the world and life are results of self-organizing processes, processes directed by God, or a combination of the two.

There are a variety of positions taken by various Christians on the question of origins. There are many whose position is shaped by a simple reading of the Bible. They understand the universe to be the product of God's creativity. God spoke the world into being. "Then God said, 'Let there be light;' and there was light" (Genesis 1:3). (All citations will be from the *New Revised Standard Version* (NRSV) unless otherwise stated.)

Two readings of Genesis shape the doctrine of creation for most Christian communities. These readings are reflected in the major biblical translations used by Christians. There are those who insist that God created *ex nihilo*, that is, completely out of nothing. For the others God speaks into being out of original chaos a world of order and variety. The former prefer the *King James Version* and related translations while the latter prefer translations with affinity to the *NRSV*. The first two verses in Genesis are rendered thus:

- *King James Version*
  Genesis 1:1-2

  1 In the beginning God created the heaven and the earth. **2** And the earth was without form and void; and darkness was upon the face of the deep. And the Spirit of God moved upon the face of the waters.

- *New Revised Standard Version*
  Genesis 1:1-2

  1 In the beginning when God created the heavens and the earth, **2** the earth was a formless void and darkness covered the face of the deep, while a wind from God swept over the face of the waters.

The crucial divide, however, in how Christians read and interpret the Bible is in the approaches they take to the dominant evolutionary account of the world, biological life, and human life (Mwase 2004). There are those who reject evolution outright. They prefer a simple creationist account of origins. For some scientifically savvy Christians, big bang cosmology provides the primary backdrop for understanding the origin of the universe and biological life. They seek to interpret scripture in light of what the best science has established. A source of much debate, often acrimonious, is a movement of scholars arguing that scientific data suggest that the universe is the product of intelligent design. Intelligent design arguments are not new in the history of thought. These arguments can be traced to thinkers such as William Paley (1743–1805). The intelligent design movement is now a well-organized and well-funded movement that currently enjoys significant support and influence in many Christian communities and among conservative politicians. It is not altogether clear what impact intelligent design positions will have on decisions by Christians about the use of genetic technologies.

A significant number of Christians have come to terms with an evolutionary understanding of the universe and history. Among the major Internet portals that showcase the work of such thinkers are the John Templeton Foundation, the Center for Theology and Natural Science, and Metanexus. Current theories of evolution by a widespread consensus of scientists have much going for them. Evolution cannot be dismissed in a cavalier fashion as just a theory. When any account in science attains the status of a theory, that means the account has substantial explanatory power and fosters productive inquiry. Such is the case with present-day insights on evolution. Human beings and all living things have evolved. Recent models offer substantial genetic data in support of a Recent African Origin (RAO)—also called the Out of Africa model (Tishkoff and Kidd 2004). RAO holds that non-African populations descended from an anatomically modern *H. sapiens* ancestor that evolved in Africa roughly 200 thousand years ago and then spread and diversified throughout the world. Genetically human populations are 99.6–99.8% identical at the nucleotide level (Appiah 1995; Clark 2002; Marks 2003).

Diversity, however, does characterize *H. sapiens*. The HapMap Project is giving us a clearer picture, whereby populations are shown to have clustered by broad geographic regions that correspond with common "racial" classification (Africa, Europe, Asia, Oceania, Americas). The story of migration, isolation, and drift is emerging from use of Y-chromosomal material, mtDNA, and autosomal markers. A better understanding of the global distribution of genetic variation is vital for biomedical diagnosis and therapy. It is now a matter of common affirmation that all individuals are genetically unique. However, given that each person is a member of what appears to be distinct ancestral groups, it is important that we develop a perspective on everyone's common nature.

The Nature of Persons

What is the nature of persons? Do all human beings share the same nature? How are we to interpret what they have in common and what differentiates one individual from another or one group from another? What are the implications of human diversity for the diagnosis of diseases and for treatment regimens? Why is it that particular populations seem to have higher incidences of sickle cell trait and disease, cystic fibrosis, breast cancer, etc? Scientists at the time of this writing are feverishly attempting to define with as much clarity as possible what we know and do not know about human beings. Three major publications should prove helpful for those seeking to develop a Christian perspective on the nature of persons in light of the best science. *Nature Genetics* in its November 2004 supplement took up the topic of "Genetics for the Human Race" (Royal, Malveaux, and Dunlap 2004). The January 2005 *American Psychologist* is a collection of ten articles that explore "Genes, Race, and Psychology in the Genome Era" (Anderson and Nickerson 2005). The Social Science Research Council has made available a web forum that explores the question, "Is Race Real?"

Development of perspectives on the nature of persons occurs in a context marked by a history of racism and patriarchy. Doctrines that promote racial hierarchy have been part of the thinking of leading Christians and scientists since the Enlightenment (a philosophical movement of the eighteenth century), if not earlier. Patriarchy, the perspective that views God and society in a way that grants males prominence and primacy, has been entrenched in most Christian traditions since their inception. Racism and patriarchy are of concern in thinking about the use of genetic technologies because dominant white male culture has often harnessed the goods of medicine in a way that resulted in health inequities (IOM 2002). Many writers in critical theory have shown that colonization, slavery, and racial eugenics and genocide at best could not have been pulled off without the participation of segments within Christianity. No believer can refute the massive evidence that conversion was often the one publicly avowed purpose of fifteenth- to nineteenth-century missions to the southern and western hemispheres. The actual goals indeed included conversion and "education" into European culture, but equally important to colonizers were enslavement or genocide, sexual adventure, theft of natural resources, and just plain old expansion of territory and world dominance. The existential problem for Christians today is not only the devastation that went along with the conversions, but the issues at the heart of such (pseudo-?) conversions themselves: learning to detest the body, especially if one were of dark skin and female; internalizing hegemonic sexism *qua* monotheism; learning to renounce one's own supportive and ritualistic upbringing (that is, losing the strength and wisdom of the symbolic that constitute a "person"); learning to perceive the teachings of the other world religions, e.g., Islam and Buddhism, as primitive, mythological, and indeed demonic; and accepting the semantics of a European language as the sole mode of truth.

Feminist Christians are wont to use the word "misogyny" instead of "patriarchy," so grave is their reservation about their faith's ability to acknowledge the human status of women. Hatred of the female body and resentment of women's existence are not Freudian ruses. They are evident from the story of Adam and Eve, on through the

New Testament writings of St. Paul. Jesus took a different view of women than had yet appeared in history; so then must the Gospel writers have done. Soren Kierkegaard was a major thinker notable for his acclamation of the feminine as integral to Christian life. Also, the feminism that is evident in the "Lost Gospels" inspires many feminists of today's church. Feminists of the twentieth and twenty-first centuries have reinterpreted and even re-written the ancient foundation myths, such as the account of Adam's rib (woman comes from bone; man, only from dust) and of biting into the apple (an act showing that Eve had the courage to take risks and to initiate history and that Adam was a stupid frontally aware sycophant). Kierkegaard deconstructed the story of Abraham, Isaac, Ishmael, and Sarah in *Fear and Trembling,* setting forth the Judeo-Christian feminist genre that looks again at Mary Magdalene, at the authority of Peter, at the intentions of the Gospel of John and the parables, and at the teachings of the early mystics known as the Desert Fathers and Mothers. The very image of God as a partriarch in the sky is itself a universal human psychosis, as noted by Kierkegaard (1983), Nietzsche (in Kaufmann 1968), Bergson (1975), and Whitehead (1967), among others. Movies, paintings, and sculptures since the Middle Ages, iconography, literature, and the liturgies make appeals to an old bearded imperious white male, and to a pliable womanhood that functions only performatively, in one or more of three roles: prostitute, wife and breeder, or witch. The last of the three categories is an emotionally charged term that, when used in its negative connotations, targets creative and courageous women: female intellectuals, artists, priests, leaders, and healers.

With a crippled "personhood" that comprises the ashes of these dehumanizing aspects of Christian activities, present-day believers now face the stunning task of remaking their humanity and community; that is, of healing, even as followers of a religion whose past advocates chose to condemn human life rather than be grateful for it. Contemporary Christians also face unprecedented decisions that can graphically challenge their concepts of personhood, their ideas of freedom and dignity, and their powers of love and forgiveness. Examples are the needs for urgent yet rational decisions about chronic and infectious diseases contracted in the wake of the colonial eras, such as: epidemic proportions of depression, of illnesses related to obesity and, in the post-colonial world, of hunger, as well as HIV/AIDS, new strains of influenza, and threats of bioterrorism. The challenges include decisions many people are not emotionally equipped to make, precisely because of the psychotic aspects of Christian "religious" history. And yet, believers must make such decisions, and soon. To name a few, these are: whether human cloning is merely a professional ethics issue or entails a newly emergent ontology of the soul; whether organ transplantation will continue to grow as a resource for organized crime or be perceived as a miraculous way for people to help one another when their lives are at an end; whether food and its attendant rites are to be produced by plastics conglomerates or by enraptured human labor qua investiture with the earth; whether women can or will resolve to perpetuate intelligence as they did before they were assigned to do the bedding and boarding.

Views that Christians hold about the diverse lives of the 6.5 billion human beings inhabiting this small planet do affect what happens in personal and collective interactions. Wars erupt because one group sees itself as entitled to privileges and as better than another. Nazi Germany was responsible for mass murder, convinced that certain populations were inferior, and a drag on the economy and a genetically superior nation. Medicine in the United States has systematically provided sub-optimal care to Blacks because of insidious and damaging views about their personhood. A recent IOM report (2002) documents health disparities among Blacks and Latinos in comparison with those regarded as White. Although Christian texts and traditions emphasize the equality of human beings, racial superiority doctrines were articulated in part by prominent Christian thinkers. The text of immediate appeal to advance an egalitarian view of all human beings is usually Galatians 3:28, "There is neither Jew nor Greek, slave nor free, male or female, for you are all one in Christ Jesus."

It is readily evident that human beings vary individually and as members of particular sub-populations. Ethiopians are different from Kenyans who in turn are different from Ashkenazi Jews, American Indians, Sri Lankans, Maoris, Han Chinese, etc. The question of scientific and theological import is whether these differences matter in substantial ways. A reductively biological way to put this question is: are these differences much like those one finds among cattle, which come in varieties such as Brahman, Afrikander, Longhorn, etc.? Recent advances in genetics, partly because of the Human Genome Project and the International Haplotype Map Project, will help scholars to assert appropriate claims about the varieties that make up the genus *Homo sapiens*. Controversy rages on about whether there are distinct races in the genus. Additionally researchers wonder whether there is a biological or genetic basis to "race" or "racial" differences. Is race a sociopolitical or biological construct? And if biological, does this mean "genetic"? The emerging consensus is that race has no basis in biology. The questions are complicated by those who seek to answer them in a way that reinforces racial superiority doctrines. Such doctrines can be traced back to nineteenth-century science, including that of taxonomist Charles Linnaeus and others such as Georges Buffon, Charles Darwin, Franz Boaz, and Francis Galton. It will suffice to adumbrate the views of Linnaeus.

Linnaeus judged *Homo sapiens* to comprise a hierarchy of organisms. In his 1735 *General System of Nature* he advanced the view that human beings are higher order mammals because they are able to reason. But he went further. Not all human beings are the same. They are different due to climate and culture. Linnaeus categorized *Homo sapiens* into four groups: (Hossain 2000):

- *Americanus.* Native American males were supposedly red; had black hair and sparse beards; were stubborn; prone to anger; "free"; and governed by traditions. Thus, this form of *Homo sapiens* was definitely inferior and uncivilized.

- *Asiaticus.* The male Asian was said to be "yellowish, melancholy, endowed with black hair and brown eyes...severe, conceited, and stingy. He puts on loose clothing. He is governed by opinion." Thus, like the aforementioned type of *Homo sapiens*, the *Asiaticus* could only be a mediocre prototype.

- *Africanus.* The male of this subset, according to Linnaeus, could be recognized by his skin tone, face structure, and curly hair. This kind was apparently cunning, passive, and inattentive, and ruled by impulse. The female of this kind was also apparently shameless, because "they lactate profusely."

- *Europeaus.* The males of this subset were supposedly "changeable, clever, and inventive. He puts on tight clothing. He is governed by laws."

Jonathan Marks (2003) explains how Linnaeus's classification system for animals shows the biologist's political bent, especially as seen in his choice of the term "mammals." Linnaeus sympathized with a back-to-breastfeeding movement that was popular in Sweden and northern Europe at the time he created the biological classification system that is still used. *Mammalia* are thus named only for one of the two sexes, and for no other characteristics than that of having breasts. Disregarded are such qualities as increased use of the brain and the senses, and warm-bloodedness. Linnaeus still has some disciples who, like him, believe that whites or Europeans are the superior sub-population of *Homo sapiens.* There are many who openly and secretly harbor similar views. One wonders about the impact of such views in clinical settings and in the development of healthcare policies. Current science is emphatic about the unity and diversity of *Homo sapiens.* Genetic and ancestral diversity have to be acknowledged for biomedical research. If differences are of a sort that medicine might not work equally well for everyone, that becomes a major issue. Christianity in recent days has equally been emphatic about the unity and diversity of all human beings. In fact some groups such as the Southern Baptist Convention that historically courted outright racists have taken a clear position that denounces racism as both sin and bad theology.

Beginning- and End-of-Life Issues

It is a commonplace that many Christians arduously defend "the right to life." These persons for the most part comprise mainstream Catholics and fundamentalist Protestants. The basic argument "for life" is that a conceptus is a human being, as is a person in a persistent vegetative state. Catholic doctrine is that a fetus or a neonate must receive the sacrament of baptism. Also important to Catholics is the fulfillment of the "natural law," in this case the natural law's demand that birthing be completed and families and religious communities be built and continued. The history of Catholic doctrine on abortion is complex; it was in the twentieth century that abortion became a significant target for abolition in the church. Although Protestants "for life" do not base their anti-abortionism on an appeal to the sacraments and natural law, they do associate the conceptus's (**and** the persistently vegetative individual's) spiritual status, i.e., that of a human being and child of God, with his or her right to go on living. Often their position is developed from a literal reading of Psalm 139:15 (*King James Version*), "My substance was not hid from thee when I was made in secret, and curiously wrought in the lowest parts of the earth."

On the other hand, many Christians believe that the human, and thus the spiritual, status of those at the absolute beginning of their biologically human lives, and at the absolute end of their cognitive and emotive lives, is at most ambivalent, and possibly a negative. With regard to the conceptus, the embryo, the prospect of pre-implantation genetic diagnosis of embryos, and the fetus, the Christian's argument is comparable to that of the "pro-choice" secular view. Like their counterparts outside the faith, these believers regard "human-ness" as a quality that may be defined in ways other than the fact of organic quickness in a particular member of *Homo sapiens*. For example, "humanity" for some encompasses the ability to have experiences, and to consider such experiences in rational, emotional, or creative ways, perhaps comparing different experiences and going on to categorize and make *judgments* about the experiences. Even if the fetus, or perhaps the viable or late-stage fetus, were to be proven human in some minimal sense, advocates for the legality of abortion say that it is a civil and human right for a woman to terminate her pregnancy. Loving fellow humans must support *her* spiritual growth, health, and safety. Many Christians (and from this juncture, the secular perspective is not taken into account) would encourage the woman to look deeply into her situation, a tragic one, and to pray for guidance on how to be ever free from such a plight in her future. Perhaps the church needs to think harder about its role in this situation, and open its arms wider to her during this struggle and all others to come.

Religious zeal was alive and well in the United States when it comes to end-of-life issues, as witnessed in the 2005 public displays of emotion regarding Mrs. Terry Schiavo. In the last weeks of Terry's life, many thousands of "pro-life" Christians rallied to her parents' pleas for (their version of) justice. Even Congress and President Bush took drastic measures to keep Terry alive. Unlike several past court rulings, in 2005 no reversals were forthcoming, and Terry died. The Schiavo case is comparable to that of Miss Karen Quinlan in the 1970s and Miss Nancy Cruzan in the 1980s. (It is notable that all three cases involved attractive white women of child-bearing age; this draws attention to the issue of the "nature of persons" as discussed above, at least regarding the perception of this concept in the general public's consciousness. With sincere respect for the three individuals and their families, even in reverend sorrow for their subjection to humiliation and strife at their times of departure, one can still be led to wonder whether the image of personhood ingrained in the public's mind, regarding the fates of these three women, was being somehow convoluted with expectations of white feminine vulnerability, passivity, and fertility.) In each of the three cases, bitter disputes among family members, between the courts and the health-care providers, or among all these parties along with the press, the clergy, and academic bioethicists, transpired over what the person's desires would have been had she remained conscious, and what her status as a person was as the woman lay comatose and unresponsive. The earlier two cases in fact helped to solidify the very concepts of "stakeholders," "interests," and "quality of life" in the emerging field of bioethics.

Some pro-choice Christians would point to the inconsistency, even hypocrisy, involved in the "pro-lifers'" passionate hatred of abortion and indeed of its advocates, when these same people are likely to defend wars and the death penalty with equal fervor. Further, the question of suffering comes into the discourses on life, as seen in the plight of an unwanted pregnancy where the woman suffers greatly, even when she denies her emotional pain, because of her circumstances or for other reasons. The Catholic view tends to support suffering as a means of impoverishing the soul to the degree that one can encounter the fullness of grace. Protestants concur that, as it is written in the Beatitudes, the unbearable burdens of life can enhance oneness with God. However, Protestants are not so likely to perceive human struggle as a sufficient reason for continuing a human life that has no discernible "quality" remaining in it. In the case of abortion, carrying the baby to term would be not so much a punishment for the woman's sin as an opportunity to consider the meaning of God's call both to her and to her future child, to live out the miracle of life. There is also the possibility that the fetus is severely defective, a reason that women often give for abortion. The suffering of this innocent one is again perceived by some anti-abortionist Christians as an "example" of an imperfect life, an imperfect bio-graphy, that is most blessed even in its infirmities.

Genetics for Health and Health Care

On the whole, Christians at the present time withhold judgment on the uses of genetics for treatment and prevention of diseases. The spectrum of opinion is as wide on this issue as it is among secular folk. The objections amount to reservations about any and all sorts of genetic *interventions*. Like their secular counterparts, Christians would be more comfortable with somatic intervention—genetic modifications that benefit only the patient—than with those regarding germ-line transformations—modifications that benefit the patient and potential progeny—and with research on genetic treatments for chronic and critical "physical" ailments (e.g., diabetes and hypertension) rather than treatments for behavioral problems such as violence and addictions. The reasons for this involve the ideas of personhood, as well as the definitions of "life" and indeed of evolution, as reviewed in this chapter. If one believes that God's will is going to prevail and ought not to be tampered with, then greater suspicion of genetic interventions will follow. It is this kind of thinking that informs arguments against interventions as instances of "playing God." Others may be less suspicious, claiming that Christians are obligated to put up a fight against sin, and can do that within the systems of scientific discourse, which are on the whole legitimate but sometimes require critical reflection from a religious perspective.

Consider for example the question of race and medical genetics. In these early years of the twenty-first century, there is intense debate about the best way, the most balanced and anti-racist way, to address genetic diseases or conditions that may be tied to "markers" specific to race. This high intensity is inevitable, given the history of racism in the United States, including racism in health care and research. A recent example is the Food and Drug Administration's approval of BiDil, a drug produced by Nitromed, Inc., and tailored to black people's apparently distinctive propensity for heart disease (FDA 2005). Some people considered this measure to be a sophisticated form of racial profiling. Others welcomed BiDil as a sign of a new awareness of the specific healthcare needs of African Americans. In a Christian ethical context, advocates would say that medical research that takes race and genetic heritage seriously is stewardship at its best, and indeed a form of reparation for past negligence of black people as patients with an absolutely equal right to full care, including innovative, focused research.

As further examples of interventions, it is well known that fundamentalists and some others categorically oppose human cloning, as well as the use of human embryonic stem cells for research and the procedure of pre-implantation genetic diagnosis (PGD). Even animal cloning and the "treatment" cloning of human cells (a proposed measure that would provide stem cells without destroying human embryos) meets raised eyebrows among Christians. All such measures, go their arguments, amount to assuming God's rightful role of giving and taking human life, with animal cloning and non-reproductive cloning of human cells amounting to holding patterns atop a slippery slope. Should somatic interventions become feasible for the prevention or treatment of chronic and critical "physical" illnesses, many Christians would argue against such therapies.

The Marxist microbiologist Richard Lewontin (2000) has argued, surprisingly, in favor of allowing important seats to be occupied by fundamentalists at the negotiating tables on matters of genetics and health. Lewontin believes that it is fundamentalist Christians who today control the debates about human reproductive choices and genetic medical science. They have amassed great wealth, political prowess, and media visibility. Their messages that abortion is murder or at least a grievous sin, that destroying embryos is abortion, etc., have settled into the American unconscious, especially the minds of young people. And yet, in the major decision-making committees on health policy, bioethics, and relations of science to religion, fundamentalists have been conspicuously uninvited. At the tables instead are analytic philosophers of "moral theory." Policy makers in bioethics who supposedly represent religious professions, states Lewontin, tend to be comparatively bland figures from middle-of-the-road denominations. Fundamentalists may not have a voice where the jargon of analytic ethics is the lingua franca, but they get heard loud and clear in the halls of Congress and indeed in the Oval Office. Denial is the order of bioethicists' day, claims Lewontin. Until the nation and culture face the facts of who wields power in questions of science and health, and for that matter, of the political nature of these decisions to begin with, and proceed to invite those parties to "converse" with others whose views are rational perhaps to a fault, no breakthroughs in genetic medicine will occur. Lewontin may have overstated the issue, but the point merits attention from well-meaning religious bioethicists.

Another area of genetics that affects health is agricultural biotechnology. On this topic, few Christian associations have spoken out. Most U.S. Christians would be willing to support the genetic modification of crops because this enterprise is part of the trend of capitalistic globalization. Some evangelicals and Catholics, the latter inspired by liberation theology, perceive humanity's health as being based on good nutrition and on right labor. According to this view, adequate food, nurturing the land, creative work, and safe housing are human rights for all persons worldwide, and would be assured for everyone through such sustainable agricultural practices as organic crops, indigenously managed markets, communities organizing to maintain sanitation and clean air and water, and the people's relentless struggle to preserve local and family farms. Indeed, these Christians tend to garner their passions in arguments, not around abortion, a bourgeois "quality of life," or the status of an embryo, but around dirt and toilets and seasons of labor, celebration, and communion.

Crucial to the debates about genetics and health are questions surrounding the specter of *eugenics* in recent U.S. and European history. The apparently straightforward ethical issues about the utility of genetics for treatment and prevention of diseases may, in a strict logical sense, be a different topic than that of the eugenic notion of genetically engineering a "better" human of the future. The two issues are *different*, but they are not so completely *separate* as today's conventional intellectualism has it. For example, when the issue arises of behavioral genetics, i.e., genetic interventions to ameliorate behavioral problems, the distinction between treatment and eugenics becomes blurred. The reason for this blurring is that altering a behavior through genetic surgery, even if it were only a somatic treatment, would affect the *relationships* of the patient with others, including the younger generations in her community. The reduction of addictions and compulsions and their related stress would have a ripple effect on the community, de-stressing the social atmosphere and allowing people more freedom to envision richer lives for themselves and one another. For example, if someone were to be cured of alcoholism or drug addiction, everyone in their family plus their social support system, including their church, and their colleagues at work, would find relief from the tension and stress of coping with the person's former habits. Granted, co-dependencies often enable addictions. Still, when one addict opts out of their habit, the likelihood increases that the enablers also can become free from *their* denial. Thus, no behavioral intervention, however beneficial, could be only somatic. Nor could it affect only the individual. In fact, one ethical objection to behavioral genetics is that it confines medicine to an individualistic mindset, while more progressive ethics would incorporate communities and the environment into the spectrum of health care. If behavioral interventions would entail communal changes, the ethical objection of excessive individualism would be refuted. Other objections might arise, however, such as the possibility of a social direction towards *groupthink*. Also, the scenario of healing through genetic intervention carries with it the reductionist assumption that genetic modifications of behaviors are or ever will be possible. No genetic correlations to behavior have yet been found despite heated and competitive efforts to discover them.

Suppose, perhaps in a utopian way, that the ethical issues of behavioral genetics have already been sorted out by means of deliberative and democratic processes. People have at long last concurred that behaviors are genetically based. One can even assume that it has been proven true beyond any doubt that genes determine behaviors; the specific genes have been traced and the causal factors observed many times over. Even assuming that all this calmness and humanistic rationality is the way things would go as the world moved into a new era of the *meaning of health* (a deterministic and materialistic era, indeed), still one little detail must be noted. This detail is that, according to Christians of all stamps, the essential teachings of Christianity would be threatened severely. A significant basis of Christianity is that one's personhood is not reducible to any "part" of her psyche or body. Rather, the person is a wholeness, and also free, paradoxically as it were, to create even more wholeness as her life unfolds. Many Christians are fervid in their devotion to the status of embryos and fetuses and the reproductive place of women, while the actual rupture to the faith takes place with nary a whimper from those who are so enraged. A Christian sociology would have it that the reason for this absence of criticism is probably that behavioral genetics would undermine the faith insidiously.

Powerful Religious Bodies Whose Positions on Ethics Provide Guidance for Adherents to the Traditions They Serve

- Baptist Joint Committee for Religious Liberty
- Southern Baptist Convention's Ethics and Religious Liberty Commission
- The Pontifical Academy
- Americans United for Separation of Church and State
- Family Research Council
- Focus on the Family
- United States Conference of Bishops

In conclusion, it is evident that many thinkers among the faithful cannot avoid worrying a bit, that the exchanges of epithets that now pass as debates on Christian ethics in genetics are glossing the profound issues of the actual meaning of health, both in its physical and psychosocial aspects. A big emptiness makes itself evident when one listens to the banter. Today's loquacious defenders of (their version of) the faith seem to be saying that all would be well after Christianity, so long as the pomp and hierarchy continued. Values that are pumped out of the mega/media orientation of some contemporary churches seem to have more appeal in the present day than does Jesus' difficult and dangerous calling to all of humanity, to love and forgive one another, and let justice roll down like water, and dwell together in peace, and create joy unto the end of their days.

References

Anderson, N. B., and K. J. Nickerson, eds. 2005. Genes, race, and psychology in the genome era. *American Psychologist* 60 (1). http://www.genome.gov/13014159 (accessed October 9, 2008).

Appiah, K. A. 1995. *In my father's house: Africa in the philosophy of culture*. New York: Oxford University Press.

Bergson, H. 1975. *The two sources of morality and religion*. South Bend, IN: University of Notre Dame Press.

Clark, M. E. 2002. *In search of human nature.* New York: Routledge, 2002.

Food and Drug Administration (FDA). 2005. *FDA approves BiDil heart failure drug for black patients.* http://www.fda.gov/bbs/topics/news/2005/new01190.html (accessed October 9, 2008).

Hossain, S. 2000. *"Scientific racism" in Enlightened Europe: Linnaeus, Darwin, and Galton.* http://serendip.brynmawr.edu/exchange/node/1852 (accessed October 9, 2008).

Institutes of Medicine (IOM). 2002. *Unequal treatment: Confronting racial and ethnic disparities in health care.* http://books.nap.edu/catalog.php?record_id=10260#toc (accessed October 9, 2008).

Kaufmann, W., ed. *The Portable Nietzsche,* New York: Viking Press, 1968. Especially *Thus Spoke Zarathustra* (1883–1885), *The Antichrist* (1888), *Twilight of the Idols* (1888). All translated by Walter Kaufmann.

Lewontin, R. 2000. *It ain't necessarily so: The dream of the human genome and other illusions.* New York: Granta.

Kierkegaard, S. 1983. *Kierkegaard's writings VI: Fear and trembling/repetition.* Trans. E. H. Hong, H. V. Hong. Princeton, NJ: Princeton University Press.

Marks, J. 2003. *What it means to be 98% chimpanzee: Apes, people, and their genes.* Berkeley, CA: University of California Press.

Mwase, I. M. T. 2004. Critical thinking and the Black Church. In *Critical thinking and the Bible in the age of new media,* ed. Charles M. Ess, 131–147. Lanham, MD: University Press of America.

Royal, C., F. Malveaux, and T. J. Dunlap, eds. 2004. Genetics for the human race. *Nature Genetics,* Supplement. http://www.nature.com/cgi-taf/dynapage.taf?file=/ng/journal/v36/n11s/index.html (accessed June 10, 2008).

Social Science Research Council (SSRC). 2006. *Is race "real"?* http://raceandgenomics.ssrc.org/ (accessed October 9, 2008).

Tishkoff, S. A., and K. K. Kidd. 2004. Implications of biogeography of human populations for "race" and medicine. *Nature Genetics 36* (11s): S21–S27. http://www.nature.com/ng/journal/v36/n11s/full/ng1438.html (accessed October 9, 2008).

Whitehead, A. N. 1967. *Science and the modern world.* New York: The Free Press.

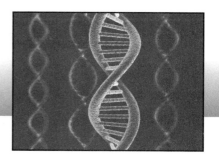

CHAPTER 13

Native American Communities: Perspectives on Healthcare Genetics

Linda Burhansstipanov, DrPH, MSPH, CHES
Lynne Taylor Bemis, PhD
Daniel G. Petereit, MD

Introduction

The purpose of this chapter is to assist nurse educators, service providers, and researchers in understanding Native American culturally relevant, but diverse, perceptions of research, technology, and genetics related to healthcare diagnostics and therapeutics. The chapter provides a brief background of why many Native American communities are resistant to participating in classical research methodology and how Native communities prefer contemporary research to be conducted (i.e., community-based participatory research). The chapter provides references for additional information about genetic issues in Native American communities and issues related to clinical trials. This chapter will focus on successful strategies to implement contemporary research studies that allow certain tribal communities access to new diagnostic and therapeutic technologies.

Background

Many of the genetic issues for Native communities have been raised prior to (1995–1997) and during "Genetic Education for Native Americans" (GENA: NHGRI Grant R25 HG01866) workshops (1998–2004) (Dignan, Burhansstipanov, and Bemis 2005). GENA was funded by the Ethical, Legal, and Social Implications (ELSI) program of the National Human Genome Research Institute (NHGRI) to provide a unique genetics education program for Native American college and university students. The decision to focus on students was based on recommendations from intertribal leaders on how to effectively integrate genetic education into Native American communities (Burhansstipanov, Bemis, and Dignan 2001).

Based upon multiple intertribal focus groups with tribal elders, the initial priority target population of GENA was Native college students. Tribal elders believed that these students would be able to return to their respective communities to help them understand genetic research requests from academic and clinical research settings. Ultimately, it was hoped that this instruction would help to improve informed decision-making about genetics and genetics research in Native American communities and to encourage students to seek genetic science career opportunities. GENA was implemented in geographically diverse settings throughout the United States, primarily in conjunction with regional and national scientific conferences that included substantial numbers of Native American attendees. The working null hypothesis was that there would be no difference in knowledge or attitudes of individuals who participated in specified education objectives (customized workshops) as compared to individuals who participated in those same objectives within the comprehensive 16-hour workshop. The pretest scores for the customized (three-to-five-hour workshops) workshops ranged from 0.3 to 4.8 and averaged 2.16. For the post-tests, the mean was 4.78 and scores ranged from a low of 3.0 to a high of 7.3. Over all customized workshops, there was a 55% increase in mean score from pretest to post-test ($p<.05$). For the comprehensive 16-hour workshops, the mean pretest score was 19.9 compared with to a mean post-test score of 27.5, a 38% increase ($p<.05$). Thus, both formats were effective ways to increase participants' knowledge and we failed to reject the null hypothesis.

Since GENA officially ended in 2003, GENA has presented 15 workshops, all of which continue to include ELSI and cultural issues. This included a total of 384 participants. The average pretest scores were 33.3% and the average posttest scores were 69.7% for an average increase of 35.2%. When pre- and post-test items are matched the p. value is .001.

There are many reasons why Native communities are resistant to taking part in research studies. These include, but are not limited to (Burhansstipanov, Christopher, and Schumacher 2005; Burhansstipanov 1999):

- Native people do not want to be "guinea pigs" (i.e., people have been used in studies without appropriate informed consent processes).
- The study findings are rarely shared with the Native communities that participated in the study.
- The study findings rarely improve local services for the Native community.
- The promised study benefits rarely reach the Native community.
- Insufficient access to resources does not allow community members to participate in the study (e.g., transportation).

There is also a history of Natives being lied to and included in studies without informed consent; this is the Native's equivalent to African Americans' Tuskegee Study. The most recent example is the forced sterilization of American Indian women in the 1970s (Staats 1976; Rodriguez-Trias 1980; American Indian Policy Review Commission 1977; Carpio 1995; Dillingham 1977; Hunter, Linn, and Stein 1984; Jarrell 1992; Larson 1977; Trombley 1988).

In addition, for the majority of Indian Health Service, Tribal, and Urban Indian healthcare programs (referred to as I/T/U programs), the physician turnover averages 18 months (i.e., loan payoff programs). Thus, there is limited trust between the patient and physician in such clinical settings. This turnover is not observed for nurses and therefore, nurses are frequently more trusted than are physicians in I/T/U programs. If a nurse is working in one of these I/T/U programs that experiences the high turnover of physicians and subsequently has low trust of those providers, one can imagine how the community feels if this same provider comes into the I/T/U programs with new technology. It is unclear whether the distrust is of the provider or the technology. Such technology needs to be explained to the Native leadership within the I/T/U programs.

In the early 1990s researchers at Stanford University proposed a project called the Human Genome Diversity Project (HGDP) (Morrison Institute 1999). This was to be a genetic catalogue of populations from around the globe. Native communities, indeed indigenous peoples from around the world, opposed the HGDP, and some communities called for an immediate halt to the project until indigenous communities had a thorough understanding of the project (the Mataatua Declaration, June

1993). Eventually components of the project went forward with a new understanding of the ethical issues related to working with these communities but not to the level of community-based participatory research (CBPR) expected by most North American Native communities. Much of the opposition to the HGDP came from the issues outlined above such as access to the information, talking down to the community, and absence of concern for cultural issues of collection, storage, and use. Another issue raised about genetic catalog projects was that the money spent on cataloging a small community could be better spent to help the community.

Largely because of the HGDP, Tribal Nations have become actively involved in meetings addressing genetic issues since 1993 (Burhansstipanov, Bemis, Kaur, and Bemis 2005). The meetings were convened in response to Native concerns about genetic patenting, genetic research,, and several other issues. Studies such as the HGDP added to concerns about tribal participation and risk to both individuals and communities. Both scientifically accurate and inaccurate information was disseminated at these early meetings as well as more recent meetings (e.g., the existence of an "American Indian gene"). Such misinformation has led to assorted fears, such as the potential annihilation of American Indians and Alaska Natives as a race. Likewise, politicians who want excuses to take over American Indian casinos have attempted to mandate that all enrolled tribal members have a blood test to prove that they are American Indian. Since there is no American Indian gene, the tests will come back negative and the Native community may lose all tribal benefits specified by both the state and the federal government.

Such misinformation contributes to great distrust by Tribal Nations of research in general, but specifically of genetic studies. Nevertheless, not all tribes are opposed to genetic research. Almost all of the tribes that the authors have worked with agree that there has been insufficient effort by scientists to understand and learn how local communities perceive genetic research.

Meetings and workshops on or related to GENA indicate that the most common genetic issues among Native communities are:

- Developing, implementing, interpreting, and disseminating genetic research in Indian Country through the use of community-based participatory research methodology;
- Following the protocols specific to each tribe to obtain appropriate tribal approvals (this includes prioritizing the topic based on health concerns that are of high priority to the specific tribe or urban Indian program and coordinating how the academic, clinic, or research setting will work and communicate with the tribe);

- Discriminating against either the Native community or the individual based on genetic research findings;

- Collecting the specimens carefully, to be respectful of local Native beliefs (e.g., using blood cells or hair follicles as the source for DNA violates several tribal beliefs);

- Storing genetic specimens (e.g., active informed consent must be obtained before specimens are used for any other study);

- Using Native DNA in cell lines (e.g., a researcher may conduct research that is contrary to Native beliefs or create structures that should be limited to the Creator only);

- Sharing of specimens without active informed consent from the participant;

- Limiting the use of specimens to the proposed study only;

- Disposing of unused specimens (for some tribes, the remaining specimens, even if anonymous, should be returned to the tribe for the traditional Indian healer to dispose of through ceremony; for other tribes, it is acceptable to dispose of the remaining blood following laboratory protocol);

- Using specimens to create patents (which are likely to result in expensive health care from which the Native people are unlikely to benefit, since so many live in poverty).

The subjection of Native communities to years of research without the benefit of study findings or perceived benefits has continued. Indeed, the communities perceive research as solely benefiting the researcher, with little or no regard for the impact on the community. Thus, for this and many other reasons the tribes who do wish to take part in research typically desire or mandate community-based participatory research (CBPR) methodology. Many scientists continue to misinterpret this methodology, yet examples of successful CBPR are well documented (Romero, Bemis, Burhansstipanov, and Dignan 2001; Orians, Erb, Kenyon, Lantz, Liebow, Joe, et al. 2004; Burhansstipanov 1998; Segal-Matsunaga, Enos, Gotay, Banner, DeCambra, Hammond, et al. 1996; Davis and Reid 1999; Israel, Schulz, Parker, and Becker 1998; Macaulay, Delormier, McComber, Cross, Potvin, Paradis, et al. 1998; Metzler, Higgins, Beeker, Freudenberg, Lantz, Senturia, et al. 2003; Minkler and Wallerstein 2003; Minkler, Blackwell, Thompson, and Tamir 2003; Cornwall and Jewkes 1995; Wallerstein and Bernstein 1994; Israel, Lichtenstein, Lantz, McGranaghan, Allen, Guzman, et al. 2001; Lantz, Viruell-Fuentes, Israel, Softley, and Guzman 2001; Israel, Schulz, Parker, and Becker 2001). Among the more common erroneous interpretations is that if Natives are study participants, then the study is a CBPR project; this can be a false conclusion. CBPR requires that the community be equal partners in all the proposed study stages (e.g., the development, refinement, implementation, assessment, interpretation, and dissemination of findings). CBPR requires for each study phase that community members and researchers have equal decision-making responsibilities. It also means that the study budget is divided equitably among all partners. This budgetary allocation is a way to begin to determine whether a study is really a partnership or CBPR.

An effective CBPR relationship among researchers and tribal leaders should exist prior to the release of the RFA. The scientists and tribal leadership typically need a few years to develop trust, agree on priorities, and establish a working relationship among the regulating entities (e.g., Tribal Review Boards and Institutional Review Boards). The following are some of the lessons learned from CBPR:

- Invest time to create the partnership team and subsequent CBPR project.
- Allocate the budget equitably among the CBPR partners.
- Create partnerships with leaders who have decision-making responsibilities from each organization.
- Provide salaries to tribal partners and project staff.
- Implement active, effective communication among all CBPR partners.
- Share raw and summary data related to the CBPR project.
- Modify standardized evaluation procedures to be culturally acceptable and respectful of the local community. (Burhansstipanov, Christopher, and Schumacher 2005).

Tribal Institutional Review Boards and Research Committees

In the early 1990s, because of repeated requests for genetic specimens with insufficient informed consent, the Alaska Native Medical Center (ANMC) took the lead in drafting Institutional Review Board (IRB) guidelines for Native communities. Dr. Bill Freeman, who at that time was with the Indian Health Service (IHS), shared the ANMC model with other communities. The Navajo Nation immediately modified the guidelines to reflect their local cultural concerns. Dr. Freeman began to offer IRB training programs to IHS Area offices and Native programs within those regions (Indian Health Service 2007). As a result there are two federally recognized Native IRBs, 12 IHS Area IRBs, and the National IHS IRB. In addition, most I/T/U programs have a research committee that must approve the project before it goes to the IHS Area IRB. IHS Area IRB approval is mandated if the research study is implemented in any clinical setting that receives IHS monies. Thus, if an urban program does not receive IHS funding, they can use the local research or academic

IRB. But any research must be approved by an IRB and the research team cannot just decide they don't need it. This includes NIH-supported research conducted in Indian Country. Still, in many I/T/U programs IRB approval has not been obtained prior to attempts to collect specimens from Natives. For example, in 2003 during a Native science conference, an individual collected specimens from high school and college students without any informed consent process. No I/T/U program had approved collection of these specimens.

The recommended IRB approval procedure for projects on Native communities is to go through a local tribal IRB or research committee, then to the academic or research facility's IRB, then to the IHS Area IRB, and finally through the National IHS IRB. Because of major reorganization of the National IHS IRB, researchers need to contact IHS in Rockville, Maryland about the current processes.

Clinical Trials and Native American Beliefs

Native American Cancer Research has been involved with clinical trials education in collaboration with the University of Colorado Health Sciences Center and Mayo clinic since 1998 (NACR 2008b). Throughout clinical trial workshops implemented within Native communities, many beliefs appear to be common:

- Native people only receive the placebo and do not get real treatments.
- Native people are used to test potentially hazardous treatments that would not be acceptable for white patients.
- The treatments are actually studying something other than the reason for which the Native patient is seeking help.
- The clinical trials are actually attempts to find ways to annihilate the race.
- The clinical trials cost a lot of money and the I/T/U programs will not pay for them.
- Only the researchers benefit from the clinical trial (i.e., they get rich, get promotions, get patents, and the Native patient continues to live in poverty).
- Native people are not really wanted on these trials (i.e., discrimination).

It is the general belief of the healthcare community that treatment provided through a clinical trial represents the best possible care that a patient can receive. Contrary to common belief, participation in clinical trials is *not* more expensive than normal standard care (Goldman, Berry, McCabe, Kilgore, Potosky, Schoenbaum, et al. 2003; Goldman, Berry, McCabe, Kilgore, Potosky, Schoenbaum, et al. 2001; Fireman, Fehrenbacher, Gruskin, and Ray 2000; Brown 1999; Wagner, Alberts, Sloan, Cha,

Killian, O'Connell, et al. 2000). Many barriers make Native populations less likely to consider enrollment:

- Lack of information about clinical trial participation and access.
- Insufficient or nonexistent provider explanations about the availability of clinical trials.
- The need for the family to be involved in decisions regarding clinical trial participation.
- Cultural practices requiring patient participation in ceremonies prior to initiating treatment (as a result, the patient does not communicate with providers until ceremonies are completed six months later and the patient is no longer eligible).
- Existing co-morbidities (e.g., high blood pressure) that render the patient ineligible.
- Clinical trials explained in jargon or terminology unfamiliar to most Native community members.
- Required co-pays for selected components of the protocols (e.g., medications that are not available through the IHS Formulary).
- Long distances between the patient's home and the clinical setting offering the trial.
- Nonexistent or insufficient housing for Native patients and their families who need to remain as outpatients throughout the care.
- Traditional Indian medicine that inadvertently interferes with eligibility criteria.

The National Native American Cancer Survivors' Support Network has been organized to improve survival from cancer and enhance quality of life after cancer diagnosis for both the patient and loved ones. However, fewer than 5 of the 240 breast cancer patients in this Native Network were provided information about cancer care clinical trials. The current literature cites numerous barriers for the recruitment and retention of women, minorities, and the medically underserved to cancer care trials (McCaskill-Stevens, Pinto, Marcus, Comis, Morgan, Plomer, et al. 1999; Wilson, Baker, Brown-Syed, and Gollop 2000; Stapleton 1999; Frank-Stromborg and Olsen 2001; NCI 2000; Friedman, Simon, Foulkes, Friedman, Geller, Gordon, et al. 1995; McCabe, Varricchio, and Padberg 1994; Blumenthal, Sung, Coates, Williams, and Liff 1995; Millon-Underwood, Sands, and Davis 1993; Swanson and Ward 1995; Chen and Hawks 1995; Uba 1992; NCI 1996; Brawley 1996; Burhansstipanov 1996; Freeman, Muth, and Kerner 1995).

Healthcare professionals often over-simplify this process and sometimes act as if identifying a precise barrier will result in a quick fix to the problem. In reality, a quick fix is not feasible. Effort needs to be directed to finding culturally acceptable ways to remove barriers in a community. The challenge remains to establish successful, practical, and culturally respectful strategies. In addition, healthcare providers must invest the time, resources, and creativity needed to tailor information about clinical trials to the intended audience. It may take five or more years before individuals are likely to have sufficient trust, knowledge, and comfort to make informed decisions about enrolling in a clinical trial. Such trust evolves as the community observes the healthcare providers' demonstration of commitment, consistency, and trustworthiness over time.

A common misconception among healthcare providers is that access to a Native American community can be achieved simply by including a respected Native on the research development team. Just because the Native representative is trusted or accepted within the intended population does not mean their endorsement is sufficient for recruitment. It may require many years before a significant increase is seen in the number of Natives who are recruited and retained in clinical trials.

A Successful But Challenging Example: The Walking Forward Program

The Walking Forward program is a collaboration among Rapid City Regional Hospital, the University of Wisconsin, the Mayo Clinic, and the American Indian community in Western South Dakota: three reservations and one urban population. Clinical practice suggests that Native American cancer patients present with more advanced stages of cancer, and hence have lower cure rates. It is hypothesized that a conventional course of cancer treatment lasting six to eight weeks may be a barrier since American Indians live an average of 140 miles from the cancer center in Rapid City (Petereit, Rogers, Govern, Coleman, Osborn, Howard, et al. 2004). The Walking Forward Program has introduced new treatment strategies through the implementation of innovative treatments, many as part of clinical trials. These new technologies include tomotherapy, a modified form of external beam radiation, and brachytherapy. Brachytherapy, also known as internal radiation, is a method of treatment where radioactive pellets, either temporary or permanent, are placed within the tumor. It is the oldest form of radiation, but can now be more precisely delivered with lower side effects by means of concurrent imaging and computerized planning systems. Brachytherapy often yields a very favorable ratio (high rates of tumor control with low side effects) since a minimal volume of normal tissue is radiated.

Tomotherapy is a novel form of external beam radiation where a conventional linear accelerator is mounted on a CT gantry. Patients are treated helically from 360 degrees, rather then from four to six stationary angles as in conventional external beam radiation. Like brachytherapy, this allows the delivery of high doses of radiation to the tumor and much lower doses to the surrounding normal tissues. Both are used for common malignancies such as prostate and breast cancer which reduce the overall treatment time by two to five weeks, thus addressing one potential barrier.

In addition, a genetic study is underway to determine the incidence of a DNA repair gene, ataxia telangiectasia mutation (ATM). The ATM gene is involved in the repair of normal tissue damage as a result of ionization or therapeutic radiation. Evidence supports a correlation between radiation toxicities and a mutation of this gene. The current study investigates this potential relationship for Native and non-Natives undergoing radiation treatments. If there is a correlation, then treatment recommendations may be altered for future patients.

Planning

The Walking Forward program required more than a year of collaborative planning among the partners prior to submitting the application to the National Cancer Institute (NCI) for funding. As part of this program, Native employees from the reservations and urban settings receive training as Community Research Representatives to work as resources and cancer educators within their respective settings. The principal investigator traveled to and met with tribal leadership in each community. The Native communities were very supportive of the project. Regardless of the support of tribal leadership, the IRB process took on a life of its own. The process of obtaining approval for these clinical trials has been published elsewhere (Rogers and Petereit 2005; Boyer, Mohatt, Lardon, Plaetke, Luick, Hutchison, et al. 2005).

As many as 14 committees, including the three reservations' Tribal Health Boards or Research Committees, four IHS service unit directors, Aberdeen Area Tribal Chairmen's Health Board (AATCHB), Aberdeen Area IHS IRB (AAIRB), Rapid City Regional Hospital IRB (RCRH IBB), University of Wisconsin IRB (UW IRB), Mayo Clinic IRB, National IHS IRB (Nat IHS IRB), and NCI reviewed each protocol before enrollment could be initiated. Four treatment modalities were addressed with a total of six clinical protocols (e.g., breast brachytherapy, prostate brachytherapy, tomotherapy for bone cancer, and tomotherapy for prostate cancer). As a result, it took over a year to activate many of these studies after initial submission to the first IRB. Each protocol had an American Indian focus (labeled "NAI" in Figure 13–1) and a general populations focus.

FIGURE 13.1
Walking Forward IRB Approval Processes

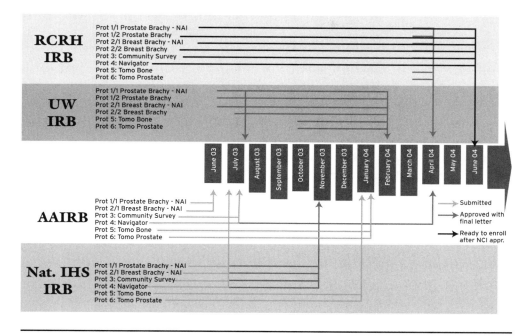

(Petereit and Burhansstipanov 2006)

Example of the Approval Process

The initial study protocols presented for review were the brachytherapy protocols for breast and prostate cancer (labeled "NAI" in Figure 13–1: clinical trial protocols #2003-305/03-R-12AA and #2003-208/03-R-11AA) that were submitted April and June of 2003. The submission process for the prostate brachytherapy protocol (2003-208/03-R-11AA) followed this sequence:

1. Submission to UW IRB in April 2003;

2. Submission to AAIRB in June 2003;

3. Submission to NHS IRB in July 2003;

4. Presentation to Rosebud Sioux and Cheyenne River Tribal Council, Pine Ridge Indian Hospital, and Cheyenne River PHS Hospital in November 2003 with immediate approval and letters of support;

5. Presentation to Rosebud IHS Hospital in December 2003 with an immediate letter of support;

6. Presentation to Oglala Sioux Tribal Council, AATCHB, and Rapid City PHS Hospital in January 2004 with immediate approval and letters of support;

7. Submission to RCRH IRB in March 2005;

8. Submission to NCI in June 2004.

The protocol received initial approval from UW IRB in July 2003, from Nat IHS IRB in November 2003, from RCRH IRB in April 2004, from AAIRB in June 2004, and from NCI in June 2004. It took four version changes to the Informed Consent and more than 12 months before a document had been negotiated that all involved decision makers could agree upon.

Every Native American Indian (NAI) *clinical* protocol took from 5 to 14 months to be approved, and almost every protocol experienced delays or was returned with requests for additional information. Issues totally beyond the study team's control included, but were not limited to, factors discussed below.

The National IHS IRB was in the process of reorganizing and subsequently had a five month interval between communications with the PI for clarification of almost every one of the protocols submitted for review. The protocols were submitted to the IHS IRB two to five times per protocol. Reasons for these delays were numerous and included delayed communication between IHS IRBs and the PI, unfamiliarity of IHS IRBs (specifically the local AAIRB to deal with clinical research and high-risk procedures), and our inexperience in dealing with IHS agencies and the whole submission process, not just to IHS but also to our own IRB in Rapid City, which was in the process of complete reorganization. Fortunately, there has been definitive improvement and progress in the overall process.

The ATM protocol was the last study submitted for approval since it was thought to be the most controversial, mainly because it involved collecting blood samples for genetic analyses. Although the other studies took an average of one year for approval, the ATM study was approved in a record time of only five months because of the trust and infrastructure that the Walking Forward program created from its first few years in the American Indian community—an excellent example of community-based participatory research.

There are no Native genetic counselors in the United States. In the current program, a non-Native PhD geneticist from the Mayo Clinic is under contract to provide counseling using a sophisticated telemedicine system from the NCI called

TELESYNERGY. In practice, the actual scheduling of appointments with the counselor proved problematic because her availability was limited and frequently could not be coordinated with the eligible patients' treatment schedules. An amendment was developed to allow patients to waive telemedicine counseling with the geneticist. This amendment was approved by the AAIRB and the RCRH IRB without hesitation. Within the first two months of the amendments being approved, 23 patients, 4 of whom are Native Americans, had enrolled in this study. The PI counseled all patients about the study, and each one declined to undergo formal genetic counseling.

Native American Perceptions about Health

Native Americans are diverse, with more than 565 federally recognized tribes and about 200 more state recognized tribes. Most tribes have specific beliefs about health, but there are some commonalities that appear to be present in most tribal cultures. Since 1985, Locust (1985) has prepared and disseminated summaries of tribal-specific health beliefs. Tribes have very unique belief systems from one another. However, *most* tribes have the following common beliefs:

- Native Americans believe in a supreme creator.
- A person is a threefold being made up of the body, mind, and spirit.
- The spirit existed before it came into a physical body and will exist after the body dies.
- Plants and animals, like humans, are part of the spirit world. The spirit world exists side-by-side and intermingles with the physical world.
- Wellness is harmony in body, mind, and spirit.
- Unwellness is caused by disharmony among the body, mind, and spirit.
- Natural unwellness is caused by the violation of a sacred or tribal taboo.
- Unnatural unwellness is caused by witchcraft (or "one who is on the bad side").
- We are each responsible for our own wellness.

A wide variety of health issues compete for attention in most Native American communities. Health priorities include alcohol and substance abuse, violence, accidents, suicide, diabetes, obesity, and cardiovascular disease. Each of the surviving federally recognized tribes has its own unique and diverse culture and many are acknowledged by Congress as sovereign nations. In addition, hundreds of tribes are recognized by individual states but not by the federal government. Many tribes no longer possess reservation or trust lands and several tribes share a single reservation.

Although each surviving Native American tribe, clan, or band (terms used to describe Native American groups) has its own unique culture, there are some generalizations which are valid for most tribal communities. The majority of Native cultures live gently and respectfully within their environment. The Indian way is to live in harmony with the Earth and with oneself and to walk with spirit, heart, mind, and body in balance as an integrated being. This concept of balance and relationship to Mother Earth, Father Sky, and all beings extends to all aspects of life and living within the family.

There are a variety of psychosocial and cultural barriers that affect the lives of older American Indians. The most powerful barrier is poverty. Poverty has multiple, confounding effects, including but not limited to having life priorities other than health (food, rent, clothing), health priorities other than cancer (alcohol or substance abuse, violence, accidents, suicide, diabetes, obesity, cardiovascular disease), lack of medical insurance or access to an IHS facility, lack of access to a working telephone, lack of transportation, and the need for child care. Many older Native Peoples respect traditional medicine and prefer it over Western medicine. There are numerous misconceptions related to cancer (e.g., a cancer diagnosis is synonymous with a death sentence). In Native cultures death is perceived as a natural and important part of the Circle of Life. Elders are respected and, when ill, are cared for in the family home (NACR 2008a).

The health status of Native American groups cannot be fully understood apart from their history or their present social conditions. As with all other minority groups in America, poverty and education play major roles. Certainly there have been many misconceptions about American Indians and Alaska Natives. All too often contemporary media carries news only of the disturbances and not the successes of Native American people. All too often the public perception is distorted, sometimes in a romanticized or negative fashion. It is time to reexamine these attitudes and to reassess the factors that determine the health and life expectancy of these groups. The cultural information supplied here is relevant to developing sensitive and acceptable health education or research programs.

All cultures, whether they be Oglala Lakota Sioux, Italian, Cambodian, etc., have positive, respected practices that helped prevent disease and contributed to the well-being of the community in the past. When Native Americans attempt to learn Native languages, dances, songs, crafts, and so on, it is to remember cultural practices that contribute to a positive, balanced lifestyle. The desire is not to give up all modern conveniences and return to living in habitats that were used in the 1400s. It is to retain the beauty and harmony of the old ways.

Basic Beliefs Systems with Regard to New Technologies

Native communities are very diverse, as are their perceptions of technology. The general perception is usually dependent on issues such as whether technology is available for isolated, impoverished communities; whether the technology will help create a healthy next generation of Native Americans; whether the technology will be too costly for I/T/U programs to purchase; whether the technology will require provider inservice training that is not available to them; and whether the technology violates any local traditional Indian beliefs (e.g., autopsy and any technology used during this procedure directly violates some tribal beliefs).

For example, the tomotherapy used in the Walking Forward study is perceived as a very positive breakthrough for Native people who are able to obtain their care from Rapid City Regional Hospital. Likewise, there is a significant shift in the percentage of Native community members who use or have access to a computer. Native American Cancer Research uses technology to evaluate workshops. At the end of most workshops the question is asked, "if these workshop slides were available as a free download from our website, would you be able to get them?" In mid-2003, 25% of the respondents said they could download the slides by themselves, 50% said they could with the help of a family member or friend, and 25% said the information would not be available to them. In the latter part of 2005, 50% of the respondents said they could download the data by themselves, 35% said they could with the help of someone, and only 15% said the information would not be available to them. These workshop participants comprise more than 560 people, of whom a third are elders. Thus, even computer technology is becoming more accepted and available. But we find that we cannot solely rely on the computer for dissemination of health-related information to community members. For a very long time, telemedicine has been accepted as a way to increase access to high quality health care (e.g., Mayo Clinic and Northern Plains tribal communities). Likewise, most providers who work in I/T/U programs indicate that they want access to new technologies. For example, providers in northern plains communities have been begging for the technology to be available, and they have already completed the inservice training. But the technology is too costly for their I/T/U clinics.

Native American Community's Perspectives on Genetic Technologies

Genetic technologies come with a different set of issues than other health technologies. Genetics can be used to identify the origins of a community, but DNA samples are not anonymous. Many communities are not averse to technology per se, but do wonder whether the genetic research or practice is practical. When, if ever, will the Native community have access to the technology in their local clinics, particularly with most I/T/U programs being under-funded by 40% to 60% of their documented healthcare needs. If the I/T/U programs cannot address current health problems using lower cost and less effective treatments, how can these I/T/U clinics justify the expense of new technologies that tend to be more expensive?

In contrast, some tribal communities have supported genetic research, such as in genetics of obesity and diabetes studies through the Center for Alaska Native Health Research (CANHR) study. This study (Mohatt, Plaetke, Klejka, Luick, Lardon, Bersamin, et al. 2007) is supported through the Centers of Biomedical Research Excellence (COBRE). This project has been developed in partnership with the Yukon-Kuskokwim Health Corporation (YKHC) of Bethel, Alaska. The center has offices at the University of Alaska Fairbanks (UAF), the University of Alaska Anchorage (UAA), and the National Institutes of Health, National Center for Research Resources. This obesity study includes multiple genetic biomarkers. Contrary to the majority of genetic studies with which Native communities do have issues, Boyer's obesity study is based on CBPR and has been sustained by the mutual respect between the investigators and community leaders. The study required more than three years of collaboration before moving forward, but community members speak of this study with pride and respect. Thus, genetic research can be implemented in a respectful manner that benefits both the community and the investigators (Boyer, Mohatt, Lardon, Plaetke, Luick, Hutchison, et al. 2005).

References

American Indian Policy Review Commission. 1977. Report on Indian health. *American Indian Journal*, 17–23.

Blumenthal, D.S., J. Sung, R. Coates, J. Williams, and J. Liff. 1995. Mounting research addressing issues of race/ethnicity in health care. Recruitment and retention of subjects for a longitudinal cancer prevention study in an inner-city black community. *Health Services Research* 30, 197–205.

Boyer, B.B., G. V. Mohatt, C. Lardon, R. Plaetke, B. R. Luick, S. H. Hutchison, G. A. de Mayolo, E. Ruppert, and A. Bersamin. 2005. Building a community-based participatory research center to investigate obesity and diabetes in Alaska Natives. *International Journal of Circumpolar Health* 64 (3): 281–290.

Brawley, O. 1996. Recruitment of minorities into clinical trials. In *Conference summary: Recruitment and retention of minority participants in clinical cancer research,* eds. National Cancer Advisory Board. U.S. Department of Health and Human Services, National Cancer Institute, National Institutes of Health (NIH Pub. No. 96–4182).

Brown, M.L. 1999. Cancer patient care in clinical trials sponsored by the National Cancer Institute: What does it cost? *Journal of the National Cancer Institute* 91: 818–819.

Burhansstipanov, L. 1996. Overcoming psycho-social barriers to Native American cancer screening research. In *Conference summary: Recruitment and retention of minority participants in clinical cancer research,* eds. National Cancer Advisory Board. U.S. Department of Health and Human Services, National Cancer Institute, National Institutes of Health (NIH Pub. No. 96–4182).

Burhansstipanov, L. 1998. Lessons learned from Native American cancer prevention, control, and supportive care projects. *Asian American and Pacific Islander Journal of Health* 6 (2): 91–99.

———. 1999. Developing culturally competent community-based interventions. In D. Weiner (Ed.), *Cancer research interventions among the medically underserved,* 167–183. Westport, CT: Greenwood Publishing.

Burhansstipanov, L., L. T. Bemis, and M.B. Dignan. 2001. Native American cancer education: Genetic and cultural issues. *Journal of Cancer Education* 16: 142–145.

Burhansstipanov, L., L. T. Bemis, J. S. Kaur, and G. Bemis. 2005. Sample genetic policy language for research conducted with Native communities. *Journal of Cancer Education* 20 (Suppl.): 52–57.

Burhansstipanov, L., S. Christopher, and A. Schumacher. 2005. Lessons learned from community-based participatory research in Indian country. *Cancer Control: Journal of the Moffitt Cancer Center* November: 70–76.

Carpio, M.F. 1995. *Lost generation: the involuntary sterilization of American Indian women.* (Dissertation). Tempe: Arizona State University Library.

Chen, M.S., and B. L. Hawks. 1995. A debunking of the myth of healthy Asian Americans and Pacific Islanders. American Journal of Health Promotion 9: 261–268.

Cornwall, A. and R. Jewkes. 1995. What is participatory research? *Social Science and Medicine* 41: 1667–1676.

Davis, S. M., and R. Reid. 1999. Practicing participatory research in American Indian communities. *American Journal of Clinical Nutrition* 69: 755S–759S.

Dignan, M. B., L. Burhansstipanov, and L. T. Bemis. 2005. Successful implementation of genetic education for Native Americans workshops at national conferences. *Genetics* 169 (2): 517–521.

Dillingham, Brint. 1977. American Indian women and IHS sterilization practices. *American Indian Journal* 3 (7): 27–28.

Fireman, B. H., L. Fehrenbacher, E. P. Gruskin, and G. T. Ray. 2000. Cost of care for patients in cancer clinical trials. *Journal of the National Cancer Institute* 93: 37–43.

Frank-Stromborg, M., and S. J. Olsen. 2001. Cancer prevention in diverse populations: Cultural implications for the multi-disciplinary team. Pittsburgh, PA: Oncology Nursing Society.

Freeman, H. P., B. J. Muth, and J. F. Kerner. 1995. Expanding access to cancer screening and follow-up among the medically underserved. *Cancer Practice* 3 (1): 19–30.

Friedman, L. S., R. Simon, M. Foulkes, L. Friedman, N. L. Geller, D. J. Gordon, and R. Mowery. 1995. Inclusion of women and minorities in clinical trials and the NIH Revitalization Act of 1993—The perspective of NIH clinical trialists. *Controlled Clinical Trials* 16: 277–285.

Goldman, D. P., S. H. Berry, M. S. McCabe, M. L. Kilgore, A. L. Potosky, M. L. Schoenbaum, M. Schonlau, J. C. Weeks, R. Kaplan, and J. J. Escarce. 2003. Incremental treatment costs in National Cancer Institute-sponsored clinical trials. *Journal of the American Medical Association* 289: 2970–2977.

Goldman, D. P., S. H. Berry, M. S. McCabe, M. L. Kilgore, A. L. Potosky, J. J. Schoenbaum, B. A. Weidmar, M. L. Kilgore, N. Wagle, J. L. Adams, R. A. Figlin, J. H. Lewis, J. Cohen, R. Kaplan, and M. McCabe. 2001. Measuring the incremental costs of clinical cancer research. *Journal of Clinical Oncology* 19: 105–110.

Hunter, K., Linn, M., and S. Stein. 1984. Sterilization among American Indian and Chicano mothers. International *Quarterly of Community Health Education* 4 (4): 343–353.

Indian Health Service. 2007. *Human research participant protection in the Indian Health Service.* http://www.ihs.gov/MedicalPrograms/Research/irb.cfm (accessed October 9, 2008).

Israel, B.A., R. Lichtenstein, P. Lantz, R. McGranaghan, A. Allen, J. R. Guzman, D. Softley, and B. Maciak. 2001. The Detroit Community-Academic Urban Research Center: Development, implementation, and evaluation. *Journal of Public Health Management & Practice* 7 (5): 1–19.

Israel, B.A., A. J. Schulz, E. A. Parker, and A. B. Becker. 1998. Review of community-based research: Assessing partnership approaches to improve public health. *Annual Review of Public Health* 19: 173–202.

———. 2001. Community–campus partnerships for health. Community-based participatory research: Policy recommendations for promoting a partnership approach in health research. *Education for Health (Abingdon)* 14 (2): 182–197.

Jarrell, R.H. 1992. Native American women and forced sterilization, 1973–1976. *Caduceus: A Museum Quarterly for the Health Sciences* 8: 45–58.

Lantz, P.M., E. Viruell-Fuentes, B. A. Israel, D. Softley, and R. Guzman. 2001. Can communities and academia work together on public health research? Evaluation results from a community-based participatory research partnership in Detroit. *Journal of Urban Health* 78 (3): 495–507.

Larson, J.K. 1977. And then there were none: Is federal policy endangering the American Indian species? *Christian Century* Jan: 61–63.

Locust, C.S. 1985. *American Indian beliefs concerning health and unwellness* (monograph series). Tucson, AZ: University of Arizona, Native American Research and Training Center.

Macaulay, A. C. T. Delormier, A. M. McComber, E. J. Cross, L. P. Potvin, G. Paradis, C. Saad-Haddad, S. Desrosiers, and R. Kirby. 1998. Participatory research with Native community of Kahnawake creates innovative code of research ethics. *Canadian Journal of Public Health* 89: 105–108.

McCabe, M. S., C. G. Varricchio, and R. M. Padberg. 1994. Efforts to recruit the economically disadvantaged to national clinical trials. *Seminars in Oncology Nursing* 10 (2): 123–129.

McCaskill-Stevens, W., H. Pinto, A. C. Marcus, R. Comis, R. Morgan, K. Plomer, and S. Schoentgen. 1999. Recruiting minority cancer patients into cancer clinical trials: A pilot project involving the Eastern Cooperative Oncology Group and the National Medical Association. *Journal of Clinical Oncology* 17 (3): 1029–1039.

Metzler, M. M., D. L. Higgins, C. G. Beeker, N. Freudenberg, P. M. Lantz, K. D. Senturia, A. A. Eisinger, E. A. Viruell-Fuentes, B. Gheisar, A. G. Palermo, and D. Softley. 2003. Addressing urban health in Detroit, New York City, and Seattle through community-based participatory research partnerships. *American Journal of Public Health* 93 (5): 803–811.

Millon-Underwood, S., E. Sands, and M. Davis. 1993. Determinants of participation in state-of-the-art cancer prevention, early detection/screening and treatment trials among African Americans. *Cancer Nursing* 16: 25–33.

Minkler, M., and N. Wallerstein, Eds. 2003. *Community-based participatory research for health.* San Francisco: Jossey-Bass.

Minkler, M., A. G. Blackwell, M. Thompson, and H. Tamir. 2003. Community-based participatory research: Implications for public health funding. *American Journal of Public Health* 93 (8): 1210–1213.

Mohatt, G. V., R. Plaetke, J. Klejka, B. Luick, C. Lardon, A. Bersamin, S. Hopkins, M. Dondanville, J. Herron, and B. Boyer. 2007. *A community-based participatory research study of obesity and chronic disease-related protective and risk factors.* http://users.iab.uaf.edu/~bert_boyer/pubs/2007_mohatt_etal.pdf (accessed October 9, 2008).

Morrison Institute for Population and Resource Studies. 1999. *Human genome diversity project.* http://www.stanford.edu/group/morrinst/hgdp/protocol.html (accessed October 9, 2008).

National Cancer Institute (NCI). 1996. *NCI reports cancer incidence and mortality rates for minorities.* Bethesda, MD: NCI Office of Cancer Communications.

———. 2000. NIH trials don't enroll enough women to allow analysis, GAO says in report. *NCI Cancer Letter* 26 (19): 3–6.

Native American Cancer Research (NACR). 2008a. *Native American palliative care and end-of-life curriculum.* http://www.natamcancer.org/ap/EOL_Obj5_Death_05-10-04b_FAC/slides.html (accessed October 9, 2008).

———. 2008b. *Our projects.* http://natamcancer.org/page5.html (accessed October 9, 2008).

Orians, C. E., J. Erb, K. L. Kenyon, P. M. Lantz, E. B. Liebow, J. R. Joe, and L. Burhansstipanov. 2004. Public education strategies for delivering breast and cervical cancer screening in American Indian and Alaska Native populations. *Journal of Public Health Management & Practice* 10 (1): 46–53.

Petereit, D. G., and L. Burhansstipanov. 2008. Establishing Trusting Partnerships for Successful Recruitment of American Indians to Clinical Trials. *Cancer Control* 15 (3): 260–268.

Petereit, D.G., D. Rogers, F. Govern, N. Coleman, C. H. Osborn, S. P. Howard, J. S. Kaur, L. Burhansstipanov, F. J. Fowler, R. Chappell, and M. P. Mehta. 2004. Increasing access to CCT and emerging technologies for minority populations: The Native American project. *Journal of Clinical Oncology* 22 (22): 4452–4455.

Rodriguez-Trias, Helen. 1980. *Women and the health care system: Sterilization abuse: Two lectures.* New York: Barnard College.

Rogers, D., and D. G. Petereit. 2005. Cancer disparities research partnership in Lakota country: Clinical trials, patient services, and community education for the Oglala, Rosebud, and Cheyenne River Sioux tribes. *American Journal of Public Health* 95 (12): 1–4.

Romero, F., L. T. Bemis, L. Burhansstipanov, and M. B. Dignan. 2001. Genetic research and Native American cultural issues. *Journal of Women and Minorities in Science and Engineering* 7: 97–106.

Staats, E. B. 1976. *Investigation of allegations concerning Indian Health Service. U.S. General Accounting Office Report on Sterilization HRD-77–3.* Washington, DC: General Accounting Office.

Segal-Matsunaga, D., R. Enos, C. C. Gotay, R. O. Banner, H. DeCambra, O. W. Hammond, N. Hedlund, E. K. Ilaban, B. F. Issell, and J. U. Tsark. 1996. Participatory research in a native Hawaiian community: The Wai'anae cancer research project. *Cancer* 78 (7): 1582–1586.

Stapleton, S. 1999. Cancer studies fail minorities. American Medical News. http://www.ama-assn.org/amednews/1999/pick_99/clta0208.htm (accessible online only to AMA members).

Swanson, G. M., and A. J. Ward. 1995. Recruiting minorities into clinical trials: Toward a participant-friendly system. *Journal of the National Cancer Institute* 87: 1747–1759.

Trombley, Stephen. 1988. *The right to reproduce: A history of coercive sterilization*. London: Weiden & Nicholson.

Wagner, J. L., S. R. Alberts, J. A. Sloan, S. Cha, J. Killian, M. J. O'Connell, P. Van Grevenhof, J. Lindman, and C. G. Chute. 1999. Incremental costs of enrolling cancer patients in clinical trials: a population-based study. *Journal of the National Cancer Institute* 91: 847–853. Also see Erratum, Journal of the National Cancer Institute 92: 164–165.

Wallerstein, N., and E. Bernstein. 1994. Introduction to community empowerment, participatory education, and health. *Health Education Quarterly* 21: 141–148.

Wilson, F. L., L. M. Baker, C. Brown-Syed, and C. Gollop. 2000. An analysis of the readability and cultural sensitivity of information on the National Cancer Institute's web site: CancerNet. *Oncology Nursing Forum* 27 (9): 1403–1409.

Uba, L. Cultural barriers to health care for Southeast Asian refugees. 1992. *Public Health Reports* 107: 544–548.

CHAPTER 14

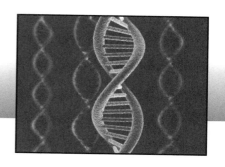

Hispanic/Latino Perspectives on Genetics and Ethics

Carmen T. Paniagua, EdD, RN, CPC, ACNP-BC
Robert E. Taylor, MD, PhD, FACP, FCCP

Introduction

This chapter explores the perspectives on genetics and ethics of the fastest growing population in the United States, the peoples of the Hispanic and Latino community. It examines their unique demographics and basic cultural values. In addition, the importance of cultural assessments when interfacing with this population and its diverse ethnicities and racial designations is highlighted. This chapter also includes trends, recommendations, and ways to prepare healthcare providers for care of these patients and families.

The cultural background of the Hispanic/Latino population has a significant influence on their perspectives on genetics and ethics. These perspectives have been given very little attention to date by healthcare providers. Understanding diversity, particularly those variations among Hispanic/Latino populations (hereafter refer to as Hispanic, to be consistent with Census Bureau nomenclature) with regard to genetics and ethics, is of major importance when providing health care to meet the needs of this growing community.

Demographics

In 2007 the Census Bureau released news indicating that Hispanics remained the largest minority group in the United States, followed by Black or African American, Asian, American Indian or Alaskan Native, and Native Hawaiians or Other Pacific Islander. Moreover, Hispanics are the fastest-growing minority group in the United States, followed by Asians (Guzmán 2001). In view of these demographic changes, it is imperative that healthcare providers increase their level of cultural sensitivity and awareness. This awareness may help to better serve this group, and an understanding of the perspectives that these populations have on genetics is pivotal in providing effective genetic care.

The term Hispanic historically denotes a relation to Spanish-speaking people from the two hemispheres. It is derived from the Latin word *Hispanicus,* from *Hispania,* Spain. Conversely, the term Latino refers to people or communities of Latin American origin and has been used interchangeably with Hispanic (*American Heritage Dictionary* 2000). In accordance with guidelines from the Office of Management and Budget, race and Hispanic origin are two different concepts, in contrast to what the media, researchers, and some organizations view (OMB 1997). Many use Hispanic origin and race as one concept, and these terms are often applied inconsistently. A person from this community can be of Hispanic ethnicity (examples include such designations as White-Hispanic, Non-White-Hispanic, Black-Hispanic, Asian-Hispanic, American Indian-Hispanic, or Native American-Hispanic), or in many cases racially mixed.

When applying genetic and genomic health care and research to the Hispanic populations, special challenges may pose limitations. The definition of racial or ethnic structure in human populations is one example. Researchers have stated that race has a geographical connotation and ethnicity takes into consideration cultural, physical, and some genetic characteristics (Burchard et al. 2003; Mao et al. 2007). On the other hand, patterns of mating and reproduction are taken into consideration when it relates to the genetic structure of human populations (Burchard et al. 2003). Biological and genetic implications are derived from these racial and ethnic differences.

The genetic admixtures within this population pose another challenge to consider when conducting population studies. A particular admixture effect will show a genetic variant to be more common in a high-incidence group than in a background population (Sweeney et al. 2007), an effect known as population stratification. Sampling bias issues may be important in studying these groups.

Population and Composition

The 2000 Census showed that there were 35.3 million Hispanics living in the United States. This represents approximately 12.5% of the total population of the country. Blacks or African Americans accounted for 12.3%, followed by 3.5% of Asians, 0.9% American Indian and Alaskan Native, and Native Hawaiian and Other Pacific Islanders with 0.1% (Guzmán 2001).

A more recent estimation by the Census Bureau (2006) showed the percentage of Hispanic to be 14.8. This estimation represents an increase of 1.9% in six years, demonstrating a fast growing trend. Moreover, the projected population by race and Hispanic origin for the year 2010 is 48.5 million and 102.6 million by the year 2050. Healthcare professionals need to take into account these trends when applying genetic and genomic health care to this population.

Of the total Hispanic population recorded in the 2000 U.S. Census, more than half (58.5%) are of Mexican origin (Guzmán 2001). Puerto Ricans accounted for nearly 9.6%, Cubans 3.5%, Central Americans, South Americans, and Other Hispanics (including Dominicans) 4.8%, 3.8%, and 2.5% respectively.

Health Beliefs and Practices

Awareness of common health beliefs and practices within the Hispanic population may help the healthcare provider understand health behaviors observed during a genetic counseling session. Attitudes of Hispanic sub-cultures toward diseases and disabilities, reproduction, pregnancy, and childbearing vary considerably.

Familiarity with certain basic cultural values that may affect their perspective toward genetics and ethics is important in determining what is applicable to the individual Hispanic patient and their family. In this chapter three of these are highlighted: *allocentrism, simpatía, and familialism.*

Allocentrism is a tendency among Hispanics to bond together, in some circumstances even by sacrificing personal needs. In other words, personal independence is not as important as the group welfare (Marin and VanOss-Marin 1991). Allocentrism may also be termed collectivism.

Simpatía values harmonic social interactions. It is the need for behaviors that encourage smooth and pleasant social interactions (Marin and VanOss-Marin 1991; Zea et al. 1994). This cultural value may be at work when a Hispanic person appears to agree with recommendations from the genetic healthcare team. In addition, they may not question genetic service providers' advice or ask for exploration of possible options in care. Because of this some patients and family members may not maximize the benefits of genetic counseling or fully participate in the treatment process. Healthcare providers who emphasize courtesy, warmth, and respect in their interactions with Hispanic families tend to be more successful in involving the patient and family members in treatment, potentially reducing non-adherence and facilitating follow-up. As healthcare providers establish a climate of respect, support, and understanding, Hispanic patients and families are more likely to talk about their concerns and sources of disagreement (Zea, Quezada, and Belgrave 1994).

Familismo is a third Hispanic cultural value that may affect the perspectives on genetics and ethics. It is described as a strong attachment to, reciprocity with, and loyalty to family members (Triandis et al. 1982). This cultural value has important implications for the perspective of genetics and ethics because extended family members are likely to be consulted and their opinions given considerable weight. Attention to this value can facilitate support and involvement during a genetic consultation and may be essential in order for the patient and family members to participate in informed decisions. Healthcare providers need to create a climate wherein genetic counseling is sensitive to the cultural values of Hispanic families.

Gender roles are delineated traditionally, with the father being the viewed as the provider, the mother as primarily responsible for the household chores and childbearing, and the children expected to be respectful to the elderly (Knoerl 2007). The efficacy of home remedies and folk medicine is a widely respected health belief among Hispanics (Giger and Davidhizer 2004). In the Hispanic population, health decisions are influenced by a diverse variety of beliefs about health and illness. Additionally, social class, the level of education, and acculturation in an individual family or kindred influence health decisions. Acculturation is the process by which changes in behaviors, norms, values, and attitudes occur when one cultural group comes into contact with another (Valentin 2001). This process takes place by observation of the new host culture, reacting to the new culture, and in the end, adjusting to the host culture in order to better function in it. For example, the movement of some Hispanic populations to the United States has resulted in the blurring of cultural values and health practices carried from countries of origin. The effects of acculturation can vary depending on several factors, and healthcare beliefs and practices may evolve as families and groups adjust to new surroundings.

Prevalence of Genetic Diseases in the Hispanic Population

The identification of genetic risks factors for disease is difficult in the Hispanic population as a result of a two-way admixture of indigenous American and European populations or a three-way admixture of indigenous American, European, and West African populations (Bertoni 2003; Tan et al. 2007). Despite this difficulty, the sub-groups within the Hispanic population are often treated as a homogenous population.

The Centers for Disease Control (CDC) listed the leading causes of death for the Hispanic population. The ten leading causes for 2004 are: (1) heart disease, (2) malignant neoplasms, (3) unintentional injuries, (4) diabetes mellitus, (5) cerebrovascular disease, (6) chronic liver disease and cirrhosis, (7) chronic lower respiratory diseases, (8) suicide, (9) influenza and pneumonia, and (10) nephritis, nephritic syndrome, and nephrosis (CDC 2004). Nearly all of these have a genetic component. As the genetic and genomic factors that underlie the major causes of population morbidity and mortality are better understood, healthcare providers will be able to offer more detailed information and counseling to Hispanic communities.

Recent findings suggest that the prevalence of hereditary hemochromatosis among Hispanics is higher than previously recorded, possibly due to the admixture of black ancestry (Mao et al. 2007; CDC 1996). Diabetes mellitus affects disproportionately the Hispanic population in the United States as well as in Puerto Rico (Flegal et al. 1991). The incidence of diabetes mellitus among subpopulations of this group (such as Cubans, Mexicans, and Puerto Ricans), can differ according to genetic factors, geographic locality, their access to care, and social and cultural factors that affect health status. Diabetes mellitus affects twice as many as among non-Hispanic Whites (9.8% versus 5.0%) (Bertoni 2003).

The incidence of asthma among Puerto Ricans in the United States is more than two times higher than Mexican-Americans (Lara et al. 2006). This suggests an ethnic group-specific genetic predisposition. We need to consider such differences in disease prevalence when offering health care to this sub-group of the Hispanic population.

A report released by the Alzheimer's Association (2004), where state and national estimates of the incidence of Alzheimer's disease are reported, indicates that Hispanics may be at higher risk to develop this disease than other racial or ethnic groups. Increased awareness of Alzheimer's disease among Hispanics could facilitate targeting of diagnostic and intervention resources for more effective care to those at risk.

A large multi-ethnic, multi-regional study found Hispanics in Texas to be at greater risk for kidney damage when diagnosed with lupus (Alarcon et al. 1999). Healthcare providers could be more vigilant and aggressive in making sure that this sub-group receives appropriate health care when offering care to those affected with lupus.

As genetic healthcare services are implemented, we need to be aware that common genetic mutations with a high prevalence in the Hispanic population can occur in other ethnic populations as well. In other words, in the genetic/genomic arena healthcare providers need to be aware that selected mutations within an ethnic population are not exclusive to Hispanic groups. Healthcare providers are ethically bound to stay informed about patterns of risk, incidence, and prevalence of genetic illness among all of the diverse ethnic and cultural groups with whom they practice.

Providing Genetic Information: Study Findings Among Hispanics

When providing genetic information, the patient's attitudes and expectations are critical. As previously mentioned, cultural values influence Hispanic attitudes and expectations and they vary among Hispanic sub-groups.

A recent study explored the values, attitudes, and beliefs of African Americans, Hispanics, and Non-Hispanic Whites with respect to genetic testing (Singer, Antonucci, and Van Hoewyk 2004). The authors did not differentiate among sub-groups (Puerto Ricans, Cubans, Mexicans, etc.) for the Hispanic population, and conducted the survey in both Spanish and English according to respondents' preferences.

Regarding attitudes to genetic testing, the study showed that Hispanics are more likely to proceed with genetic testing than Whites. This response was the same for prenatal testing and adult genetic testing although Hispanics knew less about genetic technology than other groups. According to the study, Hispanics feel a greater obligation towards others than Whites. These findings corroborate the value of allocentrism as embedded in the Hispanic culture.

In this study, Hispanics and African Americans had lower average income and were less likely to have private medical insurance, which reduced their access to genetic services. Furthermore, Hispanics and African Americans expressed religious views that might reduce the use of genetic testing. In addition, both cohorts appeared to be less sensitive to some possible abuses of genetic testing but more concerned about genetic information misuse than Whites.

A point of interest in the Hispanic cohort was that they felt that all pregnant women had a responsibility to be tested if a test was available to detect a serious genetic defect in the baby. It also showed that Hispanics tend to be less restrictive regarding disclosing genetic information to others than Whites. This finding also affirms the *familismo* value found in the Hispanic population.

The attitudes and beliefs about genetics and genetic testing in underserved, culturally diverse populations were explored in a small multiethnic focus group study (Catz et al. 2005). Positive attitudes toward genetic studies and testing were expressed by the Hispanic cohort. The main advantage for genetic testing and studies expressed by this cohort was prevention; concerns were raised regarding medical insurance, pre- and post-testing results anxiety, and test safety. The perspectives toward genetics and genomics are confirmed by this recognition that Hispanics have limited knowledge in this subject area and by the limited access to genetic information and services.

A multiethnic, multi-center survey was recently conducted in a study to include Hispanics. The authors explored predictors that genetic testing information about hemochromatosis should be shared with family members (Tucker et al. 2006). Hispanics agreed that genetic information should be shared with family members, and that genetic testing is a good idea. For the Hispanic cohort, surveys were conducted in Spanish and English, depending on respondents' preferences. The English-speaking participants were less likely to share genetic test information with family members than the other racial or ethnic groups, but still positively regarded genetic testing. Among the Spanish-speaking participants, there was a correspondence between opinions on sharing the genetic information and the belief that genetic testing is a good idea. Some speculation on possible explanations for these results was given but none were conclusive.

Concerns about insurance discrimination and psychological distress after testing were mentioned as limiting factors in the study. Another concern was that Spanish-speaking Hispanics who live away from families outside the United States might be less likely to share risk information. Explanations for this behavior included; (1) worry about communicating "bad news," (2) long-distance communication expenses, and (3) perceptions that family members would probably not be able to obtain clarification or services to reduce their risk. These findings are supportive of the familialism value.

Attitudes and beliefs of Hispanics will be a major concern for healthcare providers providing genetic information. The limited studies available open up the research arena as well as reinforce the conclusion that Hispanics are sensitive to this topic but at the same time eager for more information.

Barriers to Providing Genetic Information

Ethnocultural factors come into play during the healthcare provider–patient interaction and communication. Given the Hispanic demographic characteristics and trends in the United States, attention to ethnocultural barriers is pivotal. In the Hispanic population, the language barrier is the most important and studied one. Other barriers, such as low socioeconomic status, education attainment, and level of acculturation have been explored (Lum 1987; Cunningham 1990; Estrada, Treviño, and Ray 1990; Punales-Morejon, and Penchaszadeh 1992; Zaid, Fullerton, and Moore 1996; Lobell, Bay, Rhoads, and Keske). For example, the impact of acculturation on the awareness of genetic testing was explored in a small national study (Vadaparampil et al. 2006). The authors concluded that acculturation factors related to language may affect the awareness of cancer genetic risks and testing in Hispanics, and taking these factors into consideration will help in delivering genetic information to this group.

Another way to convey genetic information to Hispanics is using an alternative counseling process, such as a visual format. In a multi-ethnic study (Eichmeyer et al. 2005), Hispanics showed a lower understanding of numerical risk estimates despite appropriate counseling techniques. The study suggested the use of a visual, qualitative format instead of quantitative (percentages or fractions).

Telephone interviews were conducted to gather qualitative information on perceived knowledge, perceived barriers, and information-seeking habits related to genetics in the Hispanic population (Carpenter, Atkinson, and Gold 2003). Among the perceived barriers to genetic knowledge, research participation, and use of genetic health services the following findings were noted: (1) lack of information and awareness, (2) traditional cultural values and religious or spiritual beliefs, (3) economic disadvantages (e.g., lack of insurance, financial constraints), (4) culturally appropriate approaches, and (5) lack of bilingual or bicultural professionals in the genetics field. In addition, a need to increase the role of genetic research in this population was determined. This study adds to the body of knowledge regarding barriers in communicating genetic information to Hispanics.

Ethical Considerations about Genetics and Genomic Health Care

Three clinical services where ethical issues can be raised are genetic testing, population-based genetics, and carrier identification (Friedman, Ross, and Moon 2001). In genetic testing, safeguarding the autonomy of the Hispanic population is important because this population may be easily attracted to public genetic testing without an adequate understanding of the implications. In the United States it is customary to address high-risk populations, often minorities, when addressing incidence of disease. Ethical practices include sensitivity to group values and beliefs with regard genetics, and population-based approaches to offering services and communicating information must be designed to avoid discrimination.

The confidentiality of genetic identification or information is a major ethical issue in all population groups. Reproductive issues and the acceptability of prenatal diagnosis, adequate informed consent for complex and potentially controversial procedures, use of genetic information in reproductive decision-making, and reproductive rights all impose major concerns (Human Genome Project n.d.).

A forum for Hispanics to identify, prioritize and disseminate information on genetics, including ethical issues, has been established. This forum is a collaborative effort between the Hispanic/Latino Genetics Consultation Network and Redes En Acción, the Baylor College of Medicine, and the National Institutes of Health (National Hispanic/Latino Cancer Network 2003). Legislation and regulatory protection against discrimination should be instituted to protect this vulnerable population. In addition, genetic and genomic health care will be held to standards and quality control measures in testing procedures that comply with appropriate public policy and industry regulations.

Summary

In genetics, ethno-cultural factors are important because healthcare beliefs vary among Hispanic sub-categories. When providing genetic health services and conducting genetic research, healthcare providers must provide culturally and ethnically sensitive care. Specifically, Hispanics have unique genetic, linguistic, cultural, and geographic characteristics that make this population more vulnerable to discrimination than other minorities. Because Hispanics are a heterogeneous group, variations within the population often pose challenges. Furthermore, healthcare providers need to be cognizant that the genetic disorders with higher prevalence in the Hispanic population can occur in many other populations.

References

Alarcon, G. S., K. Brooks, J. D. Reveille, and J. R. Lisse. 1999. Do patients of Hispanic and African-American ethnicity with Lupus experience worse outcomes than patients with lupus from other populations? The LUMINA study. *SLE in Clinical Practice* 2 (3).

Alzheimer's Association. 2004. *Hispanics/Latinos and Alzheimer's disease.* http://www.alz.org/national/documents/report_hispanic.pdf (accessed October 9, 2008)

The American Heritage Dictionary of the English Language. 2000. 4th ed. Boston: Houghton Mifflin.

Bertoni, B. 2003. Admixture in Hispanics: Distribution of ancestral population contributions in the United States. *Human Biology* 75 (1): 1–11.

Burchard, E. G., E. Ziv, N. Coyle, S. L. Gomez, H. Tang, A. J. Karter, J. L. Mountain, et al. 2003. The importance of race and ethnic background in biomedical research and clinical practice. *New England Journal of Medicine* 348 (12): 1170–1175.

Carpenter, C. M., N. L. Atkinson, and R. S. Gold. 2003. *Using in-depth telephone interviews to conduct a needs assessment of genetics issues confronting the Hispanic/Latino community.* Presentation at the University of Maryland, Graduate Research Interaction Day, April 11, 2003, College Park, MD.

Catz, D.S., N. S. Green, J. N. Tobin, M. A. Lloyd-Puryear, P. Kyler, A. Umemoto, J. Cernoch, R. Brown, and F. Wolman. 2005. Attitudes about genetics in underserved, culturally diverse populations. *Community Genetics* 8: 161–172.

Centers for Disease Control and Prevention (CDC). 1996. Iron overload disorders among Hispanics. *Morbidity and Mortality Weekly Report* 45 (45): 991–993. http://www.cdc.gov/mmwr/preview/mmwrhtml/00044494.htm (accessed October 9, 2008).

———. 2004. Prevalence of diabetes among Hispanics—Selected areas, 1998–2002. *Morbidity and Mortality Weekly Report* 53 (40): 941–944. http://www.cdc.gov/mmwr/preview/mmwrhtml/mm5340a3.htm (accessed October 9, 2008).

Cunningham, G. C. 1990. An overview of barriers to care. *Genetic Service for Underserved Populations/Birth Defects Original Article Series* 26 (2): 87–93.

Eichmeyer, J. N., H. Northrup, M. A. Assel, T. J. Goka, D. A. Johnston, and A. T. Williams. 2005. An assessment of risk understanding in Hispanic genetic counseling patients. *Journal of Genetic Counseling* 14 (4): 319–328.

Estrada, A. L., F. M. Treviño, and L. A. Ray. 1990. Health care utilization barriers among Mexican Americans: Evidence from HHANES 1982–84. *American Journal of Public Health* 80 (suppl): 27–31.

Flegal, K. M., T. M. Ezzati, M. I. Harris, S. G. Haynes, R. Z. Juarez, W. C. Knowler, E. J. Perez-Stable, and M. P. Stern. 1991. Prevalence of diabetes in Mexican Americans, Cubans, and Puerto Ricans from the Hispanic health and nutrition examination survey, 1982–1984. *Diabetes Care* 14: 628–638.

Friedman Ross, L. and M. R. Moon. 2001. Ethical issues in pediatric genetics. In *Genetics in the clinic: clinical, ethical, and social implications for primary care,* eds. M. R. Mahowald, A. S. Sheuerke, V. A. McKusick and T. J. Aspinwall, 153–166. St. Louis, MO: C.V. Mosby.

Giger, J., and R. Davidhizer. 2004. *Transcultural nursing: Assessment and intervention.* Fourth ed. St. Louis: Mosby.

Guzmán, B. 2001. *The Hispanic population. Census 2000 brief.* Washington, DC: U.S. Census Bureau. http://www.census.gov/prod/2001pubs/c2kbr01-3.pdf (accessed October 9, 2008).

Human Genome Project. n.d. *Ethical, legal, and social issues.* http://www.ornl.gov/sci/techresources/Human_Genome/elsi/elsi.shtml (accessed October 9, 2008).

Knoerl, A. M. 2007. Cultural considerations and the Hispanic cardiac client. *Home Health Nurse* 25 (2): 82–86.

Lara, M., L. Akinbami, G. Flores, and H. Morgenstern. 2006. Heterogeneity of childhood asthma among Hispanic children: Puerto Rican children bear a disproportionate burden. *Pediatrics* 117: 43–53.

Lobell, M., R. C. Bay, K. V. Rhoads, and B. Keske. 1998. Barriers to screening in Mexican-American women. *Mayo Clinic Proceedings* 73: 301–308.

Lum, R. G. 1987. The patient–counselor relationship in a cross-cultural context. *Birth Defects Original Article Series* 133–143.

Mao, X., A. W. Bigham, R. Mei, G. Gutierrez, K. M. Weiss, T. D. Brutsaert, F. Leon-Velarde, et al. 2007. A genome-wide admixture mapping panel for Hispanic/Latino populations. *American Journal of Human Genetics* 80: 1171–1178.

Marin, G., and B. VanOss-Marin, B. 1991. *Research with Hispanic Population.* Newbury Park, CA: Sage Publications.

National Hispanic/Latino Cancer Network. 2003. *Nationwide Latino genetics conference held June 22–24, 2003.* http://www.redesenaccion.org/Files/News/item20030624.html (accessed October 9, 2008).

Penchaszadeh, V. B., and D. Punales-Morejon. 1998. Genetic services to the Latino population in the United States. *Community Genetics* 1 (3): 134–141.

Punales-Morejon, D. and V. B. Penchaszadeh. 1992. Psychosocial aspects of genetic counseling: Cross-cultural issues. *Birth Defects Original Article Series* 28 (1): 11–15.

211

Singer, E., Y. Antonucci, and J. Van Hoewyk. 2004. Racial and ethnic variations in knowledge and attitudes about genetic testing. *Genetics Testing,* 8 (1): 31–43.

Sweeney, C., R. K. Wolff, T. Byers, K. B. Baumgartner, A. R. Giuliano, J. S. Herrick, M. A. Murtaugh, W. S. Samowitz, and M. L. Slattery. 2007. Genetic admixture among Hispanics and candidate gene polymorphisms: Potential for confounding in a breast cancer study? *Cancer Epidemiology Biomarkers Prevention* 16: 142–150.

Tan, H., S. Choudhry, M. Rui, M. Morgan, W. Rodríguez-Cintrón, E. González Burchard, and N. J. Risch. 2007. Recent genetic selection in the ancestral admixtures of Puerto Ricans. *American Journal of Human Genetics* 81 (3): 626–633.

Triandis, H. C., G. Marin, H. Betancurt, J. Lisansky, and J. Chang. 1982. *Dimensions of familism among Hispanic and mainstream navy recruits.* Urbana: University of Illinois.

Tucker, D. C., R. D. Acton, N. Press, A. Ruggiero, J. A. Reiss, A. P. Walker, L. Wenzel, et al. 2006. Predictors of belief that genetic test information about hemochromatosis should be shared with family members. *Genetic Testing* 10 (1): 50–59.

U.S. Census Bureau. (2006). *Hispanics in the United States.* http://www.census.gov/population/www/socdemo/hispanic/files/Internet_Hispanic_in_US_2006.pdf (accessed June 10, 2008).

———. 2007. *Minority population tops 100 million.* http://www.census.gov/Press-Release/www/releases/archives/population/010048.html (accessed June 10, 2008).

U.S. Office of Management and Budget (OMB). 1997. *Revisions to the standards for the classification of federal data on race and ethnicity.* http://www.whitehouse.gov/omb/fedreg/1997standards.html (accessed June 10, 2008).

Vadaparampil, S.T., L. Wideroff, N. Breen, and E. Trapido. 2006. The impact acculturation on awareness of genetic testing for increased cancer risk among Hispanics in the year 2000: National Health Interview Survey. *Cancer Epidemiology Biomarker & Prevention* 15: 618–623.

Valentin, S. 2001. Self-esteem, cultural identity, and generation status as determinants of Hispanic acculturation. *Hispanic Journal of Behavioral Sciences* 23 (4): 459–468.

Zaid, A., J. T. Fullerton, and T. Moore. 1996. Factors affecting access to prenatal care for U.S./Mexico border-dwelling Hispanic women. *Journal of Nurse Midwifery* 41 (4): 277–284.

Zea, M.C., T. Quezada, and F. Z. Belgrave. (1994). Latino cultural values: Their role in adjustment to disability. *Journal of Social Behavior and Personality* (9): 185–200.

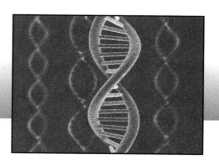

CHAPTER 15

African American Perspectives on Genetics and Ethics

Ida J. Spruill, PhD, MSN, RN, LIWS
Bernice Coleman, PhD, ACNP

Introduction

The genomic era, filled with the possibility of new discoveries and clinical testing strategies for seemingly incurable single-gene and complex trait diseases, has arrived. Many believe the availability of genetic testing and counseling for African Americans may hold the key to significantly improved care for diseases such as sickle cell (Gustafson et al. 2007), prostate cancer (Ahaghotu, Baffoe-Bonnie, Kittles, Pettaway, Powell, Royal, et al. 2004), and breast and ovarian cancer (Halbert et al. 2005). The challenge of these genomic times is to correct the racial disparities in health evident in the African American population and other groups (Communities of Color 2002; Dunston 2000) compared to the non-Hispanic Caucasian population. The magnitude of health disparities will continue to increase according to the U.S. Department of Health and Human Services (U.S. DHHS 2000). The Census Bureau reports that, by the year 2050, Hispanics and African Americans alone will comprise over one third of the total U.S. population, and non- Hispanics whites will have fallen to below 50% of the population for the first time since the nation's founding (U.S. Census Bureau 1992).

One needs only to look at the prevalence of breast cancer among ethnic groups for an example of the potential benefits of genetic education, risk assessment, and counseling. In African American women across income strata, breast cancer is the second most common, surpassed only by lung cancer, according to the National Institutes of Health National Cancer Institute (NIH/NCI 2000). While the incidence of breast cancer is lower in African Americans—119 cases per 1000 versus 141 cases per 100 among non-Hispanic Caucasians (Ries et al. 2001)—breast cancer among African Americans is often estrogen receptor negative, is discovered at later stages (Laino 2007), and demonstrates greater mortality (ACS 2005). These disparities have been attributed to lack of access to care (Armstrong 2005; IOM 2002), lower use of genetic resources (Peters, Domcheck, Rose, et al. 2005), and differences in tumor biology (Laino 2007). These outcomes seem to suggest that genetic testing, education, and counseling would benefit this population. Nevertheless, barriers to the use of these services persist.

In exploring why many African American individuals and families may not use genetic services, the social–cultural dynamic that has created and sustained health disparities cannot be overlooked. Historical contributors to these health disparities include African ancestry, the impact of race, and the legacy of unethical medical experimentation, all of which have led to mistrust of the healthcare system among many African Americans. Despite the benefits of preventive genetic intervention and early treatment, the availability and willingness of African American clients to participate in testing and counseling still influence utilization of care. This chapter offers an overview of the major barriers between African Americans and new genetic technology, and strategies that may overcome them.

African Americans: Definition and Race

African Americans are an ethnic group with a unique heritage derived from a predominantly sub-Saharan African ancestry. The majority of African Americans are descendants of the more than eight million Africans captured on the West coast of Africa during the American slave trade of the seventeenth through the nineteenth centuries (Hines and Boyd-Franklin 1996; Locks and Boateng 1996). They were brought to the United States where they were sold for the purpose of forced labor. This African American definition does not include Caucasian Africans or those of African descent who entered the United States voluntarily from Africa, the Caribbean, or South America.

The taxonomic classification of the term African American has a connotation of historic and present-day racial stratification in American society. Historically, African Americans were categorized by race based upon physical characteristics. Commonly, this group affiliation was determined by self-report, skin color, facial attributes, cranial profile, and hair texture (Fuchs et al. 2002). These characteristics have implied greater meaning than the observed phenotypical likeness. These differences, known as racial characteristics, have a greater social implication. The concept of race dates back to seventeenth-century colonial America. It originated as the rationale to justify hierarchical inequality of enslaved people such as those of African and Indian descent. Physical phenotypical traits became the grounds for socially exclusive status and inequality. Thus, race came to define cultural, behavioral, and physical characteristics. Persons of European descent were the superior race. Persons of African or Indian descent were associated with the negative qualities of an inferior race. These race beliefs were integrated institutionally and became embedded in the national belief systems. This was evident not only in U.S. society, but in Europe as well. Today the term used to describe U.S. citizens who are descendents of African slaves is African American. For a person who self-reports as an African American, this term has more than cultural or historical meaning. It connotes pride, kinship, and solidarity with an extended family network of others whose ancestors survived the Middle Passage and slavery in America (Hines and Boyd-Franklin 1996).

For many African American families, privacy is the most important ethical issue in genetics. African American concerns about confidentiality stem from a long and tortured battle with heredity-based, socially sanctioned tyranny. This legacy and ongoing struggle has led to a strong cultural suspicion of the motives of those collecting genetic information. Exacerbating this general unease is the contrast between how African Americans define family and the traditional family definition of mainstream American society.

Genetics Is a Family Affair: The African American Family

Genetic counseling uses family history and pedigree as an important tool in the process of determining risk assessment. The usefulness of family history as a tool is predicated on gathering information about the proband's parents, siblings, and other relatives who constitute their family. One might expect that both parents of the proband would also be able to provide health history information for their parents and siblings. Gathering this information about African American families often presents different challenges.

Key to the accurate collection of African American genetic information is an understanding of the family structure as broader and more diverse than that of the mainstream Euro-American family. Within the African American ethnic group, biological relatedness and legal marriage does not constrain the domain of kinship. In addition to consanguinity and legally sanctioned descendency, membership within an African

American family may be organized by family group consensus. For example, the family may decide to consider a close friend as a family member. Other family members reinforce this decision by treating the individual in ways indistinguishable from blood or legally related relatives. The person may assume the title of "cousin," "auntie," or "sister." They may have the same privileges and responsibilities as any other member of the family. This is such a central tenet of African American family life that relatives often forget over time. Or the individual's genetic relation to the family is not known. Matters of paternity, sibling status, or even maternity may be socially ascribed rather than fixed by genetic or legal criteria.

Another social dynamic often complicating African American genetic counseling is that African American culture allows greater flexibility in the roles of family members. The social norms and social scripts that determine the roles people should play in the family are more amenable to emotional and financial connections. For example, after the death or disappearance of a mother, an older sister may assume the role of mother and raise her younger siblings because she is an adult with a job. She may have a significant male friend who is a "father" figure and the family constellation changes accordingly.

The initiation of the African American family often begins with birth of a child. Census data reports that 62% of African American children are born into a matrilineal family organization where the mother is not married to the biological father (U.S. Census Bureau 2000). Therefore, while roles within the family are more flexible, the designation of family membership is an inviolable trust vital to the effective operation of the family. As one probes for pedigree relationships to determine risk, it is useful to inquire as to the biological lineage. However, taking time to explain the rationale for knowing biological connections to the client to assist in a clinical prediction sets the context of the questioning without devaluing the relationship of "family membership." Instead of the more traditional question "Who lives in your household?", one might ask "What are the names of blood relatives and your birth parents?"

African Americans and Health Disparities

For African Americans in the United States, health disparities can mean earlier death, decreased quality of life, loss of economic opportunities, and perceptions of injustice. For society, these disparities translate into reduced productivity, higher health-care costs, and social inequity. Multiple factors contribute to racial and ethnic health disparities, including socioeconomic factors, lifestyle behaviors, social environment, racial and ethnic discrimination, neighborhood work conditions, and access to preventive healthcare services (Williams, Neighbors, and Jackson 2003).

The first attempt at an official definition of *health disparities* emerged in 1999 from a National Institutes of Health (NIH) working group. They defined *health disparities* as those differences in the incidence, prevalence, mortality, and burden of diseases and other adverse health conditions that exist among specific population groups in the United States (CRCHD 2008).

In 2000, U.S. Public Law 106–525, the Minority Health and Health Disparities Research and Education Act, provided a legal definition of health disparities: a significant disparity in the overall rate of disease incidence, prevalence, morbidity, mortality, or survival rates in the population compared to the health status of the general population. Since the passage of the law, public and private agencies have used different definitions for their own purposes, but these definitions tend to have several things in common. For example, the Office of Minority Health website provides a general definition of disparities as the differences between one population and another in "the overall rate of disease incidence, prevalence, morbidity, mortality or survival rates" (Office of Minority Health 2005).

The term *health disparity* is used almost exclusively in the United States, while *health inequality* and *health equity* are mainly found outside of the United States (Carter-Pokras and Banquet 2002). Even though there is continuing debate about the causes of health disparities, the three generally accepted causes are:

- Personal, socioeconomic, and environmental characteristics of different ethnic groups,

- Structural barriers such as transportation, scheduling, language, and health literacy that ethnic groups encounter when trying to enter healthcare delivery systems, and

- The quality of health care and health outcome received by racial and ethnic groups.

Other reasons in addition to the above are lack of diversity in the healthcare workforce and cultural differences.

The Henry J. Kaiser Family Foundation (KFF) reports that only 4% of physicians practicing in the United States are African American (KFF 1999). Important considerations regarding disparity between health caregiver, client culture, and ethnicity are potentials for miscommunication, patient dissatisfaction with the delivery of appropriate and effective care, and impact on access to health care (Cooper et al. 2003; Saha et al. 1999). Miscommunication can lead to incorrect diagnosis, improper medications, inaccurate pedigree, ineffective genetic counseling, and failure to follow up. Similarly, provider discrimination either unconsciously or consciously can affect the quality of health care as documented by IOM (2002). This report documents that:

- A consistent body of research demonstrates significant variation in the rates of medical procedures by race, even when insurance status, income, age, and severity of conditions are comparable.
- U.S. racial and ethnic minorities are less likely to receive even routine medical procedures and experience a lower quality of health services.
- A large body of research underscores the existence of health disparities.

They conclude that minorities are less likely to be given appropriate cardiac medications, undergo bypass surgery, or receive kidney dialysis or transplants, and are more likely to receive certain less desirable procedures such as lower limb amputations for diabetes and other conditions. Although, the nation's health has greatly improved in the past century, large gaps in health status for many still exist. Thus the burden of illness and death weighs heavier on racial minorities compared to the U.S. population as a whole. As a result, African Americans, Alaska Natives, American Indians, Asian Americans, Hispanic Americans, and Pacific Islanders are more likely than whites to have poor health, to be uninsured, and to die prematurely (U.S. DHHS 2001).

Inequality, Equity, and Inequity

There are semantic differences among the terms health disparities, inequality, equity, and inequity. A formal definition of health inequality refers to a broad range of differences in both health experience and health status between regions or socioeconomic groups. Most inequalities are not biologically inevitable but reflect population differences in circumstances and behavior that are socially determined. Health inequalities can be defined as gaps in the quality of health and health care across racial, ethnic, and socioeconomic groups (U.S. DHHS 2001).

Equity is an ethical value and conveys a sense of fairness. Human rights activists Braverman and Gruskin (2003) define equity as:

> ...an ethical concept grounded in the principle of distributive justice...Equity in health reflects a concern to reduce unequal opportunities to be healthy [which are] associated with membership in less privileged social groups, such as poor people; disenfranchised racial, ethnic or religious groups; women and rural residents. Pursuing equity in health means eliminating health disparities that are associated with underly-

ing social disadvantage or marginalization. Equity focuses attention on socially disadvantaged, marginalized, or disenfranchised groups within countries, but not limited to the poor. (p. 539)

Carter-Pokras and Banquet (2002) report that disagreements over which term should be used and whether a judgment is unavoidable or unfair continue and can affect programs and policies. Nonetheless, a basic ethical issue in genetics is equity or fairness for African American families and other minorities: equal access to genetic testing and genetic counseling and treatment. However, until affordable gene-engineered medical advances are developed and distributed equitably, genetics will be a specialty serving the "haves" rather than the "have nots" (Wertz and Fletcher 2004).

The Human Genome Project (HGP)

Historically, African Americans and other minorities have been the last to benefit from medical advances and innovations from the Human Genome Project (HGP). Even though the HGP provided some opportunities to reduce health disparities via targeted preventive programs and increased understanding of common polygenic and single-gene disorders, African Americans continue to be over-represented in deaths and under-represented in genetic testing, counseling, and clinical trials. The HGP formally began in 1990 as a 13-year effort coordinated by the Department of Energy (DOE) and the National Institutes of Health. Its goals (U.S. DOE 2004) were to:

- "*identify* all the approximately 20,000–25,000 genes in human DNA,
- *determine* the sequences of the 3 billion chemical base pairs that make up human DNA,
- *store* this information in databases,
- *improve* tools for data analysis,
- *transfer* related technologies to the private sector, and
- *address* the ethical, legal, and social issues (ELSI) that may arise from the project."

The Ethical, Legal and Social Implications (ELSI) division of the National Human Genome Research Institute (NHGRI) at NIH is an innovative outgrowth of the HGP as it sought to educate professionals and the public through literature, conferences, workshops, and multimedia presentations. An array of programs were funded by DOE and ELSI; these consisted of educational materials for physicians, educators, students, clergy, judges, and other legal professionals (U.S. Department of Energy 2004).

Completion of the HGP offered significant opportunities for African Americans. According to the African American Social Worker's Social Policy working group, the human genomic sequence disproves all assertions that African American are genetically different from other groups. The human genome sequence gives us a view of the internal genetic scaffold around which every human life is molded. This scaffold has been handed down to us from our ancestors, and through it we are all connected. From a genetic perspective, "all humans are therefore Africans, either residing in Africa or in recent exile; ...from the few studies of nuclear DNA sequences, it is clear that what is called 'race,' although culturally important, reflects just a few continuous traits determined by a tiny fraction of our genes" (Pääbo 2001). Thus, it is important to note that because of the HGP findings, the observed differences in a patient's ability to metabolize a drug is clustered in genotype markers and not the patient's socially-ascribed race.

Similarly, Bowman (2000) argues that the HGP refutes separation based on race and that race is a social and cultural phenomenon. Bowman asserts that the HGP dispels the myth that African Americans (Cooper et al. 2003) or any other ethnic groups are genetically inferior. Dunston (2001) agrees:

> "Each of us is unique, and only differ in DNA sequence by about one base in every thousand. While these differences underlie uniqueness, as individuals, it should be clear that we are about 99.9% the same as everyone else and this is true regardless of race, gender, or anything else. Thus, the 0.1% differences accounts for much of what makes us individuals in addition to other non-genetic environmental input."

Another significant implication of the HGP for African Americans is the exciting opportunity to address health disparities in both single- and multiple-gene disorders that disproportionately affect them (sickle cell disease, type 2 diabetes, prostate and breast cancer, and cardiovascular disease). Genetic information will allow providers to create medical interventions targeted on the disease at the molecular level rather than to a "race of people." Genetic counseling provided by culturally competent healthcare professionals with specialized degrees and experiences in genetics and counseling can increase patient–provider concord. Genetic counselors are the link between clinical genetics and genetic testing and they work with clients throughout the life cycle. The term was coined in 1947 to replace *genetic hygiene* and *genetic advisor*. Currently, the profession uses a non-directional approach to counseling to provide:

- Accurate, full, unbiased information that patient and family may use to make decisions, and

- Understanding, empathetic relationships that offer guidance to help the patient work and make their own decision (NSGC 2004; Whitehead 1990).

Because less than 5% of genetic counselors are African Americans, the National Society of Genetic Counselors (NSGC) launched an initiative to increase the number of minority counselors. In a speech to the Education, Labor, and Pension committee of the U.S. Senate, NSGC's president reported an increase in the number of educational programs but a decrease in the number of minority applicants, citing that there were 2,100 practicing genetic counselors and greater than 95 % were Caucasian (NSGC 2004).

Similarly, the American Society of Healthcare in Genetics reported that only 1.1% of members were African Americans and 7% Hispanic. In spite of the small numbers of African American genetic counselors and the lack of genetic counseling studies on racial or ethnic minority group, some researchers have attempted to develop culturally sensitive genetic counseling. Mittman (1998) advocated the use of a community empowerment model for genetic education to minority communities. Mittman argued that members of ethnic minorities face formidable cultural, financial, educational, and physical barriers to receiving medical services based on new understanding of genetics. In addition to advocating an increase in minority counselors, she cited three barriers to care:

- Lack of culturally competent educational materials available to families;
- Lack of health providers with the skills to provide culturally competent care, and
- Lack of culturally diverse providers.

Armstrong (2005) studied 408 African American women to assess the association between race and genetic counseling and testing for women at risk of the BRAC1/2 mutation. The goal was to evaluate the influence of risk perception, worry, and socioeconomic attitudes on genetics. The study found that African American women are much less likely (78%) to undergo genetic testing for BRAC1/2 than non-Hispanic Caucasian women with a history of breast or ovarian cancer. However, she noted that this could not be explained with socioeconomic statistics, cancer risk perception, worry, or primary care physicians' discussions about BRAC1/2 testing. The study concluded that these disparities in counseling highlight the need to develop public policies to ensure that all segments of the population can benefit from the HGP.

Singer, Antonucci, and Hoewyk (2004) also studied African Americans' and other minorities' response to genetic testing in 2004. By telephone they surveyed African Americans, Latinos, and non-Hispanics Whites in order to shed light on differences in utilization of genetic testing. The study explored values, attitudes, and beliefs of the three groups, and found that African Americans and Latinos are less knowledgeable about genetic testing, less likely to have financial resources to facilitate testing, and more concerned about personal privacy than Non-Hispanic Caucasian responders.

The final significant implication from the HGP for African Americans is that genetics has confirmed that humanity originated in Africa. This places the continent of Africa at the center of the genetic analysis for the entire human species, altering how Africa is viewed by the world. "We are one human family over multiple generations and the findings from HGP reinforce the significance of the importance of African people to the world. Most importantly, the HGP will stimulate positive thinking in how African Americans view themselves" (Dunston 2000). Genetic research that backs negative perceptions of group origin, ancestry, or composition could lead to a catastrophic assault on certain groups still contending with the evils of racism and bigotry. However, findings from the HGP not only provide scientific evidence against racism, but prove that specific ethnic groups are not exclusive carriers of certain genetic alleles and diseases.

Most inherited diseases are rare, but taken together the more than 3,000 disorders known to result from single genes stifle many potentially healthy and productive lives. The HGP allows scientists to study the structure of genes and characterize the molecular alterations, or mutations, that result in diseases. Mutations play a role in many of today's most common diseases, such as heart disease, diabetes, immune system disorders, and birth defects. These diseases are believed to result from complex interactions between genes and environment and are not population-specific. When genes for diseases are identified, scientists can study how they and specific environmental factors such as economic inequalities interact to cause diseases.

Scientists can then determine which gene or combination of genes may contribute to single-gene disorders or diseases that involve several complex traits. These discoveries have implications for pharmacogenomics, proteomics, gene therapy, and genetic counseling. Despite findings from the HGP and the trends toward improved health care, minority scientists, especially African Americans, continue to be underrepresented as both scientists and research participants at the National Institutes of Health (NIH) and the HGP. Consequently, many African Americans believe that the sequenced human genome contains genes primarily from Northern Europeans, leading to the suspicion that the findings will benefit mostly Caucasians.

HGP and Historical Unethical African American Research

The Tuskegee Syphilis Study is frequently mentioned as the primary reason African Americans do not participate in medical research and distrust medical institutions and public health programs (Katz et al. 2007). However, Gamble (1993) notes that this distrust of the medical community predated public revelation about the Tuskegee study.

Washington (2006) agrees and provides documentation of African American suspicions of exploitation by medical profession dating back to the antebellum period when slaves and free Blacks were used as subjects for dissection and medical experimentation. She finds that physicians also used poor whites, but slaves were used more often because the state considered them property and denied them the legal right to object, and physicians needed the bodies. Both Gamble and Washington cite evidence of two antebellum experiments: one physician (Thomas Hamilton) in Georgia used slaves to test remedies for heatstroke, and another (Marion Sims) from Alabama used slave women to test an operation to repair vesicovaginal fistulas.

Medical exploitation during slavery and after the Civil War moved African American leaders to protest these abuses and prompted the establishment of African American-controlled hospitals. Thus the Tuskegee Study merely confirmed the long held beliefs in the African Americans community. Gamble suggests that these historical beliefs may explain delayed or inadequate treatment of AIDS in African American communities, and she cautions that these beliefs must not be dismissed as the views of a few. A 1990 survey by the Southern Christian Leadership Conference revealed several prevalent beliefs (Quinn 1997):

- Thirty-five percent of 1,056 church members believed that AIDS was a form of genocide.
- White Americans have historically been and continue to be indifferent to the existence of African Americans.
- African Americans are devalued by white society.

She further states that these beliefs influence the relationship and trust between African Americans and modern society and continue to shape perceptions about research. For example, the current perspective on heredity is shaped by the legacy of the "one drop rule," a colloquial term for laws in some states indicating that a person with any trace of African ancestry (however small or invisible) cannot be

Caucasian. Therefore, unless that person can claim an alternative non-Caucasian ancestry such as Native American, Asian, Arab, or Australian aboriginal, they are of African descent. This rule has influenced the thinking and socialization of African Americans in that having even one African Americans ancestor would still mandate African American ethnicity. Jackson contended that social dictates such as the one drop rule tended to make African Americans socialization inclusive rather that exclusive (Jackson 2000).

Other studies also document African American mistrust of the medical community. Wertz and Fletcher (2004) cited a study by Thomas with 500 African American participants. The study reported that 36% of the sample was distrustful of medical research and subjects were less likely to participate in research because they likened their participation to that of "guinea pigs." Thomas concludes that African Americans are more difficult to locate, need more time to recruit, and are more costly as research subjects than Caucasians. In contrast, Spruill (2004) found that when research studies are designed to be culturally sensitive, as with the Gullah population in South Carolina, and research information is provided along with compensation, African Americans will participate in genetic research.

A study by Achter, Parrot and Silk among 858 Americans in four community settings indicated that African Americans were significantly more likely to believe that clinical trials might be dangerous. Additionally, they found that the federal government knowingly conducted unethical research, including studies in which risky vaccines were administered to prisoners. This research concluded that most Americans trust government to act ethically in sponsoring and conducting research, including genetics research, but that African Americans are particularly likely to see government as powerfully protective in some settings yet disingenuous in others (Achter, Parrot and Silk 2004).

Despite the potential that the HGP holds for dismantling racial and health disparities, it remains in the shadow of the Tuskegee syphilis study. Genetic discoveries from the HGP will continue to have a major impact on society, but challenges to improve health care for all remain. Genetic advances can close gaps in health care for African Americans with better trust and communication, information management, and participation in research.

African Americans, Education, and Community Outreach

Although, there have been some attempts to understand how African Americans feel about genetic literacy, testing, and counseling, overall the literature remains scarce. In an effort to remedy both the reality of genetic literacy and perceptions of health-care inequity, ELSI and the DOE funded an array of projects to provide genetic education to minority communities.

- The Communities of Color and Genetics Policy Project is a consortium of three universities: University of Michigan, Michigan State University, and Tuskegee University. They were charged with developing a process for engaging communities of color and diverse socioeconomic levels in dialogues relating to genomic research and its resulting technology. These dialogues resulted in recommendations for laws, professional standards, and institutional policies regarding the use and application of genomic research and technology. In the initial project, community participants represented some of the racial and ethnic groups. However, the absolute numbers of minority groups in communities were small. Consequently, a renewal project was funded, similar to the initial project but incorporating important modifications, and was more successful in engaging people of color. The project closed at the end of 2002 (Communities of Color 2002).

- The Zeta Phi Beta sorority was the first Greek letter organization to address the impact of the HGP in the African American community. Its National Education Foundation planned and conducted five major conferences on the challenges and impacts of the HGP: New Orleans in 1999, Philadelphia in 2000, Atlanta and Washington, DC in 2001, and Los Angeles in 2007 (Zeta Phi Beta Sorority). In 2003, the Sigma Nu Zeta chapter, in partnership with the Abyssinian Baptist Church Health Ministry, presented a panel of experts to the Central Harlem community.

- In 1998 over 150 leaders from the Baltimore minority community attended a meeting organized by the Center for Minority Health. The goals of the meeting were to inform the community about the potential benefits of the HGP and to make the aspirations and interests of the African American community known. The attendees perceived that scientists had been involved in the HGP since 1986, but minorities had not been sufficiently aware of the research or aware of how diseases would be diagnosed and treated in the future. Furthermore, the group reported that the project could enable unscrupulous organizations to discriminate against persons defined as having "less-than-optimal" genetic profiles. The group consensus was that findings from the HGP could also significantly enhance the health status of all persons, including minorities, and that informed groups have the option of acting on genetic information to make certain that their communities share equitably in the new resources (Human Genome News 1998).

- At Tuskegee University in 1996, Plain Talk about the Human Genome Project brought together international recognized scientists, bioethicists, and legal scholars from government, industry, and academia to discuss the use and misuse of genetic information. Concerns ranged from the fear of actuarial classifications of "genetic exceptionalism" to the burden African Americans would face if they were among those labeled by some as a biological underclass (Plain Talk about the Human Genome Project 1997).

- The National Human Genome Center at Howard University in Washington, DC conducted a workshop in 2003 entitled Human Genome Variation and Race. It was sponsored and financially supported by the genome programs of DOE's Office of Science, the Irving Harris Foundation, the NIH's NHGRI, and Howard University.

Despite these initiatives by ELSI and DOE, the perspectives of African Americans about genetics and ethics remain insufficiently studied, especially as they affect African American nurses. Spruill, Coleman, McNeil, and Johnson (2006) surveyed nurses attending the National Black Nurses Association annual convention. Seventy-seven attendees at a business meeting at the conference completed a 19-item survey, the goal of which was to assess their knowledge, beliefs, and interest in genetics.

The response rate for the survey was 100% (see the three tables on pages 229 and 230). Over 41% of the respondents worked in the hospital setting, yet 61% did not feel comfortable explaining genetic information to patients. Moreover, only 42% described their genetic knowledge as good, and 59% had never had a course in genetics. The nursing school curriculum of 63% had not included a course in genetics, 68% reported that they knew someone with a genetic condition, and 85% knew how to complete a family health history. When asked about their beliefs, 96% agreed that family health history could help to identify at-risk families. Further, 96% agreed that family history could be used as a tool to teach patients and family about the importance of genetics. However, questions regarding perceptions of barriers to gaining this information were not asked. Of this professional sample, 77% voiced concerns regarding the potential of genetic testing information to discriminate against minorities. Questions related to interest and practice level revealed that 93% would be willing to teach their families how to complete the health history, 93% believed that the organization should have in role in genomic education, and 88% favored an institute in 2008 on genetics.

Results from the survey indicate that there is an opportunity to both further explore this issue and provide African American nurses with genetic education to improve their competency as health providers. It is interesting that this small homogeneous sample did voice concerns about discrimination based on genetic information intended to improve health outcomes in the African American population.

Closing the Gaps: Genetic Discovery and Utilization in the African American Community

Eliminating disparities in minorities' utilization of genetic health care is imperative. Unfortunately, overcoming a history of mistrust remains an issue for today's clinician. Communication between patient and provider is a first critical step. Research suggests that interactions are improved with patient–provider racial concord. Cultural competence and sensitivity in providers promotes longer visits, greater satisfaction with quality of communication and care, and greater physician participation in care (Cooper et al. 2003; Saha et al. 1999).

The National Coalition of Ethnic Minority Nurse Associations (NCEMNA) is made up of five minority nursing organizations joined in a unique mission to give voice to more than 350,000 ethnic minority nurses:

- Asian American/Pacific Islander Nurses Association (AAPINA)
- National Alaska Native American Indian Nurses Association (NANAINA)
- National Association of Hispanic Nurses (NAHN)
- National Black Nurses Association (NBNA)
- Philippine Nurses Association of America (PNAA)

NCEMNA's goal is development of culturally competent ethnic nurses who reflect the diverse national populations receiving care. It provides a unique basis for cultivating nurse leaders qualified to influence health policy, practice, education, and research of minority populations.

On all accounts, this ethnic concord will take some time to grow. Thus, for all clinicians the first step is to provide culturally sensitive and competent interactions particularly in gaining family information. The providers need to pose questions in a way that elicits the information needed to construct a pedigree without seeming to devaluing an apparently unconventional family structure. To this end, culturally sensitive communication styles along with appropriate educational material are crucial to gaining the needed trust and genetic information (Kessler et al. 2005).

Nurturing the trust of minority populations will need to extend beyond the provider–client dyad. Management of sensitive genetic information by insurance companies and health institutions remains a major concern of the African American community and its professionals. African Americans genetics professionals will need to be present at public policy venues to advocate for protecting the rights of all persons when genetic information is collected, to preserve future benefits for all.

Lastly, benefits for African Americans from the HGP will remain limited until participation in research provides better direction for individualized treatment plans. Researchers must seek collaborative alliances with other minority researchers when studying subjects of disparate ethnicity. Such collaborative links between ethnic and non-ethnic minority researchers provides rich culturally sensitive insight into the development, recruitment, and implementation of research projects. The ultimate goal is to increase trust and participation in research by African American and all ethnic communities. Eliminating health disparities will require new knowledge about the determinants of disease, causes of health disparities, and effective culturally appropriate interventions designed for prevention and treatment.

Summary

There remains a need in the African American community to heighten awareness of benefits from the HGP. Reassuring minorities that obtaining information perceived as sensitive is warranted by the benefit of improving outcomes remains the fundamental goal for the use of genetic services in minority communities. The HGP has great potential to revolutionize medicine with the prospect for medical treatment that is based on an individual's genetic uniqueness. However, communities of color should support initiatives that strive for answers to the following ethnic, social, and legal issues:

Ethnic and Social Issues:

- The confidentiality and sharing of individual genetic information
- The equity issues surrounding available and affordable genetic testing
- Diverse pool of genetic counselors to increase cultural competency
- Minority researchers in the HGP, and increasing minorities in clinical trials
- Informed consent in genetic counseling and testing
- Genetic research used as a tool to perpetuate racism
- Overemphasizing genetics and downplaying environment injustice and social inequality.

Legal Issues:

- Protection against genetic discrimination by employers and insurance companies
- Affordable health insurance for genetic counseling
- Title 1 of the Americans with Disabilities Act (protection against employment discrimination as genetic testing become more available)
- DNA proofing replacing racial profiling, and minorities with same access to genetic evidence after conviction as others in the criminal system

Communities of color must continue to make the African American voice heard, maintain visibility, be present when policy is discussed and decisions are made that affect African American lives. Additionally, African Americans must define their own issues, acknowledge the history of medical mistrust, and ensure their input into the resolution of genetic issues so that African American interests are served along with the majority.

TABLE 15-1
Selected Knowledge Questions about Genetics (N=77)

Knowledge Level	Course	Curriculum	Referral	Genetic C.
Fair 32.5%	Yes 40.3%	Yes 35.1%	Yes 39%	Yes 68.8%
Poor 23.4%	No 59.7%	No 63.6%	No 61%	No 29.9%
Good 42.9%				

Comfort Level	Can Complete	Has Completed	Like to Learn
Yes 36.4%	Yes 85.7%	Yes 84.4%	Yes 77.9%
No 61. %	No 13%	No 14.3 %	No 11.7%

TABLE 15–2
Selected Questions about Family Health History and Beliefs (N=77)

ID at Risk F.	Teach Genetics	Discrimination
Yes 96.1%	Yes 96.1%	Yes 77.9%
No 3.9%	No 1.3%	No 11.7%

TABLE 15–3
Selected Questions about Interest and Practice (N=77)

Teach	Support	NBNA	2008
Yes 93.5 %	Yes 90.9%	Yes 93.5 %	Yes 88.3 %
No 1.3 %	No 5.2%	No 1.3%	No 7.8 %

References

Ahaghotu, C., A. Baffoe-Bonnie, R. Kittles, C. Pettaway, I. Powell, C. Royal, H. Wang, S. Vijayakumar, J. Bennett, G. Hoke, et al. 2004. Clinical characteristics of African-American men with hereditary prostate cancer: the AAHPC study. *Prostate Cancer and Prostate Disease* 7 (2): 165–169.

Achter, P., R. Parrot, and K. Silk. 2004. African Americans opinions about human genetic research. *Politics and Life Science* 23 (1): 60–66.

American Cancer Society (ACS). 2005. *Breast Cancer Facts & Figures 2005–2006*. Atlanta: American Cancer Society.

American Society of Healthcare in Genetics. 2007. A study underlying the study about ASHG membership: No surprise that minority members comprise low percentage. Rockville, MD.

Armstrong, K. 2005. African American women are less likely to undergo genetic testing than White Women. *Journal of the American Medical Association* 293: 1729–1736.

Bowman, J. 2000. The study of African American problems: W. E. B. Du Bois's agenda, then and now. *Annals of the American Academy of Political and Social Science* 568: 140–153.

Braverman, P., and S. Gruskin. 2003. Poverty, equity, human rights, and health. *Bulletin of the World Health Organization* 81: 539–545.

Carter-Pokras, O., and C. Banquet. 2002. What is a "health disparity"? *Public Health Reports* 117: 426–434.

Center to Reduce Cancer Health Disparities. (CRCHD) 2008. Health disparities defined. http://crchd.cancer.gov/definitions/defined.html (accessed October 7, 2008).

Communities of Color and Genetics Policy Project. 2002. *Project summary.* http://www.sph. umich.edu/genpolicy (accessed October 7, 2008).

Cooper, L., D. Roter, R. Johnson, D. E. Ford, D. M. Steinwachs, and N. R. Powe. 2003. Patient-centered communications, rating of care, and concordance of physician and patient race. *Annals of Internal Medicine* 139 (11): 907–915.

Dunston, G. 2000. The implications of human genome research for minority health issues. http://www.ornl.gov/sci/techresources/Human_Genome/publicat/zetaphibeta/dunston.s html (accessed October 7, 2008).

Fuchs, S., S. Guimaraes, C. Sortica, F. Wainberg, K. O. Dias, M. Ughini, J. A. S. Castro, and F. D. Fuchs. 2002. Reliability of race assessment based upon the race of ascendants: A cross-sectional study. *BMC Public Health* 2: 1–5.

Gamble, V. N. 1993. A legacy of distrust: African Americans and medical research. *American of Journal of Preventive Medicine* 9: 35–38.

Gustafson, S. L., E. A. Gettig, M. Watt-Morse, and L. Krishnamurti. 2007. Health beliefs among African Americans women regarding genetic testing and counseling for sickle cell disease. *Genetic Medicine* 9 (5): 303–310.

Halbert, C., L. Kessler, A. Collier, E. P. Wileyto, K. Brewster, and B. Weathers. 2005. Psychological functioning in African American women at an increased risk for hereditary breast an ovarian cancer. *Clinical Genetics* 68: 222–227.

Hines. P., and N. Boyd-Franklin. 1996. African American families. In, eds. M. McGoldrick, J. Giordana, and N. Garcia-Preto, *Ethnicity and family therapy* (2nd ed.). New York: The Guilford Press.

Henry J. Kaiser Family Foundation (KFF). 1999. *A synthesis of the literature: Racial and ethnic differences in access to medical care.* http://www.kff.org/minorityhealth/upload/A-Synthesis-of-the-Literature-Racial-Ethnic-Differences-in-Access-to-Medical-Care-Report.pdf (accessed October 7, 2008).

Institute of Medicine (IOM). 2002. *Unequal treatment: Confronting racial and ethnic disparities in health care.* Washington, DC: National Academics Press.

Jackson, F. 2000. *Scientific and folk perspectives on heredity.* http://www.ornl.gov/sci/techresources/Human_Genome/publicat/zetaphibeta/jackson.shtml (accessed October 7, 2008).

Katz, R. V., B. L. Green, N. R. Kressin, C. Claurdio, M. Q. Wang, and S. L. Russell. 2007. Willingness of minorities to participate in biomedical research studies: Confirmatory findings from the Tuskegee Legacy Project questionnaire. *Journal of the National Medical Association* 99 (9): 1052–1060.

Laino, C. 2007. Deadly breast tumors higher in blacks. http://www.webmd.com/breast-cancer/news/20070906/deadly-breast-tumors-higher-in-blacks?src=rss_cbsnews (accessed October 7, 2008).

Locks, S., and L. Boateng. 1996. Black/African Americans. In G. J. Lipson, L. S. Dibble, and P. A. Minarik (Eds.), *Culture and nursing care: A pocket guide.* Berkeley: University of California Press.

Minority Health and Health Disparities Research and Education Act. 2000. *United States Public Law* 106–525.

Mittman, I.S. 1998. Genetic education to diverse communities employing a community empowerment model. *Community Genetics* 1 (3): 160–165.

National Coalition of Ethnic Minority Nurse Associations (NCEMNA). (n.d.). What is NCEMNA? http://www.ncemna.org/ncemna/whatisncemna.asp (accessed October 7, 2008).

National Institutes of Health, National Cancer Institute (NIH/NCI). 2000. Cancer statistics. http://www.cancer.gov/statistics/ (October 7, 2008).

National Society of Genetic Counselors (NSGC). 2004. *Letter to Senator Mike Enzi.* http://www.nsgc.org/news/mediakit/letters/111204.cfm (accessed October 7, 2008).

Office of Minority Health. 2005. *What Are Health Disparities?* http://www.omhrc.gov/templates/content.aspx?ID=3559 (accessed October 7, 2008).

Pääbo, S. 2001. The human genomic and our view of ourselves. *Science,* 291, pp.1219–1220.

Peters, N., S. Domchek, A. Rose, R. Polis, J. Stopfer, and K. Armstrong. 2005. Knowledge, attitudes, and utilization of BRCA1/2 testing among women with early-onset breast cancer. *Genetic Testing* 9 (1): 48–53.

Quinn, S. R. 1997. Belief in AIDS as a form of genocide: Implications for HIV preventions programs for African Americans. *American Journal of Health Education* 28 (6 Supp): S6–S11.

Ries, L., M. Eisner, C. Kosary, B. Hankey, B. Miller, L. Clegg, and B. Edwards (Eds.). 2001. *SEER Cancer Statistics Review, 1973–1999.* Bethesda, MD: National Cancer Institute.

Saha, S., M. Komaromy, T. Koepsell, and A. P. Bindman. 1999. Patient–physician concordance and the perceived quality and use of health care. *Archives of Internal Medicine* 159: 997–1004.

Singer, E., T. C. Antonucci, and J. Van Hoewyk. 2004. Racial and ethnic variations in knowledge and attitudes about genetic testing. *Genetic Testing* 8: 31–46.

Spruill, I. 2004. Project Sugar: A recruitment model for successful African American participation in health research. *Journal of National Black Nurses Association* 15: 48–53.

Spruill, I., B. Coleman, J. McNeil, and S. Johnson. (2006). *Knowledge, attitudes, and interest of African American nurses toward genetics.* Unpublished manuscript.

U.S. Census Bureau. 1992. *1992–2050 Population projections of the United States by age, race, sex, and Hispanic origin.* Washington, DC: Government Printing Office.

U.S. Census Bureau. 2005. *African Americans by the numbers.* http://www.infoplease.com/spot/bhmcensus1.html (accessed August 19, 2008).

U.S. Department of Energy (DOE). 2004. Minorities, race, and genomics. http://www.ornl.gov/sci/techresources/Human_Genome/elsi/minorities.shtml (accessed August 19, 2008).

U.S. Department of Health and Human Services (DHHS). 2000. *Healthy People 2010: Publications.* http://www.healthypeople.gov/Publications/ (accessed October 7, 2008).

Washington, H. A. 2006. *Medical apartheid.* New York: Doubleday.

Wertz, D. C., and J. C. Fletcher. 2004. *Genetics and ethics in global perspective.* New York: Springer.

Whitehead, M. 1990. *The concepts and principals of equity and health.* Copenhagen: World Health Organization.

Williams, D., H. Neighbors, and J. Jackson. 2003. Racial/ethnic discrimination and health: findings from community studies. *American Journal of Public Health* 93: 200–208.

Zeta Phi Beta. 2000. *Human genome project.* http://www.zphib1920.org/nef/genome.html (accessed August 19, 2008).

PART 3

Applications of Genetics and Genomics in Health Care

This section of the monograph discusses selected applications of genetic and genomic technologies, particularly the current patterns of mutational testing that are widely available today. While these chapters present the more common tests, the reader should know that additional mutational analyses are being transferred from the laboratory to the clinical setting. We are moving quickly to the place in our history when we will be able to study the interplay of several genes as well as environmental factors that result in conditions of health and illness.

One of the most rapidly advancing areas of research is expected to broaden our understanding of the appearance of such population level causes of morbidity and mortality as heart disease, cancer, and diabetes. We can expect to learn more about specific environmental conditions and their influence on sets of genes that result in metabolic processes that lead to chronic illnesses in the future. At the moment, how we might avert or reverse these abnormal processes is not imaginable, but our children and grandchildren may live in a world where some of these questions will be commonplace. This monograph is designed to make a contribution to the cultural traditions that could guide their future lives.

PART 3 ⮹ CONTENTS

CHAPTER 16

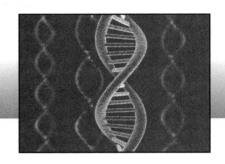

Concerns of Patients and Families Surrounding Genetic Testing

Janet K. Williams, PhD, RN, PNP, CGC, FAAN

Individuals and families participate in genetic testing for a variety of clinical reasons. Concerns of individuals and families include an understanding of the purposes of genetic testing, potential benefits, risks, limitations, and consequences of the test for themselves, their family member, and their community. Regardless of the reasons, though, the results can affect the health and well-being of the individual being tested, as well as the person's biologic family.

Nurses ensure that the rights of individuals and their families are protected throughout the genetic testing process, regardless of the purpose of the test. Knowledge of the potential benefits, limitations, and risks of genetic information, such as that obtained through genetic testing, is a component of the core competencies for all healthcare professionals (NCHPEG 2005). This responsibility is also reflected in the code of ethics for nurses (ANA 2001). This chapter discusses the concerns that individuals and families may have regarding genetic testing. These concerns include: What is the purpose of the test? How can the test help me? What are the limitations of genetic testing? How could having a genetic testing harm me? What can I do to relieve my concerns?

What Is the Purpose of the Test?

A genetic test can be any assessment method that identifies biologic information that is contained in the person's cells. This term often refers to a chromosome analysis or a molecular genetic test, but can include human DNA, RNA, chromosomes, proteins, and some metabolites (Holtzman and Watson 1999).

Diagnosis

Genetic tests are conducted for the purposes of establishing or clarifying a clinical diagnosis. An example is the use of a molecular genetic test to determine if a child with developmental delay has the diagnosis of Fragile X syndrome, the most common inherited form of mental retardation in males (Bailey, Skinner, and Sparkman 2003). This condition is caused by a mutation on the X chromosome that can be identified through molecular genetic testing. When a test is conducted for the purpose of diagnosis, family members may not complete the full informed consent process. One component of that process is to review the potential outcomes of a test. In this instance, because the test is attempting to establish the diagnosis of a condition that can be inherited within families, nurses share responsibilities with other healthcare providers to ensure that persons agreeing to the test understand its purpose and the potential implications of the result for other family members.

Carrier Status

Genetic tests are also conducted to determine if persons who are not ill could be carriers of inherited conditions. A person consenting to a carrier test may wish to know if he or she has an increased likelihood to have a child with an inherited condition. Some conditions have an autosomal recessive pattern of inheritance, meaning that a mutation must be present in each of the two copies of the gene in order for the condition to be present. Certain inherited diseases are only manifested if the person has a mutation in each gene for an autosomal recessive disorder, or, in males, if the mutation is on the X chromosome. Carrier testing can determine if persons have only one copy of the mutation. An example of an autosomal recessive condition is cystic fibrosis (CF). In this case it is important for the individual, or couple, to understand that a carrier does not have the disease, but when they are each carriers, their children could have CF.

Future Likelihood to Develop Disease

Genetic testing is possible for some conditions where the causative mutation is known, such as Huntington disease (HD), to determine if the person has a high likelihood of developing the condition in the future. This type of testing is referred to as presymptomatic testing (Secretary's Advisory Committee on Genetic Testing 2000). When the purpose is to determine if a person has inherited a genetic susceptibility that increases the likelihood they will develop a disease in the future, this is referred to as predictive or susceptibility testing. When a person has a relative with a mutation in the BRCA1 or BRCA2 gene, which are associated with an increased chance to develop breast and ovarian cancer, the test could provide information about their future likelihood to develop these diseases. These testing terms may not be used consistently by healthcare providers. Thus, it is essential that people considering genetic testing to provide information about future chances of developing a disease have a clear understanding of what type of information the test can provide for them.

How Can The Test Help Me?

Accuracy

One aspect of answering this question is the clinical validity of a test. This refers both to the sensitivity, i.e., the proportion of people with the disease who have a positive test, and the penetrance of the gene mutation identified. Penetrance is the proportion of people who have the mutation who will also have signs and symptoms of the disease (Burke 2004). Individuals and families may need help in understanding what kind of information the test will provide. In one survey of parents of children who had a genetic test to diagnose Fragile X syndrome, the majority of parents found the test helpful because it provided a reason for their child's problems (Bailey et al. 2003).

Use in Healthcare Decisions

In other circumstances, the result of a genetic test can provide information that can be useful for making clinical decisions about a person's health promotion or disease management. It is important to note that results from a genetic test are only one factor in clinical decisions. Usefulness of results in predicting future disease or selecting management options will vary for each test and clinical situation. One example of use of a genetic test to guide screening decisions is familial cancer genetic testing. For those who are at risk for certain inherited forms of cancer, such as hereditary nonpolyposis colorectal carcinoma (HNPCC), persons who had a positive genetic test were found to be more likely to have colonoscopy screening, than those whose test was negative. In this situation, the gene test results were used to help determine which persons should continue this screening. It was also reported in this study that some persons who had a negative gene test continued to have colonoscopy screenings. Factors other than the actual test result also influence how people use genetic testing information. This is consistent with a holistic approach to patient care, when nurses consider the entire range of factors, including prior beliefs, advice from other family members or healthcare providers, extent of understanding of test results, and other sociocultural factors that contribute to how each person uses genetic test information.

Personal or Family Benefits

One benefit of genetic testing is to obtain information that parents would like to give to their children. People who completed carrier testing for an autosomal recessive or x-linked recessive condition reported that learning their own carrier status was important in understanding if their own children could be carriers or develop the disease (Williams and Schutte 1997). Information from one person's test may be useful to others in the family. If one person in a family has a mutation in a gene for hereditary breast and ovarian cancer, this information would identify the specific mutation that would be sought in tests to determine if the person's siblings or children also have the mutation. Other uses of genetic testing information include decisions regarding family planning or prenatal diagnosis. When both parents have carrier testing for an autosomal recessive condition such as CF, this information may be used in reproductive decisions.

One hoped-for benefit of genetic testing is the ability to use genetic information in the selection of the most appropriate treatment when a person has a disease. Much of this work remains at the research level, with some findings being implemented in clinical practice. An example is genetic testing to determine HER2 status (human epidermal growth factor receptor-2) for women with breast cancer to guide selection of chemotherapy (Dendukuri, Khetani, McIssac, and Brophy 2007).

For other conditions, such as HD, the identification of a gene mutation is not yet linked to any new treatment options. However, some people who receive genetic testing find the results helpful in making decisions regarding what activities they intend to complete prior to the anticipated time of onset of the illness, or other lifestyle decisions (Codori and Brandt 1994). Genetic test results can also be helpful to people who believe that actually knowing if they have a gene mutation for a specific condition is better than not knowing.

What Are the Limitations of Genetic Testing?

Uncertain Findings

Some genetic tests yield results that do not allow definitive interpretations. When a person has a genetic test for HD, this test measures the size of the gene mutation. When the gene mutation is between the normal and the abnormal range, it is not possible to predict if the person will develop HD. This situation can also happen with other tests, such as a test in a gene for hereditary breast and ovarian cancer, when a result has not been reported to be associated with that disease.

Accessibility to Genetic Testing

Studies of people who request genetic testing for familial cancers report that people who have higher education and socioeconomic status and are not of a minority ethnic ancestry more often ask for genetic tests. Possible reasons include differences in exposure to genetic information, cost, nature of interactions with healthcare providers, and perceived genetic risk (Honda, 2003; Hughes, Gomez-Caminero, Benkendorf, Kerner, Issacs, Barter, and Lerman 1997). Assuring that each person who may benefit from genetic testing information is informed about it, as well as enabling healthcare providers to provide socioculturally sensitive information regarding genetic testing, is a component of nursing practice.

How Could I, My Family, or My Community Be Harmed By Genetic Testing?

Possible Genetic Discrimination

Loss of privacy of one's genetic information is a situation that can lead to loss of societal benefits, such as insurability or employability. Although state anti-discrimination laws and federal laws including the Health Insurance Portability and Accountability Act (HIPAA) prohibit a clinician from disclosing medical information without the signed consent of a patient (U.S. Department of Health and Human Services 2004), the risk of genetic discrimination remains for some people. Over half of women in one survey reported that fear of insurance discrimination was an important factor in their decision about having a genetic test for familial breast and ovarian cancer

(Armstrong, Weber, FitzGerald, Hershey, Pauley, Lemaire et al. 2003). The potential for loss of societal benefits is a component of the informed consent process for many presymptomatic, predictive, and carrier genetic tests. The Genetic Information Nondiscrimination Act (GINA) was signed into law on May 21, 2008 (GINA 2008; NHGRI 2008). This legislation was intended to decrease the likelihood that individuals will experience discrimination in either their health insurance coverage or employment based on their risk for or the presence of a genetic condition (Coalition for Genetic Fairness, 2008).

Family Disruption

When a person learns that they have a mutation in a gene that could lead to disease in that person or that person's children, this information has implications for the health of others in that family. One of that person's parents is presumed to have the same mutation, and the persons' siblings and children may also have it. Those who get genetic testing for hereditary breast and ovarian cancer or for HD may be selective regarding which biologic relatives they inform of their test results. This may reflect an attempt to protect the relative from news that may lead to feelings of guilt and sadness, a perception that the relative may not be receptive to hearing the genetic test information, or a reluctance to risk losing bonds that the person felt had kept the family together (Hamilton, Bowers, and Williams 2005).

Direct-to-Consumer Marketing

Most genetic tests are not included in current oversight provided by the U.S. government. Thus, there is the potential for false and misleading claims by organizations that offer genetic testing online or through other direct consumer contact. The full impact of public use of genetic tests without explanation and interpretation by health professionals is not known. The number of referrals for further information increased more than 240% in one city when direct advertising to consumers was initiated for genetic testing for inherited mutation in genes associated with breast cancer (Mouchawar, Hensley-Alford, Laurion, Ellis, Kulchak-Rahm, Fincane, et al. 2005). Concerns expressed by healthcare professionals regarding direct marketing of genetic testing include varying opportunities for genetic counseling among companies, and profit for the company being linked with selling a test (Wolfberg 2006). Nurses who are informed about the accuracy and purposes of specific genetic tests, and the possible benefits, limitations, and risk for harm, can act as advocates for their patients and their patients' families, and can assist them to receive information from knowledgeable sources (Williams, Skirton, and Masny 2005).

Cultural Issues in Specific Native or Cultural Communities

Respect for autonomy and privacy may take on different meanings when genetic testing for purposes of research is requested from members of a group that is relatively stable, remains geographically settled, and marries within the group. Native American Indians or Amish are examples of communities in which genetic research may be requested (Bowekaty and Davis 2003). Partnership by persons from the community in decisions about research that includes genetic testing is an important strategy to address concerns of the community that may differ from those of the researcher.

What Can I Do to Relieve My Concerns?

The opportunity to participate in informed consent is important for all involved in genetic testing, one component of which is a discussion of the benefits and risks associated with the test (ISONG 2000). The Genetic Alliance's brochure on understanding the informed consent process for genetic testing in research is another excellent resource (2001). Portions of the discussion may involve healthcare providers such as geneticists, genetic counselors, or advanced practice genetic nurses who can help the individual or family understand the genetic aspects of the test. The discussion may also include other healthcare providers, especially primary care providers and nurses, with whom the patient and family have an ongoing relationship. Educational resources, such as a continuing education program on Ethics and Genetic Testing, currently in production at the University of Iowa (The University of Iowa, College of Nursing 2007) is one resource that can prepare nurses to explain genetic testing.

Summary

Genetic tests are conducted for a variety of purposes. Adherence to principles of respect for dignity of the individual, family, and community underlies the nursing care in response to concerns raised by genetic testing. Knowledge of the purpose and accuracy of a specific test, the potential benefits, limitations, and harms is an essential component of professional nursing practice. This knowledge enables nurses to provide information on expert genetic testing resources, as well as nursing care that helps persons, families, and communities to benefit from genetic testing information.

References

American Nurses Association (ANA). 2001. *Code of ethics for nurses with interpretive statements.* http://nursingworld.org/ethics/code/protected_nwcoe813.htm (accessed October 11, 2008).

Armstrong, K., B. Weber, G. FitzGerald, J. C. Hershey, M. V. Pauly, J. Lemaire, K. Subramanian, and D. A. Asch. 2003. Life insurance and breast cancer risk assessment: Adverse selection, genetic testing decisions, and discrimination. *American Journal of Medical Genetics, Part A* 120 (3): 359–364.

Bailey, D. B., D. Skinner and K. L. Sparkman. 2003. Discovering fragile X syndrome: Family experiences and perceptions. *Pediatrics* 111 (2): 407–416.

Bowekaty, M. B., and D. S. Davis. 2003. Cultural issues in genetic research with American Indian and Alaskan Native People. *IRB: Ethics & Human Research* 25 (4), 12–15.

Burke, W. 2004. Genetic testing, in *Genomic Medicine,* eds. A. E. Guttmacher, F. S. Collins and J. M. Drazen, 14–27. Baltimore: Johns Hopkins University Press.

Coalition for Genetic Fairness. What does GINA Mean? A Guide to the Genetic Information Nondiscrimination Act. http://www.geneticalliance.org/ksc_assets/publications/gina publication.pdf (accessed October 11, 2008).

Codori, A., and J. Brandt. 1994. Psychological costs and benefits of predictive testing for Huntington disease. *American Journal of Medical Genetics* 54: 174–184.

Collins, V., B. Meiser, C. Gaff, D. J. St. John, and J. Halliday. 2005. Screening and preventive behaviors one year after predictive genetic testing for hereditary nonpolyposis colorectal carcinoma. *Cancer* 104: 273–281.

Dendukuri, N., K. Khetani, M. McIssac and J. Brophy. 2007. Testing for HER2-positive breast cancer: A systematic review and cost-effectiveness analysis. *Canadian Medical Association Journal* 176 (10): 1429–1434.

GINA 2008. (Genetic Information Nondiscrimination Act of 2008; HR 493). http://frwebgate. access.gpo.gov/cgi-bin/getdoc.cgi?dbname=110_cong_bills&docid=f:h493enr.txt.pdf (accessed October 11, 2008).

Hamilton, R. J., B. Bowers, and J. K. Williams. 2005. Disclosing genetic test results to family members. *Journal of Nursing Scholarship* 37 (1): 18–24.

Holtzman, N., and M. Watson. 1999. *Promoting safe and effective genetic testing in the United States: Final report of the task force on genetic testing.* Baltimore, MD: Johns Hopkins University Press.

Honda, K. 2003. Who gets the information about genetic testing for cancer risk? The role of race/ethnicity, immigration status, and primary care clinicians. *Clinical Genetics* 64: 131–136.

Hughes, C., A. Gomez-Caminero, J. Benkendorf, J. Kerner, C. Isaacs, J. Barter, and C. Lerman. 1997. Ethnic differences in knowledge and attitudes about BRCA1 testing in women at risk. *Patient Education and Counseling* 32: 51–62.

International Society of Nurses in Genetics (ISONG). 2000. Position statement: Informed decision-making and consent: The role of nursing. http://www.isong.org/about/ps_consent.cfm (accessed October 11, 2008).

Mouchawar, J., S. Hensley-Alford, S. Laurion, J. Ellis, A. Kulchak-Rahm, M. L. Fincane, R. Meenan, L. Axell, R. Pollack and D. Ritzwoller. 2005. Impact of direct-to-consumer advertising for hereditary breast cancer testing on genetic services at a managed care organization: A naturally-occurring experiment. *Genetics in Medicine* 7 (3): 191–197.

National Coalition for Health Professional Education in Genetics (NCHPEG). 2005. *Core competencies in genetics for health professionals.* Third edition. http://www.nchpeg.org/core/Core_Comps_English_2007.pdf (accessed October 11, 2008).

National Human Genome Research Institute. (NHGRI). 2008. Genetic Information Nondiscrimination Act: 2007–2008.

Secretary's Advisory Committee on Genetic Testing. 2000. *A public consultation of oversight of genetic tests.* National Institutes of Health. http://www4.od.nih.gov/oba/sacgt/reports/Public%20Consultation%20Summary.pdf (accessed October 7, 2008).

University of Iowa College of Nursing. 2007. Ethics and genetic testing for nurses. Continuing Education. (CE offering; can be ordered online (accessed October 10, 2008) http://www.nursing.uiowa.edu/continuing_ed/Online_CE_Courses2.htm

U.S. Department of Health and Human Services Office for Civil Rights. 2004. *HIPAA, Medical Privacy: National standards to protect the privacy of personal health information.* http://www.hhs.gov/ocr/hipaa/ (accessed September 10, 2008).

Wolfberg, A. J. 2006. Genes on the web: Direct-to-consumer marketing of genetic testing. *New England Journal of Medicine* 355 (6), 543–545.

Williams, J. K., and D. L. Schutte. 1997. Benefits and burdens of genetic carrier information. *Western Journal of Nursing Research* 19 (1): 71–81.

Williams, J. K., H. Skirton, and A. Masny. 2005. *Ethics, policy, and education issues in genetic testing* 38 (2): 119–125.

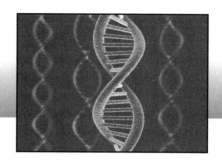

CHAPTER 17

Parental Request for Advanced Directives: Decision Making in Evolving Environments

Robin R. Leger PhD, MS, RN, CCRP

Introduction

Today, we see numbers of children born with congenital anomalies and those who develop serious, life-threatening genetic illnesses despite advances in prevention, screening, and treatment developed over the past century. The questions surrounding the quality of life for these children and their families have generated debate. New discussions of how best to support these families have gathered parents, nurses, other healthcare professionals, lawmakers, policymakers, and philosophers to search for answers.

The common worldview is that children should and will outlive their parents. Sadly, this is not always the case. Parents of children with genetic conditions may need to participate in decisions regarding their child's dying. For family members, neighbors, healthcare providers, and society the dialog regarding decisions to forego therapeutics that would prolong life is challenging. During these difficult times, nurses are in key roles to provide information, anticipatory guidance, and comfort, and to be present with families. Nightingale believed that nursing is care of patients and of the environments of care. These environments include acute and critical care, home, schools, group homes, long-term care and rehabilitation facilities, and hospices. Nurses provide clinical care as well as leadership in facilitating the development of formal and informal guiding principles and infrastructures for making decisions.

Nurses provide care to families who are at different developmental stages when faced with a child's condition incompatible with prolonged or quality life. Decisions may need to be made prior to birth, when the condition is identified by prenatal screening, or during their child's infancy, childhood, adolescence, or adulthood. The context of care varies depending on the setting, severity of illness, genetic condition, professionals involved, and differing social, political, spiritual, and ethical backgrounds. Families may interface with one key professional, a clinical team they have known for years, or a lead representative of a bioethical committee they're meeting with for the first time. They may find themselves leading the establishment of end-of-life care plans with staff from the hospital, school, emergency medical teams, or long-term care facility. Decisions may be made with or without considerations of faith, and in the presence or absence of religious or spiritual support systems. Different criteria for describing their child's condition and future quality of life may be presented by health professionals or these discussions may take place away from families. Policies, guidelines, and protocols for withholding or withdrawing treatments and technology may be in place or there may be a need for guidelines for individual situations and environments.

Rather than providing answers, this chapter will examine guiding principles and reference selected literature that illustrates current policies; a single case scenario would be extremely limiting. Other topics include:

- A review of some of the historic and current literature that has guided decision making.
- The uniqueness of each individual's and family's situation, considering the environment of care.
- Ethical, social, and political contexts of care.
- Peripheral coverage of the extensive literature on palliative care and end-of-life decision making.

The scope of content is this chapter will be limited to genetic conditions that are thought to be lethal, have progressed, or have a changing prognosis incompatible with prolonged quality of life. With growing knowledge of genomic issues and the outcomes of illness, nurses today are even more challenged when caring for these families (Feetham, Thomson, and Hinshaw 2005).

Historical Perspectives

Families, healthcare professionals, and practices in environments of care are influenced by cultural, religious, and political mores as well as scientific and editorial accounts in the literature and public press. The context of this historical review will be limited to practices in the West rather than worldwide, and primarily to events and practices in the last 50 years. Why revisit our history? Alexis de Tocqueville warned us in the 1840s about *historical amnesia,* an abiding weakness of democracies so focused on the excitement of the future that past experiences are forgotten (de Tocqueville, 1956). As a society and as nurses, we may need to revisit our history concerning children with profound genetic conditions, bearing in mind that this background is but one portion of our evolving clinical practice.

Congenital anomalies and selected genetic conditions with visible phenotypic deformities were once thought to be the results of magic, myths, demons, and curses (Curran and Graille 1997). Denis Diderot, the editor of the Encyclopedie (1751–1777), rationally characterized congenital anomalies apart from the understanding of the time as "monstrosities" into a lexicon where anomalies were recognized as natural occurrences. Although he demystified these "products" of life in the supplement "*Monstre,*" Diderot reduced individuals to their anatomical defect (Curran and Graille 1977).

Over the centuries, the arts and society have continued to use those with congenital anomalies as metaphors of subhuman, surreal, or fantastic imagery and for political ends such as to endorse the practice of institutionalization and limit financial resources and services for those affected. Genetic mapping is the newest lexicon to identify human differences and indeed may not be the last in this century. The lexicons, taxonomies, and severity of illness criteria used by healthcare professionals and society may be both an aid in making difficult decisions and a risk for "sliding down slippery slopes" where there is increasing erosion of respect for human dignity.

In the twentieth century, criteria were published that dictated practices in healthcare institutions; these continue to be debated and analyzed from a bioethics prospective. The Harvard Criteria of 1968 were devised as a rigorous means of determining and defining brain death and choices for removing life support. Neurological capacity and sensory motor potential were recognized as defining life rather than heartbeats and respirations (Farrell and Levin 1993).

Scholars continue to be concerned with the role of transplant physicians on decision-making committees that focus on the new aspects of organ transplantation and the emerging value of resuscitation and EEG (electroencephalogram) technology

(Wijdicks 2003). The committee was also praised for its diligence and foresight that led to an array of criteria in other countries. The Harvard Criteria continue to spark ongoing questions about their ethical and utilitarian goals (Wijdicks 2003). Questions continue as to whom or what new science or advances in technology might have been gained by the early decisions over the risks of those experienced by the patients and families.

A landmark article published in Great Britain influenced decisions about treatment of newborns with spina bifida to various extents worldwide. Many clinicians practicing in those years referred to these decision-making guidelines as Lorber's Criteria, named for the physician who noted that babies born with "total paralysis of the legs, a high level of spinal cord lesion, sever kyphosis, hydrocephalus and other major malformation have a poor prognosis" (Lorber 1971). The practice was highly controversial; it drew media attention and, in some cases, legal punitive action. In the 1970s and 1980s, primarily in Europe, there were cases of newborns left untreated; they did not receive shunts for hydrocephalus and surgical closure of the myelomenigocele (Dunne, Bishop, Wright, and Menelaus 1992). Although reports of "non-aggressive treatment" are not readily available, a retrospective study of 120 infants born with open spina bifida between 1971 and 1976 in Great Britain revealed that 71 infants had adverse criteria at birth and were not treated. Of these, 90% died within six months of birth (Lorber and Salfield 1981).

Although this practice was not formally implemented in the United States, it is known in the medical community that untreated children died in the newborn period or later in long-term care facilities, or were later admitted to hospitals with advanced sequalae due to lack of surgical care. Having survived the newborn period, these children would be seen in pediatric specialty centers with large head circumferences, symptoms of chronic hydrocephalus, significant developmental delay, and in need of neurosurgical, orthopaedic, and plastic surgical repair to their spines and other increasing deformity.

In the late 1970s and early 1980s the first articles in the U.S. media appeared regarding cases that sparked the need for professional, institutional, and political policy formation. The first highly publicized case of separating twins joined at the heart included Dr. Koop as a member of the surgical team, which colored his lifelong and somewhat controversial commitment to families and the disabled (U.S. National Library of Medicine, n.d.). Newspapers reported "The twin decision: One must die so one can live… an agonizing choice; parents, doctors, rabbis in dilemma," highlighting the hours and weeks of discussions around ethical issues (Drake 1977). The case of "Baby Doe" in 1982 focused on the parental decision not to surgically correct the obstructed esophagus in their son born with Down syndrome, and the ensuing dilemma involved the courts and U.S. Department of Health and Human

Services regulations over withholding treatment and nutrition in medical institutions. In 1983, the case of "Baby Jane Doe," a neonate with spina bifida, microcephaly, and hydrocephalus brought to light the erratic implementation of Lorber's criteria in the United States and prompted further dialog on the definitions under Section 504 of the Rehabilitation Act of 1973 forbidding discrimination based on a handicap by any person or entity that receives federal funds.

The selection and allocation of medical treatment, the family's level of participation in decisions, and the "rightful" use of societal resources were topics for the agenda. Parental rights and privacy was discussed as issues in the context of the right of the public to have access to their stories. The media reports, sensationalized or sensitive, were often superficial accounts that captured fragments of reality and tried to generalize or validate a particular point of view. In these selected cases—the conjoined twins, "Baby Doe," and "Baby Jane Doe"—the infants died in an atmosphere of care, publicity, and uncertain policy.

Recent reports in the international press and medical journals continue to discuss the extent of euthanasia of severely ill newborns. The "Groningen Protocol," named after a university in the Netherlands, is used for cases in which a decision is made to actively end the life of a newborn (Verhagen and Sauer 2005). There are five criteria in this protocol:

- Suffering must be so severe that the newborn has no prognosis for the future.
- There must be no possibility of a medical or surgical cure.
- Parents must give their consent.
- A second opinion must be provided by an independent and uninvolved physician.
- The ending of life must be meticulously carried out with an emphasis on aftercare.

Issues include defining infant suffering, policymaking and political agendas, the need for honest reporting, and media references to such notorious figures as Doctors Jack Kevorkian (an American physician who has championed a terminal patient's right to die via physician assistance; known as Dr. Death) and Josef Mengele (a German SS officer and physician in Nazi concentration camps who supervised human experimentation without consent; known as the Angel of Death).

The hesitancy of the research and clinical community to develop health status measures for spina bifida and other genetic conditions may be based in our historic experience where treatment and resource allocations were based on prognosis (Leger 2005). Scores for severity of illness and prognostic measures for most genetic conditions do not exist. Even if developed, severity-of-illness scores and quality-of-life criteria are dependent on the sophistication, stability, and sensitivity of the measures used. Often families do not have this information or it is not readily understood. Clinical information for today's decision making consists of laboratory tests of genotyping, blood levels for different disease states (e.g., renal failure), diagnostic imaging that reveals profound neurological or other life-threatening conditions, and pulmonary and other critical organ function tests. These measures and parameters each have their own strengths and limitations when providing guidelines for families and professionals in decisions about withholding or withdrawing life-sustaining technology, and they are only one part of the algorithm. Bioethical debates continue in peer-reviewed journals and inflame dialog in public forums (Singer 1993). One recurring premise is that, in the presence of uncertainty, the benefit of the doubt should be given to survival (Cook 1996).

Guiding Principles within an Ethical, Legal, and Social Context

Individual- and Family-Centered

Decisions need to be patient- and family-centered. The individual's and family's developmental status and needs, cultural and religious backgrounds, and presence of social supports should be assessed and validated. A variety of scenarios demonstrate unique challenges. They include but are not limited to:

- prenatal (in vitro and prenatal screening);
- newborns at the threshold of viability (with select genetic problems that are lethal or complex congenital anomalies and those not responding to intensive care therapeutics);
- childhood conditions with disease progression; and
- the aging adult with a chronic and potentially disabling genetic condition experiencing advanced pathology.

The impact of prenatal diagnosis (early maternal serum screening, chorionic villus sampling of tissue taken from the developing placental tissue, often 10–12 weeks into the pregnancy, and mid-trimester amniocentesis for DNA analysis to screen for genetic conditions) has influenced choices for electing termination or continuing the pregnancy. Therapeutic interventions for women who continue pregnancy include advanced pharmaceutical and surgical treatments where maternal side effects and long-term effects on growth and development in the child are as yet unknown (Alving and Gunther 2004). Nurses in advanced pediatric specialty or genetic programs provide anticipatory guidance and information to women carrying a fetus identified with a genetic condition. Nurse need to be experienced and trained in genetics and counseling, and knowledgeable about the condition and its various prognostic potentials (Beery and Hern 2004; Horner 2004; Jenkins, Grady, and Collins 2005; Lewis 2001; Loescher and Merkle 2005). Sensitivity is needed in providing information in unbiased terms and in a private and unhurried environment to the parents and their support system.

Seamless Across Environments of Care

Advances in the healthcare delivery system (especially neonatal and pediatric critical care settings) and the transfer of care from medical institutions to the community have further influenced end-of-life choices and the withholding and withdrawing of technical, medical, or therapeutic supports (Caitlin and Carter 2002). Community environments include (but are not limited to) schools, emergency medical teams, home care, medical day care, respite programs, and group homes. Many of these settings are responding by developing protocols and standards of care, establishing parameters and committees for bioethics, and creating resources for families.

In 1991, the federal Patient Self-Determination Act (PSDA) required hospitals and nursing homes participating in Medicare/Medicaid programs to inform adult patients of their rights for advance directives and to document that they had done so. The PSDA guidelines include: 1) the right to participate and direct one's own health care, 2) the right to accept or refuse medical or surgical treatment, 3) the right to prepare an advance directive, and 4) information on the provider's policy that governs the utilization of these rights. PSDA prohibits institutions from discriminating against a patient who does not have an advance directive and requires institutions to document and provide ongoing community education on advance directives. The PSDA guidelines facilitated practice changes in a number of environments, for children as well as adults. Today, advance directives are in place in settings as varied as delivery rooms (Toce 2001; Toce, Leuthner, Dokken, Carter, and Catlin 2004), neonatal intensive care units (Catlin and Carter 2002), pediatric emergency rooms (Walsh-Kelly, Lang, Chevako, Blank, Korom, Kirk, et al. 1999), operating rooms (Fallat and Deshpande 2004), schools (AAP 2000), and pediatric palliative care and hospice programs (Himelstein, Hilden, Boldt, and Weissman 2004; Rushton 2004; Sandler, Kennedy, and Shapiro 2004).

Pre-hospital advanced directives (PHADs) are implemented in some states and provide critical policies for the community environments of care, first responders and EMTs, and emergency departments (Walsh-Kelly et al. 1999). Physicians may include a "Comfort Care Order" with a DNR (Do Not Resuscitate) order that includes what, if any, individualized comfort measures should be given to a child or adult, where they should be moved if in a public area such as in school, who of their family and social supports should be notified, who should make the pronouncement of death, and how to make funeral arrangements. Comfort Care and DNR orders often include a medical bracelet and arrangements with pre-hospital emergency care providers. Professional associations have developed protocols for DNR orders to be integrated into the student's individual education plan (IEP) with Individual Healthcare and Emergency Care Plans (IHP, IECP) for students covered under Section 504 of the Rehabilitation Act or Public Law 94–142 (AAP 2000; Himelstein, Hilden, Boldt, and Weissman 2004). The American Academy of Pediatrics (AAP) recommends that parents of children at risk of dying at school who desire an advance directive meet with their IEP or school health team and pediatrician to develop DNR orders; review as needed and at a minimum of every 6 months; utilize and collaborate with the board of education, local emergency response services, and legal counsel as needed; and include educational and support services about death and dying for the student community (AAP 2000). A guide to multidisciplinary team assessment, planning, and management for pediatric palliative care is available for promoting proactive critical decisions. *Essential Elements in the Approach to Pediatric Palliative Care* includes five practice spheres: physical concerns, psychosocial concerns, spiritual concerns, advance care planning, and practical concerns which align with assessment and planning options (Himelstein, Hilden, Boldt, and Weissman 2004).

Awareness of the Quality of Life Debate

Quality of life remains a key consideration in choosing between aggressive, limited, or no treatment (Rushton 2004). Does severity of illness influence how we measure an individual's goal of independence and productivity? Each individual's understanding of quality of life and quality of death depends on many variables—their developmental and cognitive levels and their social, emotional, cultural, and spiritual experiences. Families of children with chronic genetic conditions are often linked to other families with the same condition and to local and national support groups that can contact them with others who have similarly witnessed the decline in health and eventual death. At times, families are better prepared for their loved one's imminent death than the healthcare providers around them. There continues to be a shortage in pediatric organ donation despite family's willingness, sense of value in donating, and the positive impact on the bereavement process (Morris, Wilcox, and Frist 1992).

Nondiscrimination in the use of lifesaving measures is considered an obligation of healthcare providers. They are in a position to assess a family's understanding of the situation and consider consent issues and proxy consents by ethical boards when needed. An understanding of autonomy and the developmental understanding of death is imperative (Himilstein, Hilden, Boldt, and Weissman 2005; Karns 2002).

Activities and initiatives are beginning to focus on a lifespan approach to "living well with a disability" (CDC 2002). The Centers for Disease Control and Prevention (CDC) reintroduced its mission to promote health and quality of life by preventing and controlling disease, injury, and disability by opening the National Center for Birth Defects, Developmental Disabilities, and Disability and Health in 2002. This groundbreaking facility provides an integrated forum for organizations and agencies concerned with disability, and does so under a lifespan model. Now, marginally funded and primarily pediatric and family- or consumer-run associations are being recognized by prominent adult disability organizations. This integration of groups allows for a critical mass effect under the umbrella benefits of the CDC, which can have implications for policy development and implementation.

The two primary goals of *Healthy People 2010* are to increase the quality and years of healthy life and to eliminate health disparities (Betz 2002). The first goal promotes initiatives and research on preventing secondary conditions, promoting health, and improving or maintaining health-related quality of life (HRQOL). The second identifies the area of disparities an area where care and research efforts are nearly nonexistent.

Preventing Disparities in Health Care: Observations at the Beginning of the Twenty-first Century

Disparities in health care include new and old orphans of health care (conditions that have not received adequate attention for diagnosis, prevention, or treatment). Some common genetic conditions (spina bifida and sickle cell disease, to name two) and many rare genetic disorders have been and remain orphans of care. Disparities in healthcare services exist for disenfranchised groups or patient populations without fiscal or political power to attract support from the healthcare insurance industry (Smedley, Stith and Nelson 2003). Today, disparities take on a new face with the aging of youth with genetic conditions. Faced with healthcare reform and cutbacks in healthcare finances, many pediatric specialty clinics across the country that provided multidisciplinary comprehensive services to children have closed some or all of their services. The mean age of the population is approaching adulthood. Yet the transition of care for adults with genetic conditions to primary and specialty care is hampered with obstacles and a lack of funding (Blum 1995; Kaufman, Terbrock, Winters, Ito, Klosterman and Parks 1994; Leger, Burke, Dunleavy, and Engelmann 1998; Rosen 1994).

Currently there is a lack of transition services to specialty adult healthcare providers. Individuals with chronic genetic conditions may be discriminated against in subtle ways but with significant impact (Turner-Henson, Holady, Corsen, Olgetree, and Swan 1994). They may need little day-to-day pharmaceuticals and little medical or surgical care, which in turn make them not an attractive investment to the pharmaceutical or insurance industries. The ethical dilemma: how do we as a society continue to care and provide resources for those living with genetic conditions while they age, and do these families experience stigmatization that continues throughout the life span?

Summary

In this evolving human genome era, ethical issues will continue to evolve and nurses are key contributors to the dialog and direct responders and participants in care. Central to the solution is a patient and family-centered, individualized, and culturally appropriate approach. Assessment of families' developmental needs and implementation of policies across care settings should be collaborative and seamless. Integration of curative and palliative care from the very beginning of diagnosis and treatment throughout the individual's lifespan may eliminate feelings of crisis and abandonment (Sandler, Kennedy, and Shapiro 2004). Bioethical reviews of international policies, clinical pathways that promote state-of-the-art pain management and comfort measures, and consumer resources need to be ongoing (Frankel, Goldworth, Rorty, and Silverman 2005; Rushton 2004).

There is a dearth of research and evidenced-based practice in this area. Follow-up family interviews (Culbert and Davis 2005; Glassford 2003; Sandler, Kennedy, and Shapiro 2004; Seecharan, Andrersen, Norris, and Toce 2004) and healthcare provider's perspectives of their understanding and experiences (Anderson, Seecharan, and Toce 2004; Schwarz 2003) are just making their way into the literature. High-risk therapeutic clinical trials for treating or curing genetic conditions have made front page news. The decision-making process in clinical research includes the concept "equipoise": randomly selecting one of several competing treatments if there is genuine uncertainty in the expert medical community—not necessarily on the part of the individual investigator—about the preferred treatment (Freedman 1987). Equipoise, an initial state of genuine uncertainty, can likewise guide nurses as they evaluate each encounter with ethical decision making in genetics.

References

Alving, E. P., and D. F. Gunther. 2004. Congenital adrenal hyperplasia. In *Primary Care of the Child with a Chronic Condition,* 4th ed. eds. P. Jackson Allen and J. A. Vessey. St. Louis, MO: Mosby.

American Academy of Pediatrics (AAP). 2000. Committee on School Health and Committee on Bioethics. Policy statement: Do not resuscitate in schools. *Pediatrics* 105: 878–879.

Anderson, E., G. A. Seecharan and S. Toce. 2004. Provider perspective of child deaths. *Archives of Pediatric and Adolescent Medicine* 158: 430–435.

Beery, T. A., and M. J. Hern. 2004. Genetic practice, education, and research: An overview for advanced practice nurses. *Clinical Nurse Specialist* 18: 126–132.

Betz, C. L. 2002. Healthy Children 2002: Implications for pediatric nursing practice. *Journal of Pediatric Nursing* 17: 153–156.

Blum, R. W. 1995. Transition to adult health care: Setting the stage. *Journal of Adolescent Health* 17: 3–5.

Catlin, A., and B. Carter. 2002. Creation of a neonatal end-of-life palliative care protocol. *Journal of Perinatology* 22: 184–195.

Centers for Disease Control and Prevention (CDC). 2002. *Introducing the CDC's newest center: National center on birth defects and developmental disabilities, disabilities and health.* Atlanta, GA: CDC.

Cook, R. E. 1996. Ethics, law, and developmental disabilities. In *Developmental disabilities in infancy and childhood: Neurodevelopmental diagnosis and treatment.* Volume I of Developmental Disabilities in Infancy and Childhood. 2nd ed. eds. A. J. Capute and P. J. Accardo. Baltimore: Paul H. Brookes Publishing Co.

Culbert, A., and D. J. Davis. 2005. Parental preferences for neonatal resuscitation research consent: A pilot study. *Journal of Medical Ethics* 31: 721–726.

Curran, A., and P. Graille. 1997. The faces of eighteenth-century monstrosity. *Eighteenth-Century Life* 21 (2): 1–15.

De Tocqueville, Alexis. 1956. *Democracy in America,* ed. Richard Heffner. New York: New American Library.

Drake, D. C. 1977. The twins decision: One must die so one can live. *The Philadelphia Inquirer,* October 16. http://profiles.nlm.nih.gov/QQ/B/B/X/Z/_/qqbbxz.pdf (accessed October 7, 2008).

Dunne, K. B., J. Bishop, S. Wright, and M. B. Menelaus. 1992. Are adults with spina bifida receiving adequate medical and rehabilitation care? *Developmental Medicine and Child Neurology* 34 (Suppl.): 6–8.

Fallat, M. E., J. K. Deshpande, American Academy of Pediatrics Section on Surgery, Section on Anesthesia and Pain Medicine, and Committee on Bioethics. 2004. Do-not-resuscitate orders for pediatric patients who require anesthesia and surgery. *Pediatrics* 114: 1686–1692.

Farrell, M. M., and D. L. Levin. 1993. Brain death in the pediatric patient: Historical, sociological, medical, religious, cultural, legal, and ethical considerations. *Critical Care Medicine* 21: 1951–1965.

Feetham, S., E. J. Thomson, and A. S. Hinshaw. 2005. Nursing leadership in genomics for health and society. *Journal of Nursing Scholarship* 37: 102–110.

Frankel, L. R., A. Goldworth, M. V. Rorty, and W. A. Silverman. 2005. *Ethical dilemmas in pediatrics*. Cambridge, England: Cambridge University Press.

Freedman, B. 1987. Equipoise and the ethics of clinical research. *The New England Journal of Medicine* 317 (3): 141–145.

Glassford, B. 2003. Ethical issues: A case study in caring: Trisomy 18 syndrome. *American Journal of Nursing* 103: 81–83.

Himelstein, B. P., J. M. Hilden, A. M. Boldt, and D. Weissman. 2004. Medical progress: Pediatric palliative care. *The New England Journal of Medicine* 350: 1752–1762.

Horner, S. D. 2004. A genetic course for advanced clinical nursing practice. *Clinical Nurse Specialist* 18: 194–199.

Jenkins, J., P. Grady, and F. Collins. 2005. Nurses and the genomic revolution. *Journal of Nursing Scholarship* 37 (2): 98–101.

Karns, J. T. 2002. Children's understanding of death. *Journal of Clinical Activities and Handouts in Psychotherapy Practice* 2: 43–50.

Kaufman, B. A., A. Terbrock, N. Winters, J. Ito, A. Klosterman, and T. S. Parks. 1994. Disbanding a multidisciplinary clinic: Effects on the health care of myelomeningocele patients. *Pediatric Neurosurgery* 21: 36–44.

Leger, R. R. 2005. Severity of illness, functional status, and HRQOL in youth with spina bifida. *Rehabilitation Nursing* 30: 180–187.

Leger, R. R., M. L. Burke, M. J. Dunleavy, and J. Engelmann. 1998. *The transition to adult living program: Health services for young adults with spina bifida*. Boston: The Genetic Resource.

Lewis, J. A. 2001. The human genome and public policy: A nursing prospective. *Journal of Obstetrics, Gynecology, and Neonatal Nursing* 30: 541–545.

Loescher, L. J., and C. J. Merkle. 2005. The interface of genomic technologies and nursing. *Journal of Nursing Scholarship* 37: 111–119.

Lorber, J. 1971. Results of treatment of myelomeningocele: An analysis of 524 unselected cases, with special references to possible selection for treatment. *Developmental and Child Neurology* 13: 279–303.

Lorber, J., and S. A. Salfield. 1981. Results of selective treatment of spina bifida cystica. *Archives of Diseases of Childhood* 56: 822–830.

Morris, J. A., T. R.Wilcox, and W. H. Frist. 1992. Pediatric organ donation: The paradox of organ shortage despite the remarkable willingness of families to donate. *Pediatrics* 89: 411–415.

Report of the Ad Hoc Committee of the Harvard Medical School to Examine the Definition of Brain Death. 1968. A definition of irreversible coma. *Journal of the American Medical Association* 205: 337–340.

Rosen, D. S. 1994. Transition from pediatric to adult-oriented health care for the adolescent with a chronic illness or disability. *Adolescent Medicine: State of the Art Reviews* 5: 241–248.

Rushton, C. H. 2004. Ethics and palliative care in pediatrics: When should parents agree to withdraw life-sustaining therapy for children? *American Journal of Nursing* 104: 54–63.

Sandler, I., C. Kennedy, and E. Shapiro. 2004. Parental grief and palliative care require attention. *Archives of Pediatric and Adolescent Medicine* 158: 590–591.

Schwarz, J. K. 2003. Understanding and responding to patients' request for assistance in dying. *Journal of Nursing Scholarship* 35: 377–384.

Seecharan, G., E. M. Andrersen, K. Norris, and S. S. Toce. 2004. Parents' assessment of quality care and grief following a child's death. *Archives of Pediatric and Adolescent Medicine* 158: 590–591.

Singer, P. 1993. *Taking life: Humans* in *Practical ethics: Second Edition*. Cambridge, England: Cambridge University Press. 175–217.

Smedley, B., A. Y. Stith, and A. Nelson, eds. 2003. *Unequal treatment: Confronting racial and ethnic disparities in health care*. Committee on Understanding and Eliminating Racial and Ethnic Disparities in Health Care, Board on Health Science Policy, The Institute of Medicine. Washington, D. C.: The National Academies Press.

Toce, S. S. 2001. Ethical decision making in the delivery room. *Focus on Pediatrics* (Spring).

Toce, S. S., S. R. Leuthner, D. L. Dokken, B. Carter, and A. Catlin. 2004. Applying palliative care principles to the care of high risk newborns. In *Palliative care for infants, children and adolescents: A practical handbook*, eds. B. Carter and M. Levetown. Baltimore: John Hopkins University Press.

Turner-Henson, A., B. Holady, N. Corsen, G. Olgetree, and J. Swan. 1994. The experience of discrimination: Challenges for chronically ill children. *Pediatric Nursing* 20: 571–577.

Verhagen, E., and P. J. J. Sauer. 2005. The Groningen protocol—Euthanasia in severely ill newborns. *New England Journal of Medicine* 352: 959–962.

U.S. National Library of Medicine. n.d. Congenital birth defects and the medical rights of children: The 'Baby Doe' controversy. in The C. Everett Koop Papers. http://profiles.nlm.nih.gov/QQ/Views/Exhibit/visuals/babydoe.html (accessed October 7, 2008).

Walsh-Kelly, C. M., K. R. Lang, J. Chevako, E. L. Blank, N. Korom, K. Kirk, and A. Gray. 1999. Advanced directives in a pediatric emergency department. *Pediatrics* 103: 826–830.

Wijdicks, E. F. 2003. The neurologist and the Harvard criteria for brain death. *Neurology* 61: 970–976.

CHAPTER 18

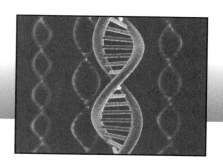

Ethical Analysis of
Genetic Testing in Children

John G. Twomey, PhD, PNP

Introduction

The increasing capacity of genetic testing technologies provides more opportunities for disease-related genes to be identified. Currently, over 1400 disease genes have been mapped (http://www.geneclinics.org accessed October 7, 2008). However, the applicability of these individual tests to clinical application and subsequent health promotion is very unclear. For example, the expression of many identifiable genetic mutations, such as variations of the Cystic Fibrosis Transmembrane Conductance regulator (CFTR) gene, can produce so many different symptoms that gene testing alone is insufficient for the health counseling that families need (McKone, Emerson, Edwards, and Aitken 2003).

What is clear is that if members of our society are going to begin to reap even some of health benefits from this ongoing flow of genomic information, healthcare professionals must be prepared to discuss options available in many areas. Recognition that genomic health information can be provided to consumers only through vigorous educational and training efforts has moved the healthcare professions to focus on varied ways of transmitting such information to its members, including integration of genetic information into basic education programs as well as ongoing education programs (National Coalition for Health Professional Education in Genetics 2005).

Role of Nursing

The nursing profession plays a critical leadership role in the genetic health of the nation. The ongoing coalition between the American Nurses Association (ANA) and the International Society of Nurses in Genetics (ISONG) has produced documents, such as *Statement on the Scope and Standards of Genetics Clinical Nursing Practice* (ANA 1998) and *Genetics/Genomics Nursing: Scope and Standards of Practice* (ANA and ISONG 2006), that lay claim to a central role for nursing in genomic health. This role is recognized by commentators outside the profession, who have noted that nurses have the most logical role in the genetic counseling process because of their numbers and presence throughout the healthcare system (Fletcher 2001).

Maternal Child Nursing and Parental Decision Making

Nurses who care for families have long been involved in advising parents about the genetic aspect of children's health because of the historic nature of genetic awareness. Genetic diseases have traditionally been recognized more in children who are diagnosed with illnesses requiring immediate symptom management, such as sickle cell disease, hemophilia, and others. While the emphasis in such areas is usually on amelioration of symptoms, the genetic aspect of such symptoms and how the etiology of the disease may affect other family members is never far from the surface of parental concerns. They may need information to pass on to other family members, and they may wonder what knowledge will be needed in the future to counsel children who are growing into their own childbearing years and may not understand how a sibling's illness may be reflected within the family genome.

Parents may also seek information from RNs when they learn about the genetic nature of their own illnesses. For example, primary concerns of parents who have been diagnosed with a cancer with possible genetic links, such as breast cancer, tend to include the risk of passing the gene to their children, as well as its impact on other family members (Patenaude 2004). But assessing such risk and helping to provide recommendations about further investigation into the family genome are very complex, depending on the genetic condition of interest and other factors, such as family constellation, ethnic heritage, and other aspects of health that impact genetic expression of symptoms. Because of the multifactorial aspect of some genetic illnesses, RNs are faced with complex sets of data as they help parents address questions that arise. Because an essential part of this nursing care may be continued genetic testing within the family, special considerations must be paid to the questions that genetic testing engenders.

Scope of Genetic Assessment in Pediatrics

It is probably a misnomer to refer to a genetic "test." Such language conjures an image akin to having a child checked for strep throat by swabbing a throat culture. Not only does the procedure sound straightforward, it suggests that the results will be clear and concise and will provide unambiguous guidelines to parents and clinicians about how to proceed. Of course, few biomedical tests are so simple. Chest x-rays, complete blood counts, even blood pressure readings, are procedures that represent only part of the assessment process of most acute and chronic health conditions. Genetic tests are no different, for the molecular testing one thinks of when referring to a chromosomal or specific gene test is usually done only as part of a larger health workup. For RNs working with families, it is more appropriate to use "genetic assessment" when referring to the process of examining the risk for or the presence of existent disease mutations.

The concept of genetic assessment becomes easier to understand and much more comprehensive when one realizes that many genetic illnesses are diagnosed without a classic genetic "test." The notion that a genetic test is an examination of chromosomes or specific genes contained in blood or tissue specimens is a very limited one. Consider that many genetic illnesses are diagnosed indirectly, such as when sickle cell disease is determined to be present by both the characteristic symptoms and the serologic testing that quantifies the types of typical hemoglobins present in the disease state. One only has to think back to the royal families of Europe in the late nineteenth and early twentieth centuries to understand that none of the forms of hemophilia present back then were found via examination of genes. Despite the lack of genetic technologies then, there was no doubt of the genetic nature of the condition.

So if we expand the concept of genetic testing to genetic assessment, we have a better base to understand how families experience the arrival of genetic illness. Consider how families encounter an illness such as neurofibromatosis2 (NF2), a disease of the acoustic nervous system that occurs when a genetic mutation causes tumors, known as schwannomas, to grow and impinge on the acoustic nerve and cause symptoms such as tinnitus, deafness, and balance problems. New mutations will often occur in young adulthood, after the patient has married and had children, who are in turn at risk for this autosomal dominant illness. The diagnosis is made by clinical examination and imaging of the tumors (Lim, Rubenstein, Evans, Jacks, Seizinger, Baser, et al. 2000). Parents must decide whether to supplement surveillance of their children with an examination of the 22q12.2 chromosome for NF2. In this case, the genetic assessment, augmented by the chromosomal analysis, will result in a parent being given information that will not be used immediately for medical benefit but instead may enable them to consider future family directions as they live with a chronic illness.

Today we have expanded the scope of genetic assessment to include many procedures that provide data about family health, including probably the most important one, the family history. Now we know can better appreciate the vast array of data about genomic health that RNs need to best counsel their patients. Even a preliminary list of occasions when parents can expect to confront opportunities to obtain genomic information should impress us with the preparation necessary to assist with the possible decision:

- The prenatal period—Parents now can access assess genomic risks both in the
  - Pre-pregnancy period, when partners may be screened for the presence or absence of disease genes or as part of the assisted fertilization process, when molecular examination of cellular components of the fertilization process can accomplish the same goal, and in the
  - Pregnancy period, when the fetus can be screened for chromosomal or individual genetic abnormalities.
- The perinatal period—Newborn children are exposed to an intense genetic scrutiny, as comprehensive newborn health assessment includes physical examinations and mandatory serological screening for batteries of illnesses that may not be immediately evident on examination.
- Infancy through adolescence—Through accepted schedules of expected health assessments throughout childhood, the genetic health of growing youth is appraised through history and physical examination to determine increasing risk for heritable illnesses such as hypertension, diabetes, and asthma.

Ethical Issues in Genetic Assessment

The essential nature of genetic information is shared data, details about individual health that have implications beyond the person being assessed. So when RNs are approached by parents about making decisions about doing further genetic assessments of their children, the situation resonates with meanings for others. Not only do RNs have the basic ethical duty their profession mandates to protect such information (ANA 2001), in addition, nurses who specialize in genetic practice have adopted special ethical recommendations for those who counsel patients about genetic assessment (ISONG 2005). Specifically, nurses must take into consideration such duties as the preservation of autonomy of the individual seeking a genetic assessment, and provide counseling of the potential benefits that may accrue by gaining more information, noting the risks that new information about one's genome may provide little medical benefit but deliver distressing news about one's health. These ethical obligations do not seem new or unique, so why should nurses working with families make such strong efforts to concentrate on ethic issues?

Who Is the Patient?

In 2001, ANA published *Code of Ethics for Nurses with Interpretive Statements,* which represented a total rewriting of past iterations of its code. One of the most important modifications made to the code was to widely define the recipient of nursing services as anyone who is the object of nursing care. This means that the concept of patient extends beyond the individual to encompass groups, such as families. This is a model of patient care that that had been adopted by the genetics nursing community and articulated within their position statement "Informed Decision-Making and Consent: The Role of Nursing" (ISONG 2000), which recognizes the role of the family in genetic health decisions. It is reiterated in the group's newly updated position statement "Privacy and Confidentiality of Genetic Information: The Role of the Nurse" (ISONG 2005), in which the autonomy of the individual is recognized while the inseparable role of that person's family members is also highlighted. The result is that nurses in any setting who are providing genomic care can never look at the individual in isolation, but must use the concept of the person-within-a-group.

This does not mean that information obtained about a single patient may be freely shared without permission. Indeed, the requirement is just the opposite. Because the nature of genetic information is an immutable mapping of individuality that provides data about both past and future health and may have multiple interpretations, the such information must be zealously guarded. The key parts of including the family while providing nursing care to the individual are explaining the implications for the synergistic nature of genetic information, and considering that family members have a strong interest in, though not necessarily rights to, any information found in a genetic assessment that may affect their health.

Theoretical Background

Bioethical thinking in genetics has followed the same theoretical framework that healthcare ethics in general has adhered to. The hierarchical principled system of moral behavior that uses the ethical theories of *deontology* and *utilitarianism* is quite familiar to healthcare professionals (Beauchamp and Childress 2001). Because the seeming contrast between the two theories—deontological thought demands that specific rules that directly lead to specific goods be followed no matter what collateral effects occur, while utilitarian thought dictates that moral decisions be based on the greatest good that derives from an act—would suggest that choices need to be made between one theory or another, principled theory appeals to both to support its dictums. For example, when the principle of autonomy, which supports individual rights over the collective and is supported by deontology, is challenged by the principle of justice, which almost always uses utilitarianism to support actions that provide health goods that are community-based rather than individual in nature, principled theory allows both considerations to be weighed and the decision made in favor of the principle which seems overriding in a given situation.

One critique of principlism derives from the dilemmas that adhering to its guidelines frequently lead to. When does one principle trump another? In genetic ethics, a frequent ethical issue involves sharing genetic information between family members. Should the autonomy of the proband found to have a serious heritable illness be honored when he refuses to share such information with at-risk family members? When would the potential benefits to having such information support the possible risk of harm that releasing such information might entail? A second critique of principlism involves the evolution of the individual in Western society. Because the concept of autonomy has come to exert much influence in our current ethical deliberations, it is difficult to weigh the other principles properly when juxtaposed to the broad model of individuality prevalent in today's society.

Despite these weaknesses, principled ethical theory is probably going to maintain its preeminent position in our health system. Because it is expressed in language that is easily understandable, it has been taught now for two generations of healthcare professional education, composes the basic language of many bioethical guidelines, and even has been written into health policy law (Evans 2000). Any examination of its role in genetic ethics should seek not to eliminate it but to determine where it fails to support our moral actions and provide some other framework to enhance it and strengthen our moral behaviors.

Parents, Children, and Genetic Ethics

The formalized parent–child ethics that RNs share with other family health professions follows a framework based on the principled theory already presented. In brief, the following interpretation (Miller and Nelson 2006) of the principles is accepted:

- Minor children (from birth until the eighteenth birthday in most societies) are not considered autonomous decision makers, legally or ethically. Instead they are seen as developing a capacity for the autonomy they will achieve with adulthood. Because children develop cognitively at individual rates, parents and healthcare professionals are urged to include them in healthcare decisions as far as their individual capacities for understanding dictates;

- Because parents are the principal protectors and decision makers for their children, their role in the developing capacity for autonomy of their children is primarily to protect and nurture it;

- In order to best serve the child's need for protection, parents are expected to make healthcare decisions that maximize benefit and minimize risks of harm. While that is a normal decisional equation for anyone, adults are allowed much more leeway in accepting risks for themselves in medical decisions than they are for their children.

A case example of this model would be the family that belongs to the Jehovah's Witnesses faith and adheres to its dictums not to accept blood product transfusions. It is clear that healthcare professionals would have to honor the parents' refusal of a transfusion for one of themselves and would have to refuse to honor refusal of a needed transfusion for one of their young children. For an older child who is nearing adulthood, his or her ability to understand the implications of agreeing with the parent's request would weigh heavily on any arbiter asked to rule whether or not to respect the family's decision to refuse.

Evolution of Ethical Thought about Children and Genetic Assessment

It is against this backdrop of ethical thinking that genetics professionals have begun to consider the possibilities of parental requests of genetic assessment for their children (Wertz, Fanos, and Reilly 1994). Because of the recognition that there were theoretical risks to children if tested for genetic illness, there was a consensus that any such risk should be at least balanced, if not outweighed, by the benefits of such a test. After a period of discussion within the genetics community, advisory statements about the genetic testing of children were issued that recommended caution when parents were requesting genetic assessments that did not seem to offer any direct benefit to the child and might be simply an attempt by a parent to access genetic information about their child (The American Society of Human Genetics Board of Directors and the American College of Medical Genetics Board of Directors 1995; Nelson, Botkijn, Kodish, Levetown, Truman, and Wilfond 2001).

Examples of how the type of assessment requested can affect the ethics of the request can be seen in two different types of cancer genetics. In colon cancer caused by familial adenomatous polyposis (FAP), children who inherit the autosomal dominant mutated gene will develop cancer sometime in the future. If the mutation is discovered, early surveillance can lead to necessary surgical intervention to avoid the certain spread of the cancer. Women with heritable breast cancer also have an autosomal dominant gene mutation. However, any relative they share the mutation with, including their children (males with this BRCA mutation also have increased breast and prostate cancer risks), has only a higher, and unknown, risk of developing related cancers, such as breast and ovarian disease. A parent seeking genetic assessment for the BRCA genes for a child would receive information that could just suggest a need for higher surveillance that will only be of benefit later in life, for young children do not develop the illnesses caused by the BRCA genes.

Another opportunity for parents to gain genetic information early in a child's life is currently being offered to an increasing number of new parents in states that choose to offer cystic fibrosis (CF) testing through their newborn screening programs (Wilfond and Gollust 2005). By testing for the most frequent of the mutations of the CFTR gene that causes CF, infants can be screened to discern if they have a mutation. This is an autosomal recessive illness that requires one copy of the gene to be inherited from each parent, and the screening will only show the presence or absence of the gene, not the characteristics of any copies that may be present. A positive screen will need to be followed by more specific diagnostic tests to see if a child with a positive test result has the illness or is simply a carrier.

There appears to a small amount of nutritional benefit from early diagnosis of CF in healthy-appearing infants by screening rather than waiting for symptoms to develop; this is the basis for the assessment. However, it appears from data that about 90% (modal) of positive screens result in the discovery of infant CF carriers and only about 10% will actually have the illness (Wilfond and Gollust 2005). Knowing that one is a carrier for a genetic illness is not immediately beneficial to children, and whether they will use such information for health promotion as they grow into adulthood has been questioned (Fanos and Johnson 1995a). So how can such screening that does not impart benefits to such a large percentage of children assessed be ethically justified?

Harms from Genetic Assessment?

One reason that people, including parents and professionals, find such decisions to be morally acceptable is because they believe that the group not incurring any benefits is also exposed to few risks when assessed, even if information about their individual genomes is discovered. But it certainly is hard to claim that the children's information gained through newborn screening programs will be protected until they mature, as the information will be passed from state labs to health clinic records to families who very well may share the information with others within and outside the family. Is this harmful, and if so, is it acceptable?

The concept of harm occurring secondary to genetic assessment has been discussed within the genetic and ethics professional groups but has been hard to quantify. This is because of the tenuous nature of risk (Hoedemaekers 1998). Most rational parents will vigorously protect their child from a known risk, such refusing to let them walk to school across a dangerous highway. But when risk is less clear or not imminent, such as allowing their children to eat less nutritious foods than recommended to avoid obesity and resultant illnesses, many parents will be less inclined to act. So if RNs are to provide counseling about genetic assessment, it would be useful to see how parents tend to behave when faced with decisions that require a balancing of benefits and risks of harm.

Risks of genetic assessment are not traditional in the medical sense of risk. Drawing blood for DNA analysis holds little risk beyond a bruise on the arm; even when imaging technologies such as magnetic resonance imaging devices are employed, safety procedures will avoid injury. So physical risks are almost absent in genetic assessment. Instead, most professionals worry about risks that derive from the assessment process that are psychosocial in nature, particularly mental health issues.

Research into Harms of Genetic Assessment in Children

Concerns about the effects on children after receiving information from a genetic assessment have focused on depression, anxiety, fear, and other related emotional reactions to the news that a genetic illness has been discovered within a family and that they are at risk. Whether the genetic assessment performed is presymptomatic, such as the test for FAP, or just predispositonal, as are the results from the BRCA gene testing, the small studies that have been done fail to show significant harm because of the testing. These studies have covered a fairly broad grouping of disease mutations:

- Twenty children aged 11–17 who lived in families with hereditary breast cancer were surveyed about feelings of stress and anxiety using a modified scale about cancer worries, and also completed standardized measures of depression (State-Trait Anxiety Inventory Scale, Reynolds Adolescent Depression Scale). The results did not show any unusual cancer worries or increased psychological adjustment problems (Tercyak, Peshkin, DeMarco, Brogan, and Lerman 2002; Tercyak, Peshkin, Streisand, and Lerman 2001).

- Two studies followed children after being tested for the adenomatous polyposis coli gene mutation (APC) that is linked with FAP. Forty-eight children were followed for 38 months and administered scales measuring anxiety, behavioral problems, and depression. In both groups, 22 positives and 26 negatives, no long-term psychological effects were found (Codori, Zawacki, Petersen, Miglioretti, Bacon, and Trimbath 2003). In another study of children tested for APC, no increases in psychological stress were found in either the positive or the negative group who completed the four measures of depression, stress, self-esteem, and anxiety (Michie, Bobrow, and Marteau 2001).

- In a study of 46 families that tested their daughters aged 5–17 for either the Duchenne muscular dystrophy or the hemophilia A gene mutations, about two-thirds of the parents notified the child of their status as either an unaffected carrier or not a carrier. This group and a group of 25 siblings tested for carrier status for a lysosomal storage disease were followed for 10–24 months after testing. They were administered a 100-item questionnaire that combined the RAND Health Survey with items developed by the investigators that queried about satisfaction with the testing process. The majority (78%) of the participants did not report feeling any harms from being tested; the most reported feeling was relief at finding that they were not a carrier (Jarvinen, Lehesjoki, Lindlof, Uutela, and Kaariainen 2000).

There may be some late effects of being tested as a child for a genetic illness and finding that one is a carrier. Fifty-four adults misinterpreted their results as having health implications that were inaccurate, such as that they had no personal risk for developing the illness or that being a carrier predisposed them to developing respiratory illnesses. Many of these siblings expressed guilt over being a healthy child with an ill sibling, but this is not necessarily related to the test (Fanos and Johnson 1995a, 1995b). Another group of 27 unaffected adults who were tested as children to analyze the pattern of mutation for ataxia-telangiectasia, a progressive neurocognitive disorder, in their siblings reported generalized anxiety about the procedure and the meaning of the test results. A lack of genetic counseling seems to have contributed to this group's feelings about the testing experience (Fanos 1999).

An Alternative Ethical Framework

If considerations of immediate benefit or harm do not seem to drive the genetic assessment decisions of parents about their children, how then can RNs provide guidance to parents when they seek counsel about the appropriateness of their alternatives? In other words, is the ethical framework currently being used in genetic health care sufficient to support current practice?

Alternative ethical frameworks for examining such issues do exist. Although there are a variety of specific theories that can be used in genetic assessment issues, there are several shared components that any adequate theory must have:

- A concept of the person that puts less emphasis on individuality and more on how the person exists within a community, particularly the family;
- Explanations of how parents can be seen to support their children when decisions are made that are more family-centered than child-centered;
- The capacity to expand the concept of benefit beyond the child-centered effects of the genetic assessment;
- Rationales for why parents may conclude that genetic information obtained from their child may or may not be shared with other family members; and
- Considerations for why children not at risk for a genetic illness may nonetheless be tested to assist in further family risk assessment.

Family-centered models of genetic ethical theories have been presented that address these components. These models tend to focus on relationships between the parties involved and see the goals of moral decision making as not strengthening or asserting the individuality of one party at the cost of another, but as an attempt to place value on the interactions between parties who have either natural relationships, such as family members, or those who are developing relationships, such as nurses and patients (Twomey 2002). When related parties are involved in a moral decision, judgments about their actions will emphasize the goods that enhance the personhood of the individuals in many ways, not just in supporting autonomy but also by examining other enriching effects of the decision.

Because attempting a genetic assessment without the background of the family is hollow and without meaning, a family ethic of genetic assessment does more than just make sense; it is essential for us to understand why families make different decisions in different scenarios. Families do not enter the genetic health setting with identical blank slates; they have individual histories and may interpret data that the RN presents through prisms that may be both shared and individual. They will have pathways of discussion, conflict management, world philosophy, and views of the individual that may at times seem incoherent and dysfunctional to outsiders. However, in the end, by the very act of presenting for genetic assessment, family members are opening their private world to outsiders to help them find a conduit through the maze of complex genomic health.

Therefore, genetic ethics will help the RN to navigate through decisions with the family that needs to resolve issues such as favoritism (just or unjust), subjugation of individuality, and tendencies to see the world completely through their shared identities without sometimes considering the importance of personal identity within familial roles (McConkie-Rosell and Spiridigliozzi 2004). Difficult actions that need to be discussed by the RN may include a conclusion that one or more of the group's members is losing too much identity and is risking being subsumed as a moral being by a family decision (Nelson and Nelson 1995).

Children certainly can be at risk for such moral subjugation. Because of the power that parents naturally wield over healthcare decisions, it is not unlikely that at times youths will be presented for genetic assessment and it is unclear how their genomic information will contribute to their health or anyone else's in the family (Ross and Moon 2000). This may occur when a parent asks to test a very young child who is healthy to ascertain carrier status for an illness already established within the family. A very careful discussion must ensue to determine why the request is being made, what the parents expect to do with the information gained, what is the child's understanding, and when will he or she be able to use the information? Families who are misinformed about the usefulness of such an assessment but do not seem willing to address such questions may be poor candidates for such a test, despite the traditional leeway given parents over their child's health information.

When one avoids treating the genetic assessment decision as an isolated event and places it within the overall family experience, there are many meanings that can be attached to it that fit well by most standards of family life. A large part of a child's life is spent with others in activities intended to enhance his moral character. Parents are expected to carefully appraise the daily activities that they provide for their children with the intention that a large part of family life is spent learning to be good citizens as well as fully functioning family members (Parker 2001). The normal continuum of this process is a gradual loosening of ties to the family unit, but rare is the expectation that a child will totally sever all connections. So pediatric genetic assessment that does not have immediate medical benefit can be viewed by parents as means of integrating the child into the family's health assessment. If an examination of the family's needs is such that the child is not being subjugated for trivial knowledge gain, then a request for an assessment may seem very natural.

Parents may seek genetic information about their child for reasons that appear to be less child-centered than one expects because they see such information as part of the family history that all members are expected to contribute to. Experiences of genetic professionals tend to support the view that parents make decisions about assessments of their own genetic risk for family reasons.

- Parents and daughters from 12 families agreed that having the genetic information about the BRCA mutations in their daughters would lead to a cure, better surveillance, or screening. (Geller, Tambor, Bernhardt, Wissow, and Fraser 1995).

- The most significant reason for 184 parents seeking genetic breast cancer testing for themselves was to get information about their children's risk (Lerman, Narod, Schulman, Hughes, Gomez-Caminero, Bonney, et al. 1996).

- Parents in nine families interviewed with NF2 wanted to be reassured about suspicions about the disease gene. Nine of ten interviewed parents considered receiving the information important for reassurance, even if no action was to result (Twomey, Bove, and Cassidy 2007).

Other parents surveyed about testing their children did not feel strongly about having their children assessed. A small percentage (18/104) of parents in a BRCA surveillance program indicated they would test their own child, though 25% wanted to leave open the possibility of allowing such testing as a policy (Hamann, Croyle, Venne, Baty, Smith, and Botkin 2000). This contrasts with professionals, up to 50% of whom would be willing to test children for similar disorders (Harman 2003; Rosen 2002).

Conclusion

RNs currently may face seemingly conflicting messages about intentions of parents who present their children for genetic assessment. Because not all requests for such assessments will contribute immediately to their child's health, it can be difficult to determine the correct pathway to suggest for the parent and child. Determination of the type of gene assessment requested can help clarify the possible ethical issues that may arise for the family if the information is provided.

- Requests for tests for autosomal dominant diseases that are late onset may or may not have direct implications for the individual child's health, but may provide familial information that will be useful for overall family integrity.

- Autosomal recessive illnesses will always leave parents with the question of whether their unaffected children are carriers. This information will rarely have immediate benefit for a child, but may provide important educational opportunities for the family at some point its development.

- Requests for linkage analysis of a specific gene within a child's genome to confirm a family's propensity for a genetic illness again will not benefit the child directly, but may provide the prospect of the child to contribute greatly to the family's health with little risk to him.

Any time that a family offers a child to a professional to have a genetic assessment, there can be the risk that the child's information is going to be used inappropriately, particularly if the data will not be used for informed education of the child at later date or if the parents do not understand the need to protect such data from people within or outside the family who could misinterpret the implications of a positive test for a disease mutation. Conversely, if they understand fully the meaning of a genetic assessment of their child and the contribution of her genomic information to their family's history, and honor her donation of information, a well informed family can make this child's gift a meaningful part of her growth within the group. To facilitate this positive meaning of the genetic assessment, the nurse should work to include the child in the decision to the degree that he or she can participate in a developmental sense. If the child's cognition is not to the level that he or she can understand, then education of the family must include letting parents know at what point in the child's life information collected now must be presented to the child and how to communicate it in developmentally relevant ways. Nurses should also be prepared to counsel children who want to refuse to be assessed, and support such dissent if suitable given the child's health status, current development, and cognitive age.

Ethical guidelines exist that may help nurses to guide families making genetic assessment decisions. Nurses should be aware that varied ethical theories provide support for families that go beyond traditional rules that seem to limit parental choice in this area. Nurses are urged to become familiar with such family-centered ethics as they counsel parents and children trying to make such decisions.

References

American Nurses Association (ANA). 1998. *Statement on the scope and standards of genetics clinical nursing practice.* Washington DC: American Nurses Publishing.

————. 2001. *Code of ethics for nurses with interpretive statements.* Washington DC: American Nurses Publishing.

————. and International Society of Nurses in Genetics (ISONG). 2006. *Genetics/genomics nursing: Scope and standards of practice.* ANA and ISONG. Silver Spring, MD: Nursesbooks.org.

American Society of Human Genetics Board of Directors and American College of Medical Genetics Board of Directors. 1995. Points to consider: Ethical, legal, and psychosocial implications of genetic testing in children and adolescents. *American Journal of Human Genetics* 57 (5): 1233–1241.

Beauchamp, T. L., and J. F. Childress. 2001. *Principles of biomedical ethics,* 5th ed. New York: Oxford University Press.

Codori, A. M., K. L. Zawacki, G. M. Petersen, D. L. Miglioretti, J. A. Bacon and J. D. Trimbath. 2003. Genetic testing for hereditary colorectal cancer in children: Long-term psychological effects. *American Journal of Medical Genetics* 116A (2): 117–128.

Evans, J. H. 2000. A sociological account of the growth of principlism. *Hastings Center Report* 30 (5): 31–38.

Fanos, J. H. 1999. The missing link in linkage analysis: The well sibling revisited. *Genetic Testing* 3 (3): 273–278.

Fanos, J. H., and J. P. Johnson. 1995a. Barriers to carrier testing for adult cystic fibrosis sibs: The importance of not knowing. *American Journal of Medical Genetics* 59 (1): 85–91.

————. 1995b. Perception of carrier status by cystic fibrosis siblings. *American Journal of Human Genetics* 57 (2): 431–438.

Fletcher, J. C. 2001. A good idea whose time will come. *American Journal of Bioethics* 1 (3): 11–13.

Geller, G., E. S. Tambor, B. A. Bernhardt, L. S. Wissow, and G. Fraser. 1995. Mothers and daughters from breast cancer families: A qualitative study of their perceptions of risks and benefits associated with minor's participation in genetic susceptibility research. *Journal of the American Medical Women's Association* 55 (5): 280–284.

Hamann, H. A., R. T. Croyle, V. L. Venne, B. J. Baty, K. R. Smith, and J. R. Botkin. 2000. Attitudes toward the genetic testing of children among adults in a Utah-based kindred tested for a BRCA1 mutation. *American Journal of Medical Genetics* 92 (1): 25–32.

Harman, L. B. 2003. Attitudes toward genetic testing: Gender, role, and discipline. *Topics in Health Information Management* 24 (1): 50–58.

Hoedemaekers, R. 1998. Predictive genentic testing and the concept of risk. In *The Genetic Testing of Children,* ed A. Clarke, 245–264. Oxford, England: Bios Scientific Publications.

International Society of Nurses in Genetics (ISONG). 2000. Informed decision-making and consent: The role of nursing. http://www.isong.org/about/ps_consent.cfm (accessed September 10, 2008).

———. 2005. Privacy and confidentiality of genetic information: The role of the nurse. http://www.isong.org/about/ps_privacy.cfm (accessed September 10, 2008).

Jarvinen, O., A. E. Lehesjoki, M. Lindlof, A. Uutela, and H. Kaariainen. 2000. Carrier testing of children for two x-linked diseases: A retrospective study of comprehension of the test results and social and psychological significance of the testing. *Pediatrics* 106 (6): 1460–1465.

Lerman, C., S. Narod, K. Schulman, C. Hughes, A. Gomez-Caminero, G. Bonney, et al. 1996. BRCA1 testing in families with hereditary breast-ovarian cancer. A prospective study of patient decision making and outcomes. *Journal of the American Medical Association* 275 (24): 1885–1892.

Lim, D. J., A. E. Rubenstein, D. G. Evans, T. Jacks, B. G. Seizinger, M. E. Baser, D. Beebe, D. E. Brackmann, E. A. Chiocca, R. G. Fehon, et al. 2000. Advances in neurofibromatosis 2 (NF2): A workshop report. Journal of Neurogenetics 14 (2): 63–106.

McConkie-Rosell, A., and G. A. Spiridigliozzi. 2004. "Family matters": A conceptual framework for genetic testing in children. *Journal of Genetic Counseling* 13 (1): 9–29.

McKone, E. F., S. S. Emerson, K. L. Edwards, and M. L. Aitken. 2003. Effect of genotype on phenotype and mortality in cystic fibrosis: A retrospective cohort study. *Lancet* 361 (9370): 1671–1676.

Michie, S., M. Bobrow, and T. M. Marteau. 2001. Predictive genetic testing in children and adults: A study of emotional impact. *Journal of Medical Genetics* 38 (8): 519–526.

Miller, V. A., and Nelson, R. M. 2006. A developmental approach to child assent for nontherapeutic research. *Journal of Pediatrics* 149 (Suppl. 1), S25–830.

National Coalition for Health Professional Education in Genetics. 2005. About NCHPEG. National Coalition for Health Professional Education in Genetics, http://www.nchpeg.org/ (accessed September 10, 2008).

Nelson, H., and J. Nelson. 1995. *The patient in the family: An ethics of medicine and families.* New York: Routledge.

Nelson, R. M., J. R. Botkjin, E. D. Kodish, M. Levetown, J. T. Truman, and B. S. Wilfond. 2001. Ethical issues with genetic testing in pediatrics. *Pediatrics* 107 (6): 1451–1455.

Parker, M. 2001. Genetics and the interpersonal elaboration of ethics. *Theoretical Medicine & Bioethics* 22 (5): 451–459.

Patenaude, A. F. 2004. *Genetic testing for cancer: Psychological approaches for helping patients and families.* Washington D.C.: APA Publishing.

Rosen, W. M. 2002. Attitudes of pediatric residents toward ethical issues associated with genetic testing in children. *Pediatrics* 110 (2): 360–363.

Ross, L. F. and M. R. Moon. 2000. Ethical issues in genetic testing of children. *Archives of Pediatrics & Adolescent Medicine* 154 (9): 873–879.

Tercyak, K. P., B. N. Peshkin, T. A. DeMarco, B. M. Brogan, and C. Lerman. 2002. Parent-child factors and their effect on communicating BRCA1/2 test results to children. *Patient Education & Counseling* 47 (2): 145–153.

Tercyak, K. P., B. N. Peshkin, R. Streisand, and C. Lerman. 2001. Psychological issues among children of hereditary breast cancer gene (BRCA1/2) testing participants. *Psycho-Oncology* 10 (4): 336–346.

Twomey, J. G. 2002. Genetic testing of children: Confluence or collision between parents and professionals? *AACN Clinical Issues* 13 (4): 557–566.

Twomey, J., C. Bove, and D. Cassidy. 2007. Presymptomatic genetic testing in children for Neurofibromatosis 2. *Journal of Pediatric Nursing* 23 (3): 183–194.

Wertz, D. C., J. H. Fanos, and P. R. Reilly. 1994. Genetic testing for children and adolescents. Who decides? *Journal of the American Medical Association* 272 (11): 875–881.

Wilfond, B. S., and S. E. Gollust. 2005. Policy issues for expanding newborn screening programs: The cystic fibrosis newborn screening experience in the United States. *Journal of Pediatrics* 146 (5): 668–674.

CHAPTER 19

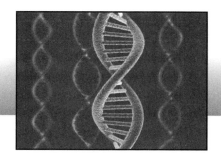

Genetics and Ethics in Nursing: Cancer Prevention for Clients with Inherited Cancer Risk

Cathleen M. Goetsch, MSN, ARNP, AOCNP

Genetic technologies and understanding of the role genes play in health and illness has expanded phenomenally in the last decade and a half. Breakthroughs in gene identification and sequencing characterized the early 1990s. The long held view of cancer as a genetic disease gained adherents. Even in acquired gene mutations, individual response to illness and risk reduction efforts may be mediated by genetic factors (Giarelli, Jacobs, and Jenkins 2002). Although most genetic changes that influence cancer development are acquired as time goes by, an important few heritable mutations are recognized in described cancer family syndromes. A small number of genes, associated with specific syndromes have been located and sequenced. Genetic testing can be used to confirm a clinical diagnosis or, in the case of cancer family syndromes, can identify potential excess risk in asymptomatic individuals (Burke 2002).

Progress in identification of individuals with inborn errors, who bear excess cancer risk, offers the possibility of intervening to moderate, reduce, and hopefully eliminate cancer risk (Reiger 2003). The essential role of the nurse in meeting the multiple needs of individuals, families, and communities with health risk related to genetic disorders is well demonstrated in the area of cancer prevention (Giarelli, Jacobs, and Jenkins 2002; Greco and Mahon 2004; Jenkins and Lea 2005; Tranin, Masny, and Jenkins 2003). This important healthcare activity is laden with potential ethical challenges for nurses and other providers of genetic services (Flach 2002).

Nursing is commonly considered an inherently ethical profession (Bishop and Scudder 1996). This is an example of virtue ethics where good intention defines morality (Flach 2002). The American Nurses Association (ANA) supports this view, defining advocacy as the primary nursing ethic (2001). Nurses have both the duty and the intention to protect and promote the health and well-being of their client, whether an individual or a group. Advocacy aids the client in gaining sufficient and appropriate information in order to make informed health decisions and then facilitates the decision-making process. The practice of advocacy and intent to improve client health is referred to as caring presence (Bishop and Scudder 1996). The caring nurse's practice of advocacy requires attention, efficiency, and efficacy.

Some systems of ethics delineate moral behavior as upholding recognized principles. Those most often used in discussions of bioethics include respect for autonomy (self-determination, the right to choose for oneself), non-maleficence (to do no harm), beneficence (good intention), and justice (equity and fairness). Respect for confidentiality and privacy, veracity (telling the truth), and fidelity (being trustworthy in performance of duty) are also important ethical principles that contribute to achievement of the prior four (Bishop and Scudder 1996; Flach 2002; Greco and Mahon 2004). For some, utility is the strongest guiding principle: a moral decision results in the best outcome. The difficulty in decision-making lies with the person or group who makes that judgment (Weed and McKeown 2003).

Under the ethical construct of casuistry, ethical behavior is determined by the individual characteristics in a situation. By contrast, normative ethics have specific precepts for what is absolutely right and wrong moral behavior (Flach 2002). Individual nurses may have such deeply held personal beliefs, but must balance them carefully against meeting the needs of their clients (Parascandola 2003). Nurses are often the moderators in the setting of multiple conflicting beliefs about what is right. Influences on ethical decisions include economic, political, socio-cultural, religious, scientific-technological, and personal experience. The nurse acts as a translator, mediator, guide, interpreter, and facilitator with the required outcome being client empowerment and the prime obligation being competency in performance (Flach

2002). Use of evidenced-based practice helps ensure competency in advocacy. Nursing activities are consistent with all of the ethical approaches described above, and each one may play a role in the cancer prevention setting with clients experiencing inherited predisposition to cancer.

Demand for and Access to Genetic Information

The consumer advocacy and patients' rights movements, along with the globalization of instantaneous communication and expanded access to data through technological advances, have all contributed to the demand for personal genetic information. The popular press complicates this demand with sensationalized reporting of inaccurate or incomplete research results. The wish to discover risk information may be based on unrealistic expectations (Greco and Mahon 2004). Most individuals seeking genetic testing do so in the hope of ruling out extreme risk.

One obvious role for nursing is in helping clients sort out the applicability and meaning of genetic information. Unfortunately, access to this information is currently limited to those with the resources to obtain up-to-date health care and who are well enough educated to request such service; typically middle- and upper-class urbanites. Reducing disparities in access to health information and health care, including genetics services, is an important ethical activity for genetic nurses. Individuals and groups whose access to genetic services is limited by geographical, social, emotional, economic, and educational disadvantage require advocacy at the national and international levels (Castiel 2003). Genetic nurses are leading efforts to relieve this inequity, a performance in pursuit of the ethical principle of justice (Cunningham 2002; Jenkins and Mansy 2003).

Communicating Risk

Nurses have an important role in assisting their clients to obtain and understand genetic risk information. Risk communication is essential but fraught with pitfalls. The probabilistic nature of risk is difficult to convey. Communicating the information that increased risk exists may cause anxiety. The intrinsic uncertainty caused by receiving notice of genetic risk may also cause worry (Greco and Mahon 2004). Since much of the risk estimation literature may not be transferable to diverse populations, even making a reasonable risk estimate may be difficult (Baltzell and Wrensch 2005; Bondy and Newman 2003; Domchek, Eisen, Calzone, Stopfer, Blackwood, and Weber 2003). Most people in the general population inaccurately estimate their risk of cancer, and this has been demonstrated in a high-risk population as well (Hass, Kaplan,

Des Jarlais, Gildengoin, Perez-Staable, and Kerlikowse 2005; Metcalfe and Narod 2005). Helping individuals with known genetic mutations understand the magnitude of their cancer risk is even more demanding.

The innate ethical challenge here is related to the principle of autonomy or self-determination. Clients with inherited cancer risk have the right to make their own informed decisions based on adequate information. The right to know as opposed to the right not to know is another part of this issue. It may be addressed before the client reaches the healthcare system, or it may be a key component of the counseling required as a genetic cancer predisposition is revealed (Greco and Mahon 1994).

In relaying information the caring nurse advocate considers the knowledge base, level of understanding, learning style, and coping skills of the client in facilitating the communication of risk. A team approach increases the number of times the learner hears the information. In addition to the client, the team may include specialty genetics providers (physician, PhD geneticist, genetic counselor, clinical nurse specialist, or nurse practitioner), radiology (physicians and radiation technologists), medical oncology, oncology nursing, radiation oncology, pathology, surgical teams (physicians and nurses specializing in breast surgery, gynecological oncology, plastic surgery, GI surgery), social workers, psychiatry and psychology specialists, financial counselors, support groups, family, friends, and employer personnel representatives. Having more than one team member provide information may help the client understand their condition and the risk for future problems.

One of the most difficult aspects of risk communication is putting risk and risk reduction in understandable terms (Jennings-Dozier and Foltz 2002; Mahon 2003). For the nurse to communicate accurately, knowledge of common ways of quantifying risk is required. Explaining the difference between the chances of developing breast cancer and the likelihood of dying from breast cancer is an important part of cancer prevention counseling. Relative risk and odds ratios are frequently used to demonstrate magnitude of cancer risk. Finding ways to personalize risk statistics promotes client empowerment. Interpreting the credibility of the sources of risk information is another important nursing activity. Are the estimates based on reliable methods? How transferable are they to the individual client? The nurse advocate can help clients clarify and give appropriate weight to conflicting information. Knowledge really is powerful if effective risk management results from the knowing.

Prioritizing Magnitude of Risk

Discussion of cancer risk in the instance of an inherited predisposition syndrome does not involve a single risk, but multiple risks. Additionally the client may be dealing with a current diagnosis of cancer. Helping the client to recognize the current cancer as the most profound threat to health assists in clarifying a sequence of actions. Putting prevention activities in this perspective aids in relieving the urge to address all risks with equal force.

Managing Risk

Once a meaningful estimate of risk has been made, the expectation is that the risk can, and should be, managed, modified, and reduced. However, as Jenkins and Lea (2005) have noted, merely having information about genetic risk does not ensure action to reduce risk even if appropriate risk reduction options exist. Communicating accurate information regarding availability and efficacy of risk reduction activities is essential to creating and individualizing a risk reduction plan. Conflicting allegiances may arise as the duty to warn family members of risk competes with maintaining privacy and confidentiality for the client of record. Fears of discrimination and stigmatization must also be addressed.

What is known about reducing risk, what is the quality of the evidence, and how does the information apply in the individual case? What are the benefits versus new problems that might be caused by the intervention? What are the likely short-term versus long-term outcomes? How will the action affect quality of life? The ethical nurse advocate acts to ensure the client has the means to answer these and other applicable questions before decisions regarding risk reduction are made or interventions instituted. If the nurse does not have the competencies necessary to fill this role, an appropriate referral must be made (Greco and Mahon 2004).

Cancer Prevention Strategies

Primary Prevention

Interventions to impede or delay the onset of cancer are primary prevention activities. Educating clients about options, efficacy, and assisting in effective behavior change is a bedrock nursing advocacy role.

Avoidance of Risk

Some activities, behaviors, and exposures are known to increase cancer risk in the general population. Individuals with inherited cancer predisposition may be more sensitive to known factors. However, those with elevated baseline cancer risk need assistance to recognize activities that add to their already excessive cancer risk.

Tobacco and alcohol are both associated with substantial epidemiological increase in cancer risk. Variations in CYP genes leave some individuals with ineffective or low levels of enzymes that function to detoxify the carcinogens in tobacco smoke, resulting in an increased risk of lung cancer (Jenkins and Masny 2003). How much incremental risk is added to baseline risk from inherited cancer predisposition mutation is unknown. However, since these are modifiable risk factors, all clients should be counseled to avoid tobacco use and that even moderate alcohol use raises risk of many cancers (Barse 2003; Schneider 2002; Stucky-Marshall and O'Brien 2002).

Radiation exposure has long been known to cause DNA damage that can lead to subsequent higher cancer risk. Some inherited syndromes are associated with increased sensitivity to radiation and require special planning for screening that limits radiation contact (Reiger 2003). Thoughtful clients will want to consider whether the increased risk associated with recommendations for more frequent screening is justified by better outcomes. Current research findings supports appropriate frequency of screening for better detection, but information about overall change in life expectancy is not yet available. Communicating uncertainty and supporting individuals living with uncertainty may be a role familiar to many nurses.

Dietary changes to diminish cancer risk have been studied by various methods. Epidemiological data suggest the benefits of low-fat, high-fiber diets for cancer risk reduction, but results from clinical trials have produced contradictory conclusions (Beresford, Johnson, Ritenbaugh, Lasser, Snetselaar, Black, et al. 2006; Prentice, Caan, Chelbowski, Patterson, Kueller, Ockene, et al. 2006). Coaching clients to make dietary changes in hope of decreasing cancer risk may be justified as an approach that may help and probably won't hurt, rather than being grounded in definitive study findings.

The effect of hormones on cancer risk has been explored in many settings. Use of either birth control pills (BCP) or hormone replacement therapy (HRT) has been shown to have both benefit and risk in average and high-risk groups (Lacey, Mink, Lubin, Sherman, Troisi, Hartge, et al. 2002; Narod, Risch, Molslehi, Dorum,

Neuhausen, Olsson, et al. 1998; Riman, Dickman, Nilsson, Correia, Nordliner, Magnusson, et al. 2002; Rossouw, Anderson, Prentice, La Croix, Kooperberg, Stefanick, et al. 2002). Some behavior choices may also modulate endogenous hormonal effect. Age at first live birth and effect of breast-feeding have both been studied as moderators of breast cancer risk (Gail, Brinton, Byar, Corle, Green, Schairer, et al. 1989; Jernström, Lubinski, Lynch, Ghadirian, Neuhausen, Isaacs, et al. 2004). Careful consideration of potential individual risk must be compared to possible benefit that may result from each of the various choices available. The timing and duration of hormone use is also controversial and should be addressed as part of a risk management plan. Clearly more research is needed in this area.

Chemoprevention

Selective Estrogen Receptor Modulators (SERMS)

Many agents have been evaluated for cancer prevention benefit. Clinical trials looking at chemoprevention effects in certain hereditary cancer risk groups have been done. The landmark National Surgical Adjuvant Breast and Bowel Project (NSAB) protocol P-1 Breast Cancer Prevention Trial with tamoxifen showed benefit in breast cancer risk reduction by 49% compared to placebo (Fisher, Constantino, Wickerham, Redmond, Kavanah, Cronin, et al. 1998). Although all participants had elevated risk ascertained by Gail model screening (a combination of family history factors and patterns of cancer), the trial started before the BRCA1 or BRCA2 genes had been identified and sequenced. Post trial testing for presence of mutations on the two genes was done. With only very small numbers of mutations found, the analysis hinted that BRCA2 mutation bearers had fewer breast cancers in the tamoxifen group, but the BRCA1 group did not (King, Wieand, Hale, Lee, Walsh, Owens, et al. 2001). Narod, Brunet, Ghadirian, Robson, Heimdal, Neuhausen, et al. (2000) reported a 50% decrease in contralateral breast cancers in BRCA1- and BRCA2-positive women with breast cancer that used tamoxifen. Discussing tamoxifen as a prophylactic agent should be part of formulating any risk reduction plan.

Raloxifene, another SERM, has data showing breast cancer risk reduction in post-menopausal women with osteoporosis (Martino, Cauley, Barrett-Connor, Powles, Mershon, Disch, et al. 2004). The NSABP P-2 STAR trial is expected to report results on raloxifene versus tamoxifen in post-menopausal women with elevated breast cancer risk. Once again the transferability of results to those with inherited breast cancer risk will not be known.

Non-Steroidal Anti-Inflammatory Drugs (NSAIDs)

This class of drugs has multiple studies showing benefit in colon polyp and colon cancer risk reduction. Low-dose aspirin has shown benefit in average risk individuals (Giovannucci, Egan, Hunter, Stampfer, Colditz, and Willet 1995; Giovannucci, Rimm, Stampfer, Colditz, Ascherio, and Willet 1994), while sulindac and celecoxib have study data demonstrating positive outcomes in individuals with familial adenomatous polyposis (Giardiello, Yang, Hylind, et al. 2002; Steinbach, Lynch, Phillips, et al. 2000). Further studies in this area are in progress. At the present time, the detrimental cardiac effects of celecoxib limit its use.

Calcium Supplementation

Reports so far have been mixed, but one large randomized study showed decreased size and number of recurrent polyps when participants took 3000 mg of calcium daily for four years (Barron, et al. 1999). Whether this benefit can be generalized to individuals with inherited colon cancer risk is yet to be elucidated. Presenting it as an element of an overall risk reduction plan may be warranted.

Exogenous Hormone Effect

Both benefit and risk data exists (Anderson, Judd, Kaunitz, Barad, Beresford, Pettinger, et al. 2003; Lacey, Mink, Lubin, Sherman, Troisi, Hartge, et al. 2002; Narod, Dube, Klijn, Lubinski, Lynch, Ghadrian, et al. 2002; Narod et al. 1998; Riman et al. 2002). Uterine and colon cancer risk may be decreased by birth control pills (BCP) and hormone replacement therapy (HRT) use (Anderson et al. 2003; Rossouw et al. 2002). Likewise BCP use may benefit ovarian cancer risk reduction in BRCA1 and BRCA2 mutation carriers, but likely increases breast cancer risk (Milne, Knight, John, Dite, Balbuena, Ziogas, et al. 2005; Narod et al. 2002; Narod et al. 1998). HRT use increases risk for both breast and ovarian cancer (Riman et al. 2002; Rossouw et al. 2002). Effects of ovarian stimulating drugs on cancer risk are not yet clear (Brinton, Lamb, Moghissi, Scoccia, Althuis, Mabie, et al. 2004). Schrag, Kuntz, Graber, and Weeks (2000) reported positive outcomes based on mathematical modeling that estimated effects of risk reduction strategies including use of birth control pills and tamoxifen in BRCA1 and BRCA2 carriers.

The complexity of hormone effects warrants careful discussion with the high-risk client in order to design the best strategy and timing of use versus avoiding exposure altogether. Once again the nurse advocate can be influential in providing information and helping clients to develop plans of risk management.

Prophylactic Surgery

Surgical intervention has been long employed for preventing the development of initial and subsequent cancer occurrences. In breast cancer risk reduction, much research has been done. Hartmann, Schaid, Woods, Crotty, Myers, Arnold, et al. (1999) in a retrospective analysis showed tremendous benefit in breast cancer risk reduction after prophylactic mastectomy in women with a family history of breast cancer. In BRCA mutation carriers benefit is also seen (Scheuer, Kauff, Robson, Kelly, Barakat, Satagopan, et al. 2002).

Preventative surgery to remove at-risk organs early in life has shown benefit in inherited cancer predisposition syndromes (e.g. colectomy for persons with familial adenopolyposis and thyroidectomy for those with MEN1-associated cancer). In instances where there is a near-100% lifetime risk of cancer occurrence (100% penetrance) and cancer onset at very young ages, the chance for preemptive surgery to be a life-saving intervention is great (Burke 2002; Greco and Mahon 2004; Niccoli-Sire, Murat, Baudin, Henry, Proye, Bigorgne, et al. 1999; Wells and Skinner 1998).

Ovarian cancer occurs in later life and its penetrance is lower in familial adenopolyposis and MEN1-related cancers. However, surgery to reduce risk of ovarian cancer occurrence has shown benefit and is advised (Burke, Daly, Garber, Botkin, Kahn, Lynch, et al. 1997; Kauff, Satagopan, Robson, Scheuer, Hensley, Hudis, et al. 2002; National Comprehensive Cancer Network (NCCC) 2006b; Rebbeck, Lynch, Neuhausen, Narod, Vant Veer, Garber, et al. 2002; Scheuer et al. 2002). These recommendations for prophylactic ovarian removal are based on the current limits of effective early detection resulting in later stage diagnosis with poor prognosis (Fields and Chevlen 2006a). If sensitive and specific screening measures become available, these recommendations will be revised.

Establishing methods of updating clients on advances in prevention methods is one of the necessary activities for the nurse providing ethical care under the advocacy model and the principle of duty. Encouraging high risk patients to enter into long-term follow-up for enhanced screening and preventative activities is another area where the nurse advocate can offer assistance.

Secondary Prevention: Screening for Early Detection

Effective screening requires several elements. The screening method should

- find what it is looking for,
- have interventions available that make a difference in outcomes,
- be cost effective,
- be acceptable to those being screened,
- be safe and easy for clients and providers,
- be accessible to the group that needs screening,
- be done in a group with a high likelihood of having the problem, and
- address a serious health threat.

Issues of accuracy and rates of false positives and false negatives must be considered. A false negative may cause harm to a person who actually has a cancer that is not identified, by providing false reassurance and delay of actual diagnosis. A false positive can lead to invasive procedures to establish that the problem is benign rather than malignant. All of these qualities are demonstrations of the ethical concept of utility. A good example of a successful cancer screening modality is mammograms for early breast cancer detection.

In the population with inherited cancer predisposition the usual screening recommendations are inadequate. Early recommendations for surveillance and intervention for individuals with known or presumed inherited cancer risk were initially based on best judgment of consensus panels of experts. (Burke, Daly, et al. 1997; Burke, Petersen, Lynch, Botkin, Daly, Garber, Kahn, et al. 1997). Guidelines for screening in groups with genetically elevated cancer risk have been updated to reflect research findings (Jarvinen, Aarnio, Mustonen, Aktan-Collan, Aaltonen, Peltomaki, et al. 2000; NCCN 2006a; NCCN 2006b; Scheuer, et al. 2002). Most recommendations include starting screening 5–10 years younger than the first cancer case in a mutation-bearing family and shortening the surveillance interval to reflect greater chance of incidence in cancer predisposition mutation carriers. Current breast cancer screening recommendations include professional breast exams every 6 months and annual mammograms and breast MRIs (Kuhl, Schrading, Leutner, Morakkabati-Spitz, Wardelmann, Fimmers, et al. 2005; NCCN 2006b). Screening for ovarian cancer even in women with elevated risk has been ineffective with our current technology (Fields and Chevlen 2006b).

Hope for better early detection is offered by promising initial results using proteomic methods for blood screening. In the absence of good screening methods, and driven by the demands of patients, many healthcare providers perform screening with a combination of transvaginal pelvic ultrasound, bimanual pelvic exam, and CA125, at varying intervals. Unfortunately, psychological risks can be associated with prevention activities. The anxiety associated with screening events can be magnified in individuals who need frequent surveillance.

Barriers to prevention activities exist in many forms. External barriers include

- insurance limits on type and frequency of screening,
- lack of any or adequate health insurance,
- lack of access to health care whether based on economics, geography, or availability,
- inability to take time off from work, have transportation or child care, and
- lack of knowledge or technology preventing providers from recommending screening.

Internal characteristics unique to each client also present barriers to screening. Healthy individuals may have less motivation to take the time to do screening. Individuals with cancer may lack the energy needed. Clients may harbor strong opinions about the acceptability of screening procedures such as colonoscopy and mammograms that are uncomfortable, at best, for many. However, those with more risk may be willing to accept more discomfort and inconvenience, feeling they have more to gain and less to lose.

Socio-cultural factors may present both external and internal barriers to screening. Education level, cultural beliefs, and even superstition have their effects. Not every client will subscribe to the belief that screening has benefit. Some clients view screening procedures as tempting fate. The meaning of illness may be culturally influenced. Detection of cancer may be seen as a "death sentence," and "not knowing is better than knowing." In situations where energy is primarily focused on day-to-day survival, some may find it difficult to see a value in future-focused activity, and other more pressing life events may take priority.

All of these barriers present challenges to the ethical nurse. Assisting the client to clarify their values and putting the recommended prevention activities in that context can provide an opportunity for changing behavior. Establishing follow-up plans and making reminder contacts can show the commitment of the nurse and provide another chance to enhance health.

Participation in a Structured High-Risk Program

Participation in a risk management program has evidence-based results. Structured programs increase compliance with recommended screening (Scheuer et al. 2002). Reduced cancer incidence has been well documented when prevention activities are maintained (Fisher et al. 1998; Harman et al. 1999; Narod et al. 2002; Narod et al. 1998; Niccoli-Sire et al. 1999; Wells and Skinner 1998). Increased early stage detection has been demonstrated (Jarvinen et al. 2000; Kauff net al. 2002; Scheuer et al. 2002). Systematic management of excess risk showed increased lifespan based on mathematical modeling (Schrag et al. 2000). Even individuals who test negative for known inherited cancer risk mutations, but have family or personal factors consistent with hereditary risk, may benefit from increased knowledge and better surveillance (NCCN 2006).

Facilitating the Activities

The first step is to form an individualized plan based on client factors such as culture, religion, age, knowledge level, literacy, language, sex, age, lifestyle, health beliefs, and level of health. The plan should include suggestions for risk reduction, a timetable for the various activities, methods of accessing the care needed, and a follow-up schedule. An interdisciplinary team can assist in formulation and enactment of a risk-reduction plan. Frequent contacts, pre-established procedures for regular follow-up, and methods for relaying advances or changes in recommendations will enhance the formation of trusting interactive relationships that are necessary for the future.

Participation in Clinical Research

Much of today's health care is based on the findings of research conducted over many years. Providing information and access to clinical trials when appropriate is key to the development of efficacious diagnostics and treatments. We are currently in the process of expanding our studies among diverse populations in order to develop more effective and individualized plans of care.

Conducting prevention research is especially problematic. The recommendation to participate in preventative screening research programs from a healthcare provider may be one of the strongest motivators for willingness to join a study. One difficulty in research for prevention is that studies require large sample sizes and extended time frames to demonstrate statistical significance that can affect public health policy. For many reasons, prevention studies are costly to conduct. These issues raise the ethical questions of equity and utility. What is the cost in comparison to other societal needs? What else could the same dollars be spent on, who will benefit, and who decides?

Summary

Genetic diagnosis of elevated cancer risk allows known preventative actions. There is easy availability of risk information but a paucity of clear, personalized interpretation. Nurses are well suited to identify, communicate, and manage genetic risk for clients. Individuals at risk must be identified and educated to facilitate prevention activities that promote their best health outcomes. The point of risk estimation is risk reduction. Reduction of risk requires designing and implementing risk management strategies. Nursing is perceived to be among the most ethical professions. Nurses are trusted to tell the truth, to do the right thing, and are recognized as knowledgeable. The intention to do good for our clients is at the core of nursing practice and defines our nursing ethic. Maintaining that tradition will require that nurses acquire up-to-date knowledge about genetics and effectively pass it on.

References

American Nursing Association (ANA). 2001. *Code of ethics for nurses with interpretive statements.* Silver Spring, MD: Nursesbooks.org.

Anderson, G., H. Judd, A. Kaunitz, D. Barad, S. Beresford, M. Pettinger, J. Liu, S. McNeeley, A. Lopez, Women's Health Initiative Investigators. 2003. Effects of estrogen plus progestin on gynecologic cancers and associated diagnostic procedures: The Women's Health Initiative randomized trial. *Journal of the American Medical Association* 290: 1739–1748.

Baltzell, K. and M. Wrensch. 2005. Strengths and limitations of breast cancer risk assessment. Oncology Nursing Forum 32: 605–616.

Barse, P. 2003. How to perform a genetic assessment. in *Genetics in oncology practice: Cancer risk assessment* eds. A. Tranin, A. Masny, and J. Jenkins. 57–76. Pittsburgh, PA: Oncology Nursing Society.

Beresford, S., K. Johnson, C. Ritenbaugh, N. Lasser, L. Snetselaar, H. Black, G. Anderson, A. Assaf, T. Bassford, D. Bowen et al. 2006. Low-fat dietary pattern and risk of colorectal cancer: The Women's Health Initiative randomized controlled dietary modification trial. *Journal of the American Medical Association* 295: 643–654.

Bishop, A., and J. Scudder. 1996. *Nursing ethics: Therapeutic caring presence.* Sudsbury, MA: Jones and Bartlett Publishers.

Bondy, M., and L. Newman. 2003. Breast cancer risk assessment models: Applicability to African-American women. *Cancer* 97 (Suppl. 1): 230–235.

Brinton, L., E. Lamb, K. Moghissi, B. Scoccia, M. Althuis, J. Mabie, and C. Westhoff. 2004. Ovarian cancer risk after the use of ovulation-stimulating drugs. *Obstetrics and Gynecology* 103: 1194–1203.

Burke, W. 2002. Genetic testing. *New England Journal of Medicine* 347: 1867–1875.

Burke, W., M. Daly, J. Garber, J. Botkin, M. Kahn, P. Lynch, A. McTiernan, K. Offit, J. Perlman, G. Petersen et al. 1997. Recommendations for follow-up care of individuals with an inherited predisposition to cancer. II. BRCA1 and BRCA2. *Journal of the American Medical Association* 277: 997–1003.

Burke, W., G. Petersen, P. Lynch, J. Botkin, M. Daly, J. Garber, M. Kahn, A. McTiernan, K. Offit, E. Thomson et al. 1997. Recommendations for follow-up care of individuals with an inherited predisposition to cancer. I. Hereditary nonpolyposis colon cancer. *Journal of the American Medical Association* 277: 915–919.

Castiel, L. 2003. Self care and consumer health: Do we need a public health ethics? *Journal of Epidemiology and Public Health* 57: 5–6.

Cunningham, R. 2002. Advancing the cancer control agenda: The role of advanced practice nurses. In *Cancer prevention, detection, and control: A nursing perspective,* eds. K. Jennings-Dozier and S. Mahon, 885–927. Pittsburgh, PA: Oncology Nursing Society.

Domchek, S., A. Eisen, K. Calzone, J. Stopfer, A. Blackwood, and B. Weber. 2003. Application of breast cancer risk prediction models in clinical practice. *Journal of Clinical Oncology* 21, 593–601.

Fields, M., and E. Chevlen. 2006a. Ovarian cancer screening: A look at the evidence. *Clinical Journal of Oncology Nursing* 10: 77–81.

Fields, M., and E. Chevlen. 2006b. Screening for disease: Making evidence-based choices. *Clinical Journal of Oncology Nursing* 10: 73–76.

Fisher, B., J. Costantino, D. Wickerham, C. Redmond, M. Kavanah, W. Cronin, V. Vogel, A. Robidoux, N. Dimitrov, J. Atkins et al. 1998. Tamoxifen for prevention of breast cancer: report of the National Surgical Adjuvant Breast and Bowel Project P-1 Study. *Journal of the National Cancer Institute* 90: 1371–1388.

Flach, J. 2002. An overview of bioethical issues and approaches in cancer prevention, detection, and control. In *Cancer prevention, detection, and control: A nursing perspective,* eds. K. Jennings-Dozier and S. Mahon, 173–210. Pittsburgh, PA: Oncology Nursing Society.

Gail, M., L. Brinton, D. Byar, D. Corle, S. Green, C. Schairer, and J. Mulvihill. 1989. Projecting individualized probabilities of breast cancer for white women who are being examined annually. *Journal of the National Cancer Institute* 81: 1879–1886.

Giardiello, F., V. Yang, L. Hylind, A. J. Krush, G. M. Petersen, J. D. Trimbath, et al. 2002. Primary chemoprevention of familial adenomatous polyposis with sulindac. *New England Journal of Medicine* 346: 1054–1059.

Giarelli, E., L. Jacobs, and J. Jenkins. 2002. Cancer prevention, screening, and early detection: Human genetics. In *Cancer Prevention, Detection, and Control: A Nursing Perspective,* eds K. Jennings-Dozier and S. Mahon, 99–142. Pittsburgh, PA: Oncology Nursing Society.

Giovannucci, E., K. Egan, D. Hunter, M. Stampfer, G. Colditz, and W. Willet. 1995. Aspirin and the risk of colorectal cancer in women. *New England Journal of Medicine* 333: 609–614.

Giovannucci, E., E. Rimm, M. Stampfer, G. Colditz, A. Ascherio, and W. Willet. 1994. Aspirin use and the risk for colorectal cancer and adenoma in male health professionals. *Annals of Internal Medicine* 121: 241–246.

Greco, K., and S. Mahon. 2004. Common hereditary cancer syndromes. *Seminars in Oncology Nursing* 20: 164–167.

Haas, J., C. Kaplan, G. Des Jarlais, V. Gildengoin, E. Perez-Staable, and K. Kerlikowse. 2005. Perceived risk of breast cancer among women at average and increased risk. *Journal of Women's Health* 14: 845–851.

Hartmann, L., D. Schaid, J. Woods, T. Crotty, J. Myers, P. Arnold, P. Petty, T. Sellers, J. Johnson, S. McDonnell, et al. 1999. Efficacy of bilateral prophylactic mastectomy in women with a family history of breast cancer. *New England Journal of Medicine* 340: 77–84.

Jarvinen, H., M. Aarnio, H. Mustonen, K. Aktan-Collan, L. Aaltonen, P. Peltomaki, A. De La Chapelle, and J. Mecklin. 2000. Controlled 15-year trial on screening for colorectal cancer in families with hereditary nonpolyposis colorectal cancer. *Gastroenterology* 118: 829–834.

Jenkins, J., and D. Lea. 2005. *Nursing care in the genomic era: A case-based approach.* Sudbury, MA: Jones and Bartlett Publishers.

Jenkins, J., and A. Mansy. 2003. In *Genetics in oncology practice: Cancer risk assessment,* eds. A. Tranin, A. Masny, and J. Jenkins, 1–12. Pittsburgh, PA: Oncology Nursing Society.

Jennings-Dozier, K., and A. Foltz. 2002. An epidemiological approach to cancer prevention and control. In *Cancer Prevention, Detection, and Control: A Nursing Perspective,* eds K. Jennings-Dozier and S. Mahon, 33–78. Pittsburgh, PA: Oncology Nursing Society.

Jernström, H., J. Lubinski, H. Lynch, P. Ghadirian, S. Neuhausen, C. Isaacs, B. Weber, D. Horsman,.B. Rosen, W. Foulkes, et al. 2004. Breast-feeding and the risk of breast cancer in BRCA1 and BRCA2 mutation carriers. *Journal of the National Cancer Institute* 96: 1094–1098.

Kauff, N., J. Satagopan, M. Robson, L. Scheuer, M., Hensley, C. Hudis, N. Ellis, J. Boyd, P. Borgen, R. Barakat, et al. 2002. Risk-reducing salpingo-oophorectomy in women with a BRCA1 or BRCA2 mutation. *New England Journal of Medicine* 346: 1609–1615.

King, M., L. Wieand, K. Hale, M. Lee, T. Walsh, K. Owens, J. Tait, L. Ford, B. Dunn, J. Costantino, et al. 2001. Tamoxifen effect on breast cancer incidence among women with mutations in BRCA1 and BRCA2: National Surgical Adjuvant Breast and Bowel Project (NSABP P-1) Breast Cancer Prevention Trial. *Journal of the American Medical Association* 286: 2251–2256.

Kuhl, C., S. Schrading, C. Leutner, N. Morakkabati-Spitz, E. Wardelmann, R. Fimmers, W. Kuhn, and H. Schild. 2005. Mammography, breast ultrasound, and magnetic resonance imaging for surveillance of women at high familial risk for breast cancer. *Journal of Clinical Oncology* 23: 8469–8476.

Lacey, J. Jr., P. Mink, J. Lubin, M. Sherman, R. Troisi, P. Hartge, A. Schatzkin, and C. Schairer. 2002. Menopausal hormone replacement therapy and risk of ovarian cancer. *Journal of the American Medical Association* 288: 334–341.

Mahon, S. 2003. Cancer-risk assessment: Considerations for cancer genetics. In *Genetics in oncology practice: Cancer risk assessment,* eds A. Tranin, A. Masny, and J. Jenkins, 77–138. Pittsburgh, PA: Oncology Nursing Society.

Martino S, J. Cauley, E. Barrett-Connor, T. Powles, J. Mershon, D. Disch, R. Secrest, S. Cummings, and CORE Investigators. 2004. Continuing outcomes relevant to Evista: breast cancer incidence in postmenopausal osteoporotic women in a randomized trial of raloxifene. *Journal of the National Cancer Institute* 96: 1751–1761.

Metcalfe, K., and S. Narod. 2002. Breast cancer risk perception among women who have undergone prophylactic bilateral mastectomy. *Journal of the National Cancer Institute* 94: 1564–1569.

Milne, R., J. Knight, E. John, G. Dite, R. Balbuena, A. Ziogas, I. Andrulis, D. West, F. Li, M. Southey, et al. 2005. Oral contraceptive use and risk of early-onset breast cancer in carriers and noncarriers of BRCA1 and BRCA2 mutations. *Cancer Epidemiology Biomarkers and Prevention* 14: 350–356.

Narod, S., J. Brunet , P. Ghadirian, M. Robson, K. Heimdal, S. Neuhausen, D. Stoppa-Lyonnet, C. Lerman, B. Pasini, P. de los Rios, et al. 2000. Tamoxifen and risk of contralateral breast cancer in BRCA1 and BRCA2 mutation carriers: A case-control study. *Lancet* 356: 1876–1881.

Narod, S., M. Dube, J. Klijn, J. Lubinski, H. Lynch, P. Ghadirian, D. Provencher, K. Heimdal, P. Moller, M. Robson, et al. 2002. Oral contraceptives and the risk of breast cancer in BRCA1 and BRCA2 mutation carriers. *Journal of the National Cancer Institute* 94: 1773–1779.

Narod, S., H. Risch, R. Molslehi, A. Dorum, S. Neuhausen, H. Olsson, D. Provencher, P. Radice, G. Evans, S. Bishop, et al. 1998. Oral contraceptives and the risk of hereditary ovarian cancer. *New England Journal of Medicine* 339: 424–428.

National Comprehensive Cancer Network (NCCN). 2006a. Clinical practice guidelines in oncology: Colorectal cancer screening. http://www.nccn.org/professionals/physician_gls/PDF/colorectal_screening.pdf (accessed September 10, 2008).

National Comprehensive Cancer Network (NCCN). 2006b. Clinical practice guidelines in oncology: Genetic/familial high risk assessment—Breast and ovarian. www.nccn.org (accessed October 7, 2008).

Niccoli-Sire, P., A. Murat, E. Baudin, J. Henry, C. Proye, J. Bigorgne, B. Bstandig, E. Modigliani, S. Morange, M. Schlumberger, et al. 1999. Early or prophylactic thyroidectomy in MEN2/FMTC gene carriers: Results in 71 thyroidectomized patients. *European Journal of Endocrinology* 121: 468–474.

Parascandola, M. 2003. Objectivity and the neutral expert. *Journal of Epidemiology and Community Health* 57: 3–4.

Prentice, R., B. Caan, R. Chlebowski, R. Patterson, L. Kuller, J., Ockene, K. Margolis, M. Limacher, J. Manson, L. Parker, et al. 2006. Low-fat dietary pattern and risk of invasive breast cancer: the women's health initiative randomized controlled dietary modification trial. *Journal of the American Medical Association* 295: 629–642.

Rebbeck, T., H. Lynch, S. Neuhausen, S. Narod, L. Vant Veer, J. Garber, G. Evans, C. Isaacs, M. Daly, E. Matloff, et al. 2002. Prophylactic oophorectomy in carriers of BRCA1 or BRCA2 mutations. *New England Journal of Medicine* 346: 1616–1622.

Reiger, P. 2003. The impact of genetic information in the management of cancer. In *Genetics in Oncology Practice: Cancer Risk Assessment,* eds. A. Tranin, A. Masny and J. Jenkins, 139–88. Pittsburgh, PA: Oncology Nursing Society.

Riman, T., P. Dickman, S.Nilsson, N. Correia, H. Nordlinder, C. Magnusson, E. Weiderpass, and I. Persson. 2002. Hormone replacement therapy and the risk of invasive epithelial ovarian cancer in Swedish women. *Journal of the National Cancer Institute* 94: 497–504.

Rossouw, J., G. Anderson, R. Prentice, A. LaCroix, C. Kooperberg, M. Stefanick, R. Jackson, S. Beresford, B. Howard, K. Johnson, et al. 2002. Risks and benefits of estrogen plus progestin in healthy postmenopausal women: Principal results from the Women's Health Initiative randomized controlled trial. *Journal of the American Medical Association* 288: 321–333.

Scheuer, L., N. Kauff, M. Robson, B. Kelly, R. Barakat, J. Satagopan, N. Ellis, M. Hensley, J. Boyd, P. Borgen, et al. 2002. Outcome of preventative surgery and screening for breast and ovarian cancer in BRCA mutation carriers. *Journal of Clinical Oncology* 20: 1260–1268.

Schneider, K. 2002. *Counseling about cancer: Strategies for genetic counseling*. 3rd edition. New York: Wiley-Liss.

Schrag, D., K. Kuntz, J. Graber, and J. Weeks. 2000. Life expectancy gains from cancer prevention strategies for women with breast cancer and BRCA1 or BRCA2 mutations. *Journal of the American Medical Association* 238: 617–624.

Steinback, G., P. Lynch, R. Phillips, M. H. Wallace, E. Hawk, G. B. Gordon, N. Wakabayashi, B. Saunders, Y. Shen, T. Fujimura, et al. 2000. The effect of celecoxib, a cyclooxygenase-2 inhibitor, in familial adenomatous polyposis. *New England Journal of Medicine* 342: 1946–1952.

Stucky-Marshall, L., and B. O'Brien, B. 2003. Gastrointestinal malignancies. In *Cancer prevention, detection, and control: A nursing perspective,* eds. K. Jennings-Dozier and S. Mahon, 445–538. Pittsburgh, PA: Oncology Nursing Society.

Weed, D., and R. McKeown. 2003. Science, ethics, and professional public health practice. *Journal of Epidemiology and Public Health* 57: 4–5.

Wells, S., and M. Skinner. 1998. Prophylactic thyroidectomy, based on direct genetic testing in patients at risk for multiple endocrine neoplasia type 2 syndrome. *Experimental Clinical Endocrinolgy and Diabetes* 106: 29–34.

CHAPTER 20

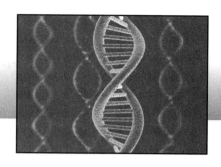

Ethical Obligations to Patients Who Engage in Lifelong Self-surveillance for Genetic Risk of Cancer

Ellen Giarelli, EdD, RN, CRNP

Genetic testing for predisposition to cancer has predictive potential and therefore has consequences different than other kinds of diagnostics. This technology transforms a person's experiences with healthcare professionals and the healthcare system. By consenting to genetic testing a patient agrees in principle to uncover information of what "is" and "what might be" in relation to the health risks of oneself and one's relatives. Such technology informs whole families of the risk for disease in living members and in future generations.

The predictive potential of genetic predisposition testing has de facto value to some people, simply because these people want the information. Value to one does not equate with value to all. A further ethical question is to determine whether the medical act of predisposition testing and the findings have de jure value and thus ought to be prized and wanted by all people.

One valuable, and therefore a "good," consequence of such technology is that once a patient is identified as having a health risk due to a genetic predisposition the patient is encouraged and advised to actively participate in enhanced surveillance for expression of the altered genotype. If in discovering and uncovering genetic nature through genetic testing we are able to "diagnose, prevent, treat, or control disease, then the technology is 'good'" (Giarelli 2003a, p. 257). We ought to want to use the technology which then can be seen as having de jure value. Access to this technology becomes a right. This raises the question, if genetic predisposition testing ought to be done, what then are the obligations to a patient once the testing is performed?

Genetic predisposition testing can become an instrumental link between best intentions and best outcomes of practice, provided professionals have a clear understanding of their obligations. The professional who conscientiously and accurately employs this "good" technology is indeed virtuous. Knowing what is good, however, is not always followed by knowing what must be done.

Knowing one's predisposition to cancer brings with it the knowledge of unpredictable expression and potential for disease. The question of the nature of professional obligation to patients is an issue after predisposition testing is conducted, risk is interpreted, and participation in lifelong surveillance—including self-surveillance—for genetic predisposition to cancer begins. Predisposition testing creates a "fact of illness" (Pellegrino 1979). A high probability or absolute likelihood of developing disease is imposed on a patient in the absence of signs and symptoms. The risk precipitates watchful waiting and raises many questions. Are there ethical issues of interest to a nurse when she or he knows a patient is engaging in self-surveillance? What is the nature of the nurse's responsibility to the patient? Who bears responsibility when self-surveillance is not done well?

Some critics are justified in claiming that healthcare providers have no ethical obligation to a patient during acts of self-surveillance because these acts are the choices made by a patient who will, to different degrees, perform these behaviors regardless of a cancer diagnosis. Self-observation of this kind results from a choice made by a patient as a direct consequence of the content and accuracy of information given by a professional. Others will argue that certain kinds of knowledge bring with them additional responsibilities.

In order to refine the nature of professional obligation in genetic health care, I will examine the theoretical phenomenon of participation in lifelong surveillance for points where ethical claims might be made and ethical problems might arise. I will propose ways that nurses might address these ethical problems to ensure that best intentions lead to best outcomes of professional practice. Only obligations related to the patient will be discussed. Another set of obligations pertain to family members; these will be the topic of another discussion. The bioethical principles of beneficence and autonomy that traditionally guide nursing practice will be considered in the context of self-surveillance.

Conceptual Model of Participation in Lifelong Surveillance

Surveillance as a cancer risk management strategy has been used in health care for the early detection of disease, for complications associated with the treatment of cancer, and for medical management of symptoms and side effects over a lifetime. Screening for cancer in the population is an example of surveillance. Individuals with a high risk for cancer, based on family history or a known inherited genetic mutation, are encouraged to engage in enhanced surveillance indefinitely. When enhanced, observations of health outcomes occur more frequently than in the general population, they begin earlier in life, and they continue over a life-time. Within the context of a socially constructed relationship between the observer and the observed, both watch and wait for a threatening event that is associated with the genetic predisposition to disease (Giarelli 2002). When the observer and the observed are different a measure of objectivity is more likely. When the observer and the observed are the same as is the case of self-surveillance, objectivity may be compromised.

People in families with cancer predisposition syndromes, such as multiple endocrine neoplasia type 2a (MEN2a) and familial adenomatous polyposis (FAP) conceptualize lifelong surveillance in broader and looser terms than do healthcare providers (Giarelli 2003b). MEN2a is a genetic cancer predisposition syndrome that causes medullary thyroid carcinoma, adrenal tumors, and parathyroid hyperplasia. FAP is another genetic cancer predisposition syndrome that causes multiple colorectal cancer and other neoplasia. Surveillance for each includes planned and incidental observations. Participation in planned surveillance means following the recommended guidelines for enhanced monitoring for signs of disease and effects of treatment. This might include visits to physicians and biochemical analyses of tissue or fluid samples. Planned surveillance is prescribed by healthcare providers and the frequency of follow-up visits depends on genotype, diagnosis, and severity of the presenting disease. Incidental surveillance is primarily self-surveillance. It is the day-to-day watching and waiting performed, largely out of the purview of professionals, by patients and sometimes by family members (Giarelli 2003b). Healthcare providers are included only when observations made by the patient are brought to the provider's attention. Categories of self-surveillance include phenotype tracking, symptom monitoring, and medication appraisal (Giarelli 2006).

Participation in lifelong surveillance is characterized by a core psychological process referred to as (Re)Minding and three psychosocial processes called Interpreting the Object, Negotiating Control, and (Re)Integration. Each incidence of self-surveillance reminds the person of the threat of cancer, loss, or disability. The reminder can be experienced as disintegrating, and it most often has a disturbing effect on one's sense of integrity. Once reminded, a person processes cognitively the surveillance event by interpreting the meaning of the observation in relation to their genetic risk for disease. The person appraises the significance of the observation and negotiates control by managing the effects of the observation. This means the person thinks about and decides how much attention should be given to what is observed, and will manage care (act on the interpretation). Finally, a person endeavors to mitigate the disintegrating effect of the surveillance event and initiates anew the cyclical psychosocial processes of: interpreting the object, negotiating control, and reintegration (see Figure 20–1).

For example, a person with FAP may see red streaks in the stool. The observation of red streaks may suggest the presence of a bleeding colorectal polyp. The person compares this observation with previous, similar observations, and health information such as personal or family history of bleeding polyps or hemorrhoids, intake of irritating foods, amount of blood, and associated physical sensations, and so on. The person may ultimately interpret the observation as unrelated to the FAP, choose to not contact the physician, and self-medicate with stool softeners. Conversely, if the person experiences the observation as especially distressing and has prior experience with this symptom being associated with polyposis, the person will contact the healthcare provider and request professional intervention.

The Giarelli model presumes that each surveillance event is unique, and one may easily imagine a number of alternative scenarios to this one. The model also illustrates the claim that all participants in lifelong surveillance experience the same complex psychosocial processes. This claim will gain support as the model is tested in different patient populations.

Examination of the Model for Points of Moral Obligation

At each juncture of the model there is opportunity for the involvement of healthcare providers who must determine what is ethically required or what is the professional obligation. The literature provides us with guidelines for structuring planned surveillance events (National Comprehensive Cancer Network 2005). Such guidelines

FIGURE 20–1
Participation in Lifelong Self-surveillance:
A Conceptual Model

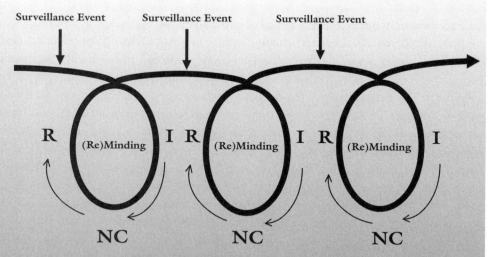

This model shows the relationship between surveillance events and the basic psychosocial problem associated with participation in life-long surveillance for genetic predisposition to cancer. See further discussion on page XX and page YY .

I = Interpretation   NC = Negotiating Control   R = (Re)Integration

Source: Giarelli, E. (2003). Bringing threat to the fore: Participation in lifelong surveillance for genetic risk of cancer. *Oncology Nursing Forum* 30 (6), 952.

Reprinted with permission of the publisher.

are available for all cancers that require follow-up care, and differ according to the natural history, stage, and grade of the cancer. The guidelines provide recommendations regarding: frequency of visits for physical exams by primary providers or cancer and other specialists; and biochemical analyses (laboratory tests), to track progression of disease, recurrence, and response to treatment. A healthcare provider is trained to identify and meet patients' educational needs. Obligations are clear in most cases with regard to the timing of and treatment during follow-up visits, recommended screening tests, medication schedules, and genetic counseling. However, there are no technical or intervention guidelines for nurses to follow vis-à-vis patient participation in incidental surveillance. Therefore, ethical obligations are also ambiguous. An examination of the psychosocial processes during self-surveillance will uncover ways in which professionals may be morally obligated to act.

Basic Psychological Problem in the Model: (Re)Minding

Once a person is informed that he or she has a genetic alteration associated with a high or absolute risk of cancer, this individual begins enhanced surveillance. Each surveillance event is noted. Planned surveillance events are prescribed by healthcare providers (HCPs) who recommend some observations over others based on clinical guidelines. For example, a patient is advised to have a colonoscopy every year for risk of colon polyps. The HCP determines which tests, visits, and other observations are needed. The HCP is obliged to share these recommendations with the patient and offer opportunities to carry them out. Patients also begin to engage in self-surveillance. They become vigilant and monitor changes in feelings and signs attributable to the cancer predisposition genotype. Self-surveillance may occur occasionally or many times per day. Self-surveillance, in most cases, occurs independent of the nurse's participation, and proceeds for nearly all patients with little or no initial guidance as to how, when, or why it should occur. If nurses are obliged to inform patients of screening and follow-up recommendations, they also have an obligation to provide guidance for self-surveillance.

At this stage of genetic cancer care, the conceptualization of ongoing self-surveillance is new. We are just beginning to identify the extent to which patients engage in these activities. We do not yet know the impact or absolute value to patients of self-surveillance. There are limited instructions or guidelines for patients, families, or nurses. However, we know that patients are engaging in such activities as a direct consequence of knowing their genetic risk, so a nurse has a professional responsibility and therefore an ethical obligation to confront this reality because any event or behavior that flows from knowing one's risk requires attention.

The individual who is informed of a genetic risk of cancer may experience emotions that range from unpleasant (worry, anger, sadness, fear) to pleasant (relief, protectiveness, certainty) (Cleiren, Oskam, and Lips 1989; Galloway and Graydon 1996; Harper and Clarke 1990; King, Dozois, Lindor, and Ahlquist 2000; Wertz, Fanos, and Reilly 1994). The healthcare provider's ethical obligation at the time of diagnosis is clear: to provide counseling to mitigate emotional distress. This is a standard of care in genetic counseling.

During lifelong monitoring, each surveillance event will generate similar feelings in affected individuals and unaffected family members who worry about their loved ones. During planned surveillance, such as a follow-up visit, a nurse must expect that

306

a patient may experience feelings ranging from relief to worry, sadness, and fear if diagnostic findings indicate recurrence of disease or further phenotypic expression. Nurses have an ethical obligation to observe the patient during planned visits for signs of emotional distress and offer counseling or emotional support. The patient's emotional state should be considered during each follow-up visit regardless of time elapsed since diagnosis.

Self-surveillance is the principle form of incidental surveillance. During these surveillance events there is equal likelihood that a patient will experience the range of negative and positive emotions. These occur out of the purview of healthcare providers, and without the benefit of emotional support and counseling. While one would not encourage a patient to contact a nurse after each and every distressing event of self-surveillance, one might expect that, based on the likelihood that patients will have these feelings, some provisions should be made to ensure that patients will have access to emotional or social support if needed. It would therefore be an ethical responsibility to address the day-to-day risk of emotional distress of knowing genetic risk for cancer. The bioethical principle of beneficence guides nurses to ensure these individuals have a means to deal with emergent distress. Support groups have been offered to patients as a way to deal with personal issues, and emergent distress can be explored in these environments. But these planned opportunities are rare relative to the frequency of self-surveillance. The challenge for nurses is to think of follow-up care in this cohort as daily and lifelong and re-conceptualize the notion of "support" without boundaries.

Interpreting the Meaning

A patient who has just been reminded of the threat of cancer, loss, or disability by the observation of some aspect of health during self-surveillance must interpret the meaning or relevance of that observation. Some observations are based on tangible evidence, for example, a patient with MEN2a might palpate a lump to the right of his trachea. After such an observation the patient must seek information, validate the threat, and assign meaning or relevance to what is found (Giarelli 2003b).

With incomplete or inaccurate information a patient's ability to interpret the meaning of the lump is impaired. If a patient has mental or emotional limitations, or has had no past experiences or only one kind of experience with such symptoms, his ability to make reasoned judgments is compromised. If past experience suggests that a lump in this location was related to pharyngitis, the patient may presume that the finding is benign and irrelevant to the genetic disorder and choose to not report this to the physician. Conversely, previous findings which are confirmed by biopsy as metastasis of medullary thyroid carcinoma will prompt the patient to assume the worst. In this case, the patient's interpretation of the relevance of the observation to the risk of cancer is biased by negative expectations. He may presume that once again this is evidence of metastasis and report these findings to the physician. If either one of these interpretations is correct, self-surveillance has been beneficial. If either is incorrect, the patient is not benefiting and may further bias his pattern of interpreting during self-surveillance.

To realize the principle of beneficence, a nurse must expand ethical obligation to the patient who is attempting to interpret the meaning of findings made during self-monitoring. Nurses do this now to some extent. For example, when a patient is discharged from the hospital after surgery he is given post-operative instructions, which often include brief descriptions of signs to watch for which might be interpreted as the onset of an infection (e.g., elevated body temperature, redness at the incision site, and so on). The patient is advised to contact the physician at the onset of these signs, at which time the nurse evaluates the relevance and need for action. The ethical obligation to do no harm is met by ensuring that the patient has sufficient information (normal versus abnormal redness), the ability (patient not visually impaired), and the equipment (thermometer) to efficiently self-monitor. The process of interpreting findings during self-monitoring for the post-operative patient is time- and object-limited, and therefore easy to design.

A nurse caring for a person with a genetic risk of cancer is ethically obligated to assure that no harm comes to the patient as a consequence of their interpretation of findings made during self-surveillance. As one would do for the post-operative patient, the nurse must ensure that the patient with genetic predisposition to cancer has sufficient information and ability to make reasoned and accurate judgments about physical and emotional signs and symptoms that suggest phenotypic expression or a problem indirectly related to the genetic risk. Also, if a patient monitors his or her blood pressure, this equipment should be evaluated to assure accuracy. At this time in our understanding of cancer predisposition and disease expression there are no standards for professionals that specifically address a patient's needs with regard to self-surveillance. We do not know all the information that is needed by a patient to self-monitor. Beside those required for the post-operative patient, there may be a need for more and different kinds of abilities to make daily, lifelong critical judgments. As for equipment, like blood sugar testing by the diabetic, there may be a need for similar biochemical screening by the MEN2a patient taking high doses of calcium because of parathyroid failure (Sijanovi and Karner 2001) when there are concurrent disorders such as renal calculi and osteoporosis. A minimum expectation of practice is that a nurse would assess the patient's self-surveillance behaviors for kinds, frequency, and emotional burden, and assess the patient's ability to critically evaluate findings. For example, a nurse should determine if a patient engages intensely and regularly in distressing self-surveillance activities. The best outcomes of the assessment would be a revision of the patient's interpretation by assisting the patient to correctly validate the threat and mitigating the negative emotional effects.

Now that we know such assessments are needed, we are faced with an ethical problem. Presently there are neither instruments to measure these variables nor criteria to aid assessment. A nurse has limited means to meet a patient's identified needs. The optimum patient outcome is impossible to achieve at this time in our understanding of self-surveillance over a lifetime. Moreover, there are innumerable factors beyond the control of the nurse. For example, we have limited influence on personality characteristics, environmental factors, limited family resources, and influence of family members. The nurse is confronted with the ethical problem of knowing what is good (best outcome) and what must be done, but lacking the ability to comply for lack of opportunity and limited empirical data to develop evidence-based practice.

Negotiating Control

Another important piece of the conceptual model is the psychosocial process of negotiating control. The patient must deal with the meaning of the observation and decide on a course of action. All patients develop some way of managing the reality of their illness and the threat of cancer, loss, or disability. The patient manages the effect and takes charge of the potential threat by identifying, for example, standards against which to measure the value of an outcome. For example, if a person is monitoring their pulse rate, they may compare the rate to a list of normal rates based on age, activity, and personal health history. Patients also manage their care in a variety of ways. Some patients actively collaborate with physicians to exchange information about symptoms, compare old and new lab values, and reach consensus on frequency of follow-up evaluations. Other patients selectively attend to recommendations and cancel appointments for office visits. Both passive and active means accomplish the same goal: managing one's care.

All patients, without exception, negotiate control to a great or lesser degree. The first moral responsibility of the nurse with regard to this phase of participation in lifelong surveillance is to accept that patients will negotiate control as a consequence of self-surveillance activities. They will, with varying intensity, style, and success, manage the effect of surveillance events on self and family, and manage their care. At this time there are no objective standards against which to measure the success of managing one's care. We presume that patient satisfaction and stable health are worthy criteria. An intuitive rule is that managing one's care should cause no harm. A nurse has a moral responsibility to ensure that while a patient is exercising the right to negotiate control by managing care he does not cause harm to either himself or others. It logically follows that this obligation should be extended to affected family members, and that managing one's own care would transition to managing the care of one's child who is similarly affected.

Negotiating control is defined in part by one's right to self-determination. A nurse must acknowledge this principle as a defining truth in self-directed health-promoting behavior. A patient's right to self-determination is a bioethical principle that pervades the complex psychosocial processes of participation in lifelong self-surveillance. A nurse must discern the patient-specific meaning of autonomy in self-surveillance and decide how to respect this basic right while negotiating control. This, like other phases of lifelong surveillance, is cyclical and ongoing; the nurse's obligations are similarly cyclical and ongoing. A nurse is obligated to apply the bioethical principle of autonomy when he or she assesses that the patient is engaging in this psychosocial process.

This is a responsibility that on the surface appears straightforward. Both nurse and patient can collaborate and negotiate the timing and kinds of follow-up interventions in response to observations that are brought to the attention of the healthcare provider. However, observations made during incidental surveillance activities will not necessarily be brought to the attention of providers. Now that we know that patients are managing aspects of their care a nurse has a moral responsibility to evaluate the likelihood that any strategies will be beneficial. She or he should determine if a patient uses idiosyncratic, unproductive, or destructive strategies to negotiate control. One such strategy may be ignoring pain. It logically follows that a nurse must arm the patient with sufficient information to make wise choices, have realistic expectations, and not make careless judgments based on inaccurate knowledge.

A common behavior among some patients with MEN2a is to adjust dosage of thyroid replacement hormone according to a collection of physical feelings (Giarelli 20003b). For example, one patient reported taking an additional dose of levothyroxine once a week to counteract a feeling of sluggishness and measured weight gain (E.T., Personal Communication, November 18, 2002). Another patient complained of feeling jittery and having rare palpitations and reported skipping a dose of levothyroxine on occasion to reduce these symptoms (B.J, Personal communication, October 2, 2002). Neither patient reported consulting their physician or nurse before managing care this way. Both patients would have benefited from additional information on drug purpose, action, and side effects. In order to help these patients to make wise choices, have realistic expectations, and not make careless judgments based on inaccurate knowledge, an ethically responsible nurse would first need to recognize the patient's absolute right to make these decisions, however ill conceived. This might be followed by an assessment of knowledge and instruction on critical problem solving.

310

Some patients will be more emotionally and intellectually equipped than others to receive such instruction. However, ethical obligations are not bound by a patient's cognitive prowess and problem-solving abilities. The ethical nurse must find a way to make such instruction relevant to any patient.

(Re)Integration

According to the Giarelli model, surveillance events may be experienced as psychologically and socially disintegrating, such that some observations if interpreted as directly related to the genetic disorder or predisposition to disease will cause changes in perceived health and self-image or as a compromise to health and wholeness. The final phase in the cyclical processes of participation in lifelong surveillance is to restore psychosocial stability in response to the perceived change. This process is called (re)integration. Most patients incorporate the effect of the observation and, ideally, move on. There are limited data on the consequences to an individual who does not effectively (re)integrate. If this does not occur, or if the person is having difficulty moving on, a healthcare provider might notice signs of (dis)-integration such as feelings of anger, hopelessness, frustration, loss of control, and being stuck. The person may increase their efforts to negotiate control, or experience enhanced distress from subsequent surveillance events. These signs indicate a disruption in the cycle (see Figure 20–1 on page 305).

I have noted that the cyclic nature of incidental surveillance causes a decrease in worry and a decreased interest in formal follow-up (Giarelli 2003b, p. 953). Incidental surveillance gives patients many years and ample opportunity to develop and refine the ability to self-assess and self-manage many aspects of their care. The burden of surveillance may shift from healthcare provider to patient as planned surveillance events like office visits become irritating and acquire a veneer of futility when check-ups offer no new information. Planned surveillance, such as lab studies, may be perceived as pointless when values are unexplainable in relation to one's symptoms and physical findings. Such experiences reinforce a patient's perception that their choice to limit contact with healthcare providers was the right choice.

It is at this juncture of reintegration when patients develop behaviors that do not promote good health. We presume that the good and valuable outcomes of reintegration are healthy adaptation and continued contact with healthcare professionals. A nurse's moral obligation to the patient during the process of reintegration is to ensure that the patient will have access to lifelong healthcare services regardless of the age at which the diagnosis was made. This obligation is especially important in the case of genetic predisposition to cancer, when such risk may be identified at birth (Knoppers and Isasi 2004; Stoffel and Syngal 2005) and health monitoring may proceed indefinitely. It is difficult to meet such an obligation when no patient has the absolute social right to healthcare services and knowledge of patients' life-long and cross generational needs varies among professionals.

Conclusion

Our quest to understand the experiences of patients who know their risk for disease has generated new knowledge about patients' feelings, behaviors, and healthcare needs. Deeper understanding brings expanded responsibilities. We know that self-management is an essential component of care in chronic illness (McLaughlin-Ren-pinning, and Taylor 2003; Ziguras 2004). We know that patients with cancer pre-disposition syndromes participate in lifelong self-surveillance. We may eventually confirm that all patients with genetic disorders perform these activities in much the same way. For patients with diabetes, for example, self-management can be as tangi-ble as blood sugar measurement. For the person whose disease is not yet, but some day will be, tangible, self-management is fundamentally different and involves largely intellectual endeavors, such as skilled observation and negotiating and critical prob-lem solving. It is not sufficient to presume that patients are capable of intelligent self-monitoring. Nor is it morally sufficient to allow all patients to participate in lifelong self-surveillance without some preparation or guidance.

A judgment of whether or not a patient should be engaging in self-surveillance is irrelevant because patients do and will continue these behaviors. More importantly, nurses and patients must reach consensus as to what extent self-surveillance can become a "good" or valuable component of lifelong surveillance. Our obligation is to understand these behaviors well enough to identify times and ways in which the value of patient self-surveillance can be optimized.

It may appear to the reader that the bioethical principles that have guided nursing practice in the past are insufficient to fully guide ethical nursing care of patients who are at increased genetic risk for disease. I have proposed that a new bioethical prin-ciple of "sustained being" is more suited to the evolving practice of genetic cancer care, and is compatible with a variety of ethical theories (Giarelli 2003a). I submit that nurses have a moral imperative to safeguard being when the potential for harm is unknown and evolving in a science. A nurse who safeguards being is mindful of real and potential dangers and believes that wholeness is intrinsically valuable.

As patients engage in self-surveillance activities the psychosocial processes previously discussed pose threats to a patient's sense of wholeness (e.g., the disintegrating effect of (re)minding. A nurse who safeguards being will search for ways to help patients maintain and restore wholeness during the processes of (re)minding and (re)integration respectively. Any action taken by the nurse to safeguard being will therefore be a professionally ethical act.

References

Cleiren, M., W. Oskam, and C. Lips. 1989. Living with a hereditary form of cancer: Experiences and needs of MEN2a patients and their families. *Henry Ford Hospital Medical Journal* 37 (3–4): 164–166.

Galloway, S. and J. Graydon. 1996. Uncertainty, symptom distress, and information needs after surgery for cancer of the colon. *Cancer Nursing* 19 (2): 112–117.

Giarelli, E. 2002 A concept model for surveillance in genetic cancer care. *Journal of Cancer Education* 17 (2): 78–82.

———. 2003a. Safeguarding being: A bioethical principle for genetic cancer care. *Nursing Ethics* 10 (3): 255–268.

———. 2003b. Bringing threat to the fore: Participation in lifelong surveillance for genetic predisposition to cancer. *Oncology Nursing Forum* 30 (6): 945–955.

———. 2006. Self-surveillance for genetic predisposition to cancer: Behaviors and emotions. *Oncology Nursing Forum* 33 (2): 221–231.

Harper, P., and A. Clarke. 1990. Should we test children for "adult" genetic diseases? *Lancet* 335, 1205–1206.

King, J. E., R. R. Dozois, N. M. Lindor, and D. A. Ahlquist. 2000. Care of patients and their families with familial adenomatous polyposis. *Mayo Clinic Proceedings* 75 (1): 57–67.

Knoppers, B. M., and R. M. Isasi. 2004. Regulatory approaches to reproductive genetic testing. *Human Reproduction* 19 (12): 2695–2701.

McLaughlin-Renpinning, D., and S. G. Taylor, eds. 2003. *Self care theory in nursing: Selected papers of Dorothea Orem*. New York: Springer Publishing.

National Comprehensive Cancer Network (NCCN). 2005. Guidelines for detection, prevention and risk reduction of colorectal cancer. http://www.nccn.org/professionals/physician_gls/PDF/colorectal_screening.pdf (accessed September 10, 2008).

Pellegrino, E. D. 1979. Toward a reconstruction of medical morality: The primacy of the act of profession and the fact of illness. *Journal of Medical Philosophy* 4: 32–55.

Sijanovi, S., and I. Karner. 2001. Bone loss in premenopausal women on long-term suppressive therapy with thyroid hormone. *Medscape General Medicine* 3 (4). http://www.medscape.com/viewarticle/408957 (accessed September 10, 2008).

Stoffel, E. M., and S. Syngal. 2005. Adenomas in young patients: What is the optimal evaluation? *American Journal of Gastroenterology* 100 (5): 1050–1053.

Wertz, D. C., J. H. Fanos, and P. R. Reilly. 1994. Genetic testing for children and adolescents: Who decides? *Journal of the American Medical Association* 272: 875–881.

Ziguras, C. 2004. *Self-care: Embodiment, personal autonomy, and the shaping of health care consciousness.* London: Routledge.

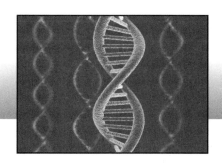

CHAPTER 21

Cystic Fibrosis: Screening, Testing, Ethics

Diane Seibert, PhD, MS, WHCNP, ANP, CRNP
Melissa H. Fries, MD, Colonel, USAF, MC

An Ancient Disease, a New Understanding: Description of the Problem

Parents of children with cystic fibrosis have recognized for centuries that the salty taste of their children was a sign of trouble. Folk tales arising during the middle ages in Central and Northern Europe warned "woe to that child which when kissed on the forehead tastes salty. He is bewitched and soon must die" (Halvorsen 2003). Many generations passed, however, before a full picture of the disorder of cystic fibrosis (CF) and the reason behind the salty taste emerged. Dr Dorothy Andersen, a pathologist at Columbia University, provided the first comprehensive pathological description of the disease in 1938. That year, the median survival for a child with CF was 12 months, and many children died so young that making the connection between respiratory disease, failure to thrive, and pancreatic disorders was virtually impossible. Andersen autopsied 49 infants and children who died from respiratory disorders characterized by thick, tenacious mucous (Andersen 1938). She found a consistent pattern of disease; all of the children had signs of pancreatic damage, chronic lung infection,

315

and malnutrition. Dr Andersen is credited with giving the disease its name, calling it "cystic fibrosis of the pancreas" because of the small cysts and fibrotic changes she noted in the pancreas.

Advances in the treatment of CF are phenomenal, highlighting the impact that basic science research can have on improving survival and quality of life for thousands of individuals. As antibiotics and vaccines against common respiratory pathogens became available in the 1950s and 1960s, targeted treatment for CF began. For the first time, a child born with CF could be expected to survive to early adolescence (Boat 1997). When the cellular defect became understood in the early 1980s, therapy was further refined and longevity improved again. In 1989, when the genetic defect was identified and early diagnosis became possible, lifespan increased again. A child born with CF in 2005 has a median life expectancy of 40 years, and CF is now considered a manageable, chronic disease, not a childhood death sentence.

Why does the CF gene remain in the human genome, if individuals homozygous for the CF gene have such a poor survival rate? The answer may lie in some protective effect for having one copy (but not two) of the CF gene. Studies (Hansson 1988; Baxter, Goldhill, Hardcastle, Hardcastle, and Taylor 1988; Rodman and Zamudio 1991) suggest that CF heterozygotes may be more resistant to bacterial toxin-mediated diarrhea, possibly protecting carriers from cholera or other chloride-ion-secreting diarrheas. This protective effect may be particularly important for infants. It has also been hypothesized that CF heterozygote individuals may have a genetic protection against typhoid fever, because *S. typhi* enters the body through GI epithelial cells, using CFTR chloride channels (Pier, Grout, Zaidi, Meluleni, Mueschenborn, Banting, et al. 1998). Whatever the benefit for carriers of a single copy of a CF mutation, a double dose of the more severe form of CF mutation has, until recently, been lethal at a very young age.

Physiology

The symptoms of CF result from a genetic defect that inactivates a large protein molecule called the cystic fibrosis transmembrane regulator (CFTR). This protein is responsible for the structure and function of epithelial chloride channels, which, when functioning normally, permit chloride channels to open and close. Typically, when chloride ions move from one side of a membrane to the other, sodium ions follow, creating an osmotic "pull" that draws water along with them. In the normal lung, chloride ions move from the interstitial tissues into the airway, pulling water in with them. This water thins pulmonary mucous, allowing cilia to sweep bacteria and mucous up and out of the lung. Normal chloride channel activity is critical to the effective functioning of epithelial cells in many body systems, but it is particularly important in lung and gastrointestinal tissues. It is the effect on the sweat glands that leads to the increased amount of surface sodium chloride, leading to the salty taste of the affected child's skin.

The CFTR gene was identified and sequenced in 1989. Located on the long arm of chromosome 7 (7q31.2), it contains approximately 250,000 base pairs and 27 exons (coding regions of the gene). To date, more than 1,300 CFTR mutations have been described, but the most common as well as the most serious mutation is a deletion of a three nucleotides encoding for phenylalynine (F) at the 508th position (DF508). Of all the patients in the United States with "classic" CF, 70% have a DF508 mutation. The wide range of mutation possibilities and severity of dysfunction is responsible for the range of symptom severity that can be seen with CF (Zeitlin 1999; Selvadurai, McKay, Blimkie, Cooper, Mellis, and van Asperen 2002). Individuals who are homozygous for DF508 or compound heterozygotes for two severe CF mutations usually present with the hallmark signs of "classic" cystic fibrosis first described by Dr Andersen: chronic respiratory infection, fat malabsorption due to inadequate pancreatic enzyme function, male infertility, and high sweat chloride levels (Knowles and Durie 200310).

Cystic Fibrosis Mutations

Cystic fibrosis mutations are classified according to how the mutation affects the CFTR protein. Class I, II, and III mutations are the most severe and typically cause symptoms associated with "classic CF," while Class IV and V are less severe because at least some chloride ions reach their target organs. Class I mutations are typically nonsense or frameshift mutations (E69X, W401X, etc.) that block CFTR protein synthesis, resulting in a complete absence of CFTR. Class II mutations (DF508, N1303K), are usually caused by a deletion or missense mutation which produces a protein that is unable to migrate from the endoplasmic reticulum to the cell membrane. In a class II mutation, CFTR protein is made, but it cannot get to its site of action. Class III (G551D) mutations are missense or substitution mutations which disrupt the regulation of CFTR at the level of the cell membrane; the protein is made, is transported, but doesn't work once it arrives. Class IV (R117H, R347P) mutations are usually missense mutations that alter the amount of chloride ions that move through the channel, reducing the overall volume. Class V (A445E) mutations are caused either by missense or alternative splicing, resulting in a reduction in the overall production of CFTR protein.

Features of Classic Cystic Fibrosis

Respiratory Tract

In the normal lung, chloride ions move freely across the epithelial cell wall via the chloride channel (from the airway epithelial cell into the mucous lining). As sodium ions move into the cell, chloride moves out and into the mucous layer in the airway, creating a concentration gradient which attracts water molecules, resulting in a thinning of pulmonary secretions, allowing for mobilization out of the airway. When the chloride channel is non-functional, pulmonary mucous becomes dehydrated and secretions become thick and tenacious. In the absence of negatively charged chloride ions, mucosal pH is also altered, creating a bacteria-friendly environment. Interestingly, it has also been hypothesized that the functioning CFTR proteins protect against *Pseudomonas aeruginosa* infection. Studies have shown that a lipopolysaccharide (LPS) in the cell membrane of *P. aeruginosa* is recognized, bound, and destroyed by CFTR protein. Lung cells with the ΔF508 mutation fail to bind and destroy *P. aeruginosa*. So, in addition to providing a healthy pulmonary environment, CFTR seems to be a critical element in lung's immune response to bacterial infection, particularly *P. aeruginosa* (Schroder, Lee, Yacono Cannon, Gerçeker, Golan, et al. 2002).

Digestive Tract

Chloride channels function in the gut by allowing pancreatic proenzymes to move from the pancreas into the bowel. When CFTR proteins are absent, proenzymes build up in the pancreatic ducts resulting initially in fat malabsorption and eventually in the destruction of the pancreas. Symptoms associated with the pancreatic enzyme insufficiency include diarrhea, malnutrition resulting in poor weight gain, and slowed linear growth. Malabsorption often begins at or shortly after birth and failure to thrive may prompt a CF workup (a series of diagnostic procedures that may indicate the presence of a specific condition, such as CF) and eventual diagnosis. As mentioned, the pancreatic damage continues throughout life, and many individuals will develop Cystic fibrosis-related diabetes mellitus (CFRD) during the second decade of life. As the pancreatic damage accumulates, physiologic changes progress from reduced insulin secretion and insulin resistance (Ratjen and Doring 2003) to a total loss of pancreatic function. A recent study has shown that poor linear growth in the first decade of life may, in fact, be related to an early reduction in insulin production (Ripa, Robertson, Cowley, Harris, Masters, and Cotterill 2002). In a study of 18 children ages 9.5 to 15, 20% had impaired glucose tolerance and among those with clinical normal glucose tolerance tests, insulin secretion was impaired in 65%. These results raise the question about whether insulin therapy should be considered in children with CF prior to the onset of CFRD (Ripa et al. 2002).

Manifestations of Non-Classic Cystic Fibrosis

CF mutations in classes other than I, II, and III (A445E, etc.) may result in a partial loss of CFTR function and thus a variety of non-classic symptoms. They may have mild or atypical disease in childhood, develop "classic" CF symptoms in adulthood, present in adulthood for an infertility workup related to congenital bilateral absence of the vas deferens (CBAVD), or remain completely asymptomatic. The relationship between CFTR, other genes, and the environment are only now beginning to be appreciated. These relationships can play a significant role in the expression of the disease; children living in a smoke-filled environment, for example, often have more rapidly progressive pulmonary disease. Danish studies have shown that individuals with a CFTR mutation and a mannose-binding lectin mutation on chromosome 10 experience more rapidly progressive lung disease (Burke 2003). Finally, for reasons that are not well understood, the phenotypic expression of even "classic" CF (ΔF508/ΔF508) varies widely, from severe disease to total absence of symptoms.

What Is the Incidence?

Cystic fibrosis is one of the most common and well-documented autosomal recessive diseases in the United States. It is estimated that over 10 million people in the United States (1 in 25–29 European Caucasians) carry a CF mutation and are completely unaware of it. These asymptomatic CF carriers are healthy, but carry one normal (or "wild type") gene and one mutated CF gene. When two asymptomatic carriers reproduce, the odds that their two mutated genes will assort together is 1:4, giving them a 25% chance of having a child with CF. This happens frequently enough that in the United States almost 1,000 people are born with cystic fibrosis each year—about 1:3,300 live births.

The Cystic Fibrosis Foundation (CFF), one of the oldest and most active disease-specific genetic support groups, was founded in 1955. The CFF supports the National Cystic Fibrosis Patient Registry, a comprehensive database with information on nearly all the 30,000 Americans living with cystic fibrosis (Cystic Fibrosis Foundation 2006), and certifies 117 Cystic Fibrosis Care Centers across the United States. The care centers provide data to the national registry annually on each one of their patients, providing critical data about patient demographics, diagnostic symptoms, genotype, survival status, primary causes of death, clinical (pulmonary) status, microbiology, anthropometric measurements, number of hospitalizations, insurance coverage, etc. (Beker, Russek-Cohen, and Fink 2001). Each patient is assigned a unique identifier, so if they are seen at a different center, they are not lost to follow-up, and information is not duplicated. The registry, established in 1955, has set a goal to recruit, track, and report on the health status of all Americans with cystic fibrosis.

Who Is at Risk?

Because CF is a recessive disorder, it is extremely unlikely that the condition would arise by two spontaneous new mutations. Most mutations have been present in carriers in population groups for many generations. Approximately 70% of the individuals living with CF are homozygous (two copies) of the ΔF508 mutation (Tinkle 2002). It is most prevalent among Caucasians. This mutation, as well as other common ones, lead to estimated CF carrier rate of 1 in 25–29 in Northern European and Ashkenazi Jewish populations (Jewish populations originating in Eastern Europe). Over 1,000 CFTR mutations have been identified, with some mutations more or less common in non-Caucasian, non-Ashkenazi Jewish populations. In a study of Hispanic individuals with CF, for example, only 46% of the chromosomes carried the ΔF508 mutation; the remainder carried a variety of different CF mutations, many of which are not included in the recommended standard CF prenatal screening panel (Grebe, Seltzer, DeMarchi, Silva, Doane, Gozal, et al. 1994). The recommended panel of DNA mutations includes approximately 24 of the most common CF mutations, and is reviewed at least annually and revised regularly by the American College of Medical Genetics to identify CF mutations that have a frequency of >0.1% in the general U.S. population (Nolen and Rhoades 2004). Many CF mutations, however, are rare and are unlikely to ever make this cutoff, making them impractical and expensive to include in routine screening.

Cystic fibrosis frequency and test sensitivity and specificity vary greatly in ethnic groups, as does the ability to detect mutations. Although the disease is relatively rare among African-Americans (1 in 60 carrier rate), only 81% of them will be identified by the standard mutation screening panel. Among Hispanic populations (1 in 46 carrier rate), although the frequency is higher than that of African-Americans, it is estimated that only 72% of the mutations in this population will be identified using the standard screening panel. Because CF is very rare among Asian-Americans (1 in 90 carrier rate) only 30% of the mutations will be identified by the standard screening panel (Tinkle 2002).

Prenatal Screening for Cystic Fibrosis

In 2001, after many years of debate, discussion, and deliberation, the American College of Obstetrics and Gynecology (ACOG) and the American College of Medical Geneticists (ACMG) made the recommendation that CF carrier screening be offered to all individuals presenting for pre-conceptual or prenatal care (American College of Obstetricians and Gynecologists, American College for Medical Genetics 2001). For higher risk couples (both from an ethnic group considered to be at high risk, a family history of CF, or one partner has CF), providers should offer additional education and counseling regarding CF screening. This recommendation quietly but significantly shifted the focus of CF screening from that of disease identification to disease prevention, because individuals are provided an opportunity to make informed reproductive decisions.

Carrier screening can be done sequentially (one individual is tested and if he or she is found to carry a mutation, the other partner is tested) or simultaneously, known as "couple-based" testing. Sequential testing is more commonly used when carrier risk is considered to be low, or where obtaining simultaneous samples from both partners is impractical. If the first person tested (often the female partner) has a CF mutation, they are informed about the result and when possible the other is counseled and offered testing (Grody, Cutting, Klinger, Richards, Watson, and Desnick 2001). Couple testing may be appropriate if a couple is considered to be at high risk for carrying a CF mutation, for example if both partners are of Caucasian or Ashkenazi Jewish descent. For an excellent review of Jewish genetic disorders, please see the Chicago Center for Jewish Genetic Disorders website at http://jewishgeneticscenter.org (Chicago Center for Jewish Genetic Disorders n.d.).

Results disclosure for couples tested simultaneously has been done in two ways. Using the Wald method (Wald, George, and Wald 1993), couples are told that they are at "high risk" for having a child with CF only if both individuals test positive for a CF mutation. If one partner is found to have a mutation, but the other does not, the couple is told they are at "low risk," but the couple is never told which partner has the mutation, unless they specifically request this information (Livingston, Axton, Gilfillan, Mennie, Compton, Liston, et al. 1994). As the limitations inherent in CF screening become better understood, the Wald method is used less frequently, a tactic endorsed by ACMG and ACOG. A 2001 policy statement by ACMG and ACOG stated "While the Committee appreciates some of the psychosocial and cost-saving advantages of the couple-testing model of Wald, we do not endorse this approach because of ethical questions surrounding nondisclosure of test results and because it deprives the positive member of the positive-negative couple the opportunity of informing his or her relatives of their risk so that they too can be tested, the so-called 'cascade effect,' an ancillary benefit of primary population screening" (Grody et al. 2001). As a result, irrespective of the order in which the testing is done (sequential or couple), individuals are provided with their individual genetic test results.

The process of DNA-based CF testing is currently being done using a pan-ethnic mutation panel that includes all CF mutations with an allele frequency > 0.1% in the general U.S. population (Grody et al. 2001). The current panel consists of 25 mutations and is projected to identify approximately 75.3% of all CF mutation carriers. The panel is reviewed at least annually and updated as mutation frequencies change. An expanded panel that includes 64 mutations and identifies approximately 81.4% of all CF mutations is available, but not recommended for population screening because the additional yield is so low. This panel may be appropriate, however, for individuals from populations with uncommon but known CF alleles, as in Pueblo and Zuni Indian populations.

It is critical for individuals being screened to understand that genetic testing does not identify 100% of all CF mutations, particularly in non-white populations. Screening reduces the likelihood that an individual carries a mutation, but does not totally exclude it. When screening is being offered to individuals, these screening variations must be carefully explained; "negative" does not mean no mutation is present: it simply means no mutation was detected by the screening. For example, a woman of Caucasian background with a 1:29 baseline risk of being a carrier undergoes standard 23 mutation prenatal screening. No mutations are identified. Her risk of being a carrier is decreased to a frequency of 1:141. If her partner (untested) were of Caucasian background with also a 1:29 carrier risk, their risk of having an affected child with CF is $1/141 \times 1/29 \times 1/4$ (the chance the child would receive both mutated genes from the parents) = 1:16,356. This is much less than the population liveborn cystic fibrosis risk of 1:3,300, but is not zero. Clarifying this point is critical for those who counsel patients considering screening. It is anticipated that as mating couples become more diverse in the United States, these statistics will change and identifying target populations for screening may become more complicated.

Evolving Genetic Screening Practices in the United States

Genetic screening is not a new concept, particularly in the prenatal and newborn care arena. In obstetrics, amniocentesis has been offered for over 40 years to screen babies for major chromosomal anomalies (Jenkins and Lea 2005). Over the past two decades an increasing number of screening tests have become available, and couples can now choose whether or not to have their fetus tested for an array of congenital and genetic conditions, including neural tube defects, cystic fibrosis, beta thalassemia, sickle cell anemia, and the cluster of disorders commonly found among the Ashkenazi Jewish population: Tay Sachs Disease, Canavan Disease, and Gaucher Disease.

Once an infant is born, a virtual plethora of genetic testing options are offered. Newborns, as a population, are routinely screened for more genetic disorders than any other group in the United States. Newborn screening (NBS) became available in 1961 when a screening test for phenylketonurea (PKU) became widely available. Since then, the number of genetic tests offered to neonates has expanded to include more than 30 disorders in some states. All infants are currently tested for PKU, congenital hypothyroidism, and galactosemia (National Newborn Screening and Genetics Resource Center 2008), and most, depending on the state of birth, are screened for at least eight to ten other genetic conditions. Recent NBS recommendations (U.S. Department of Health and Human Services, 2005) propose that all states conduct a uniform NBS panel of at least the recommended 30 tests, which also includes newborn hearing testing. The criteria used to decide which condition to screen were: a) a condition identifiable at a phase where it is not ordinarily clinically detected; b) an available sensitive, specific test; and c) demonstrable benefits to the patient from early detection, timely intervention, and efficacious treatment of the condition. The last disorder to make this "cut" was newborn screening for cystic fibrosis.

Newborn Screening for Cystic Fibrosis

It is estimated that in 2004 approximately 800,000 Americans were tested for CF at birth (Grosse, Boyle, Botkin, Comeau, Kharrazi, Rosenfeld, et al. 2004). Universal newborn screening for cystic fibrosis was instituted in Colorado, Wisconsin, and Wyoming as early as 1997, and by the end of 2004 it was expected that 12 states would include CF on their routine NBS panels. Screening via NBS does not involve a DNA test for CF; newborns are tested by performing a heel stick between days 1 and 5 of life and the dried blood specimen is analyzed for immunoreactive trypsinogen (ITR). This is a pancreatic enzyme that is converted from trypsinogen to its active form trypsin in the duodenum. In individuals homozygous for CF, serum trypsinogen levels are elevated because pancreatic contents cannot exit normally through pancreatic ducts blocked by thick, tenacious secretions. As a result, pancreatic enzymes build up in the ducts and eventually leak into the bloodstream, resulting in elevations in serum trypsinogen levels. If ITR is elevated on a NBS panel, further testing is warranted. The next step in screening varies from state to state; in some states, a second blood spot specimen is obtained and serum ITR levels are repeated, while in other states DNA analysis is done on the original blood spot specimen.

NBS algorithms for CF routinely produce both false positive and false negative results, and false positive rates are estimated to be approximately 9.5:1; comparing favorably with other NBS tests whose false positive rates can be as high as 50 times the number of disorders identified (Grosse et al. 2004). Genetic counseling should therefore be provided to families whose children have elevated ITR on NBS tests. In many cases, confirmatory testing will reveal that the child is a CF mutation carrier, which has familial implications that genetic counseling will address.

Sweat Chloride Testing

If CF is suspected, a DNA test might be ordered to assist in the diagnosis. DNA tests have their limitations, however, in that they only identify approximately 70% to 80% of people with disease and provide little information about disease severity. Sweat chloride testing is the diagnostic tool clinicians use to gauge the extent of chloride channel dysfunction. Sweat chloride testing measures the amount of sodium chloride present in sweat. The test is simple to perform; topical pilocarpine is applied to the skin, and a mild electric current is added to stimulate sweating. The area is wrapped with plastic and sweat collected on an adsorbent pad. Abnormal levels vary by age: chloride levels above 60 mmol/L is diagnostic in children older than three months, above 80mmol/L is diagnostic for adults, and although newborns are usually not tested (they don't produce enough sweat), if a sweat chloride test is done on an infant younger than three months, chloride levels above 40 mmol/L is indicative of CF. The sweat chloride false positive rate is estimated to be 10% to 15% because other conditions can cause elevated sweat chloride tests. All positive tests should be repeated, and if not done previously DNA testing should be offered.

Nasal Potential Difference (NPD) Measurement

As sodium and chloride ions move across cell membranes, they generate an electric potential gradient. This gradient in the upper airway (nasal passages) is known as the nasal potential difference which is easily measured using a surface electrode. The test is very dependent on the skill of the person administering it, however, so individuals should be referred to a CF center for NPD testing. People with CF have very different NPD values than people without CF. Although NPD is not commonly performed, it can be a very useful adjunctive test when sweat chloride or DNA tests are inconclusive.

While newborn screening has great value in identifying affected children early, it may also detect unaffected carrier children, leading to parental anxiety and confusion. For this reason newborn screening for CF has not been recommended as a replacement for prenatal parental screening.

Genetics, Policy, and Nursing

The influence of science on public policy and politics has never been more complicated. As genetic tests and therapies become available, policies advising who is the most appropriate group to be tested have emerged. Population genetics and targeted screening for common genetic disorders have become hotly debated topics, with issues like ethnic discrimination, abortion, cloning, and stem cell use at the center of the political and policy storm. The demand for well informed providers has increased dramatically, but the number of medical geneticists and genetic counselors remains woefully inadequate (Varmus 2002). Currently slightly less than 3,000 genetic providers are licensed to provide genetic health care in the United States (Cooksey 2000), and most of them are concentrated in large urban academic and medical centers to ensure access to the greatest number of patients. As genetic information moves into the public domain, more people are expected to consult with their primary care providers with questions such as: Can I be tested to see if I will get breast cancer? Will my baby inherit a genetic condition? Is there a test to tell if I'm at risk for a heart attack? It is becoming increasingly clear that that everyone—the public, nurses, physicians and many other types of healthcare providers (dentists, veterinarians, optometrists, etc.)—will have to expand their understanding in order to keep abreast of genetic information (Varmus 2002).

Registered nurses (RNs) compose the largest group of healthcare providers in the United States (U.S. Department of Labor 2004). As a group they have direct contact with the public because they are present in virtually every healthcare setting. In addition, an RN's education and training in holistic care, emphasis on wellness, and focus on patient education make them uniquely suited to provide basic genetic health care and genetic information to the general public. Nurses prepared at the graduate level (as Nurse Practitioners, Nurse Anesthetists, Nurse Midwives, and Clinical Nurse Specialists, or other advanced practice specialists) can provide more expanded and detailed genetic education. The bottom line is that nurses are at the front line in patient care, and have the potential to change the face of health care by making genetic information accessible to the general public.

Ethical Issues

Informed Consent

Individuals must know about the risks, benefits, effectiveness, and alternatives to testing in order to understand the implications of genetic testing. Testing for CF places unique educational demands on healthcare providers because there are so many different scenarios in which CF testing questions arise. Some people request testing because they have an affected family member; some will first learn about the disease when their infant is identified through NBS; and others are anticipating a normal, uncomplicated pregnancy and then learn that they are in a high-risk group. Each situation demands a different approach to education and providers must be prepared to tailor information to meet individual patient and family needs.

Individuals with affected family members may know a great deal more about cystic fibrosis than their primary care providers and may not need information about the natural course of the disease. They are often focused on finding out if they carry a CF mutation. Providers need to provide a risk assessment and order testing, but are also obligated to explain the limitations of genetic testing and explore the wide range of emotions many people experience when they receive genetic test results (Jenkins and Lea 2005).

Newborn screening also can result in significant anxiety for parents and families. Newborns with elevated ITRs will be referred for confirmatory testing because false positive and false negative results are possible. In the false negative situation, a child with CF has a normal (or borderline normal) ITR and the NBS report is negative. Parents and providers may spend many frustrating months seeking answers for the child's healthcare problems and unexplained illnesses. In the false positive situation, ITR is elevated (or borderline high), but the child is not affected (although many may be CF carriers) and families endure weeks of stress awaiting confirmatory tests. Both situations may cause long-term negative consequences for both the child and the family. Healthcare providers should carefully review the benefits and limitations of newborn screening with family members prior to testing, and ensure that support and education is available in the case of abnormal results.

Carrier testing is DNA-based, making false positive results highly unlikely. False negative results are certainly possible, however, because the standard pan-ethnic panel includes only the most common 25 known CF mutations. The possibility of a false negative test result must be carefully and fully explained to all individuals prior to

326

testing. An ancillary benefit of carrier testing is that relatives can be alerted to their risk for carrying a mutation and may also seek testing: the so-called "cascade effect" (Grody 2003).

Privacy and Insurability

Genetic testing identifies individuals who carry a genetic mutation that may put them or their offspring at risk for acquiring or developing a disease. Many people refuse genetic testing or hide important family history information in fear that this information will not remain private, putting them at risk for employment or insurance discrimination. Some countries already have genetic discrimination laws, and steps have recently been taken in the United States to provide some protection from discrimination. The Genetic Information Nondiscrimination Act of 2007 (GINA) passed in the U.S. House of Representatives on April 25, 2007 by a vote of 420–3, the Senate passed it unanimously on April 24, 2008, and President Bush signed it into law on May 21, 2008. The bill is intended to protect individuals against insurance and employment discrimination, and supports genetic testing as part of routine medical care. The bill prohibits employers from using genetic information when making employment decisions and prevents insurance companies from denying coverage or basing premium rates on genetic information. The bill also prohibits a group health plan or an issuer of a health insurance group health plan from "requesting or requiring" an individual or family member to undergo a genetic test and establishes privacy protections for genetic information held by employers, employment agencies, and labor organizations.

Confidentiality

Genetic information is sensitive and access should to limited to those authorized to receive it. Federal healthcare confidentiality and privacy measures, like the Health Insurance Portability and Accountability Act (HIPAA) and its 2003 Privacy Rule, provide some measure of protection, but many questions about confidentiality remain. Questions about how long genetic samples should be kept (newborn blood spots, military blood specimens), who owns them, who has access to them, and who can conduct research on them remain unanswered.

Final Thoughts

As population screening for genetic conditions becomes more common, primary care providers will increasingly be challenged to gather a genetic history, provide appropriate education, interpret genetic test results, and support patients with common genetic conditions. Cystic fibrosis is one of the first genetic disorders to transition into the primary care community and primary care providers must be aware of and comfortable addressing the ethical issues that commonly accompany genetic screening. Counseling those worried about CF is uniquely challenging because of the number of known mutations, the polymorphic diversity within ethnic groups, the increasing heterogeneity of the U.S. population, the array of testing options, and the disconnect between genotype and the phenotypical expression of the disease. Since ACOG and ACMG recommended that all couples presenting for preconceptual or prenatal care be offered CF screening, many individuals are currently being offered CF screening during the prenatal period when reproductive options are limited. If both partners are found to carry a CF mutation, couples are often forced to make rapid decisions about the acceptability of prenatal testing or pregnancy termination. Over time, CF carrier screening may be offered in primary care and non-GYN settings, eliminating some of the ethical challenges imposed during pregnancy. Primary care providers would be well served to stay informed about changes in CF testing, and always keep the principles of justice, beneficence, autonomy, and non-malfeasance in mind whenever genetic testing is being offered.

References

American College of Obstetricians and Gynecologists, American College of Medical Genetics. 2001. *Preconception and prenatal carrier screening for cystic fibrosis: Clinical and laboratory guidelines.* Atlanta, GA: ACOG/ACMG.

Andersen, D. 1938. Cystic fibrosis of the pancreas and its relation to celiac disease: A clinical and pathological study. *American Journal of Diseases of Children* 56: 344–399.

Baxter P. S., J. Goldhill, J. Hardcastle, P. T. Hardcastle, and C. J. Taylor. 1988. Accounting for cystic fibrosis. *Nature* 335: 211.

Beker, L., E. Russek-Cohen, and R. Fink. 2001. Stature as a prognostic factor in cystic fibrosis survival. *Journal of the American Dietetic Association* 101 (4): 438–446.

Boat, T. F. 1997. Cystic fibrosis in the post-CFTR era. In *Genetic Testing for Cystic Fibrosis, NIH Consensus Development Conference,* ed. Health No. 15–7. April 14–16, 1997. Bethesda, MD: National Institutes of Health.

Burke W. 2003. Genomics as a probe for disease biology. *New England Journal of Medicine* 349 (10): 969–974.

Chicago Center for Jewish Genetic Disorders. n.d. *Jewish Genetic Diseases.* http:// jewishgeneticscenter.org (accessed October 7, 2008).

Cooksey, J. 2000. *The genetic counselor workforce: Training programs, professional practice, and issues affecting supply and demand.* Chicago: Illinois Center for Health Workforce Studies.

Cystic Fibrosis Foundation. 2006. *Patient Registry Annual Report.* http://www.cff.org/ UploadedFiles/research/ClinicalResearch/2006%20Patient%20Registry%20Report.pdf (accessed October 7, 2008).

Grebe, T., W. Seltzer, J. DeMarchi, D. K. Silva, W. W. Doane, D. Gozal, S. F. Richter, C. M. Bowman, R. A. Norman, S. N. Rhodes, et al. 1994. Genetic analysis of Hispanic individuals with cystic fibrosis. *American Journal of Human Genetics* 54: 443–446.

Grody W. 2003. Molecular genetic risk screening. *Annual Review of Medicine* 54: 473–490.

Grody, W., G. Cutting, K. Klinger, C. Richards, M. Watson, and R. Desnick. 2001. Laboratory standards and guidelines for population-based cystic fibrosis carrier screening. *Genetics in Medicine* 3 (2): 149–154.

Grosse, S., C. Boyle, J. Botkin, A. M. Comeau, M. Kharrazi, M. Rosenfeld, and B. S. Wilfond. 2004. Newborn screening for cystic fibrosis: Evaluation of benefits and risks and recommendations for state newborn screening programs. *Morbidity and Mortality Weekly Report* 53 (RR-13): 1–36.

Halvorsen, J. 2003. Despite breakthroughs, cystic fibrosis answers remain elusive. *Medical College of Wisconsin Healthlink.* http://healthlink.mcw.edu/article/1031002244.html (accessed October 7, 2008).

Hansson, G.C. 1988. Cystic fibrosis and chloride-secreting diarrhoea. *Nature* 333: 711.

Jenkins, J., and D. Lea. 2005. *Nursing care in the genomic era: A case-based approach.* Sudbury, MA: Jones & Bartlett.

Knowles, M., and P. Durie. 2002. What is cystic fibrosis? *New England Journal of Medicine* 347 (6): 439–442.

Livingston, J., R. Axton, A. Gilfillan, M. Mennie, M. Compton, W. A. Liston, A. A. Calder, A. J. Gordon, and D. J. H. Brock. 1994. Antenatal screening for cystic fibrosis: A trial of the couple model. *British Medical Journal* 308 (6942): 1459–1462.

National Newborn Screening and Genetics Resource Center. 2008. *National Newborn Screening Status Report.* http://genes-r-us.uthscsa.edu/nbsdisorders.pdf (accessed September 10, 2008).

Nolen, A., and E. Rhoades. 2004. Population-based preconception and prenatal cystic fibrosis carrier screening: Clinical implication challenges. *The Female Patient* 29: 28–31.

Pier G. B., M. Grout, T. Zaidi, G. Meluleni, S. S. Mueschenborn, G. Banting, R. Ratcliff, M. J. Evans, and W. H. Colledge. 1998. Salmonella typhi uses CFTR to enter intestinal epithelial cells. *Nature* 393: 79–82.

Ratjen, F., and G. Doring. 2003. Cystic fibrosis. *Lancet* 361: 681–689.

Ripa, P., I. Robertson, D. Cowley, M. Harris, I. Masters, and A. Cotterill. 2002. The relationship between insulin secretion, the insulin-like growth factor axis and growth in children with cystic fibrosis. *Clinical Endocrinology* 56 (3): 383–389.

Rodman, D. M., and S. Zamudio. 1991. The cystic fibrosis heterozygote—Advantage in surviving cholera? *Medical Hypotheses* 36: 253–258.

Schroeder, T., M. Lee, P. Yacono, C. L. Cannon, A. A. Gerçeker, D. E. Golan, and G. B. Pier. 2002. CFTR is a pattern recognition molecule that extracts Pseudomonas aeruginosa LPS from the outer membrane into epithelial cells and activates NF-kB translocation. *Proceedings of National Academy of Sciences of the United States* 99 (10): 6907–6912.

Selvadurai, H., K. McKay, C. Blimkie, P. Cooper, C. Mellis, and P. van Asperen. 2002. The relationship between genotype and exercise tolerance in children with cystic fibrosis. *American Journal of Respiratory and Critical Care Medicine* 165 (6): 762–765.

Tinkle, M. 2002. Cystic fibrosis carrier screening: Are nurses ready to be on the front line? *AWHONN Lifelines* 6 (2): 135–139.

U.S. Department of Health and Human Services. 2005. *Advisory committee on heritable disorders in newborns and children.* http://www.hrsa.gov/heritabledisorderscommittee/reports/default.htm (accessed October 7, 2008).

U.S. Department of Labor. 2004. *Registered nurses.* http://stats.bls.gov/oco/ocos083.htm#training (accessed October 7, 2008).

Varmus, H. 2002. Getting ready for gene-based medicine. *New England Journal of Medicine* 347 (19): 1526–1527.

Wald, N., L. George, and N. Wald. 1993. Couple screening for cystic fibrosis. *Lancet* 342: 1307–1308.

Zeitlin, P. 1999. Novel pharmacologic therapies for cystic fibrosis. *The Journal of Clinical Investigation* 103 (4): 447–452.

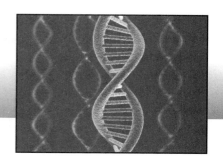

CHAPTER 22

Genetic Testing and Counseling in Huntington Disease

Heather Skirton, PhD, MSc, RGN

Introduction

The advent of recombinant DNA technology made it possible for the first time to predict the future onset of a genetic condition, prior to the appearance of any signs or symptoms. These developments enabled persons at risk for a genetic disease to see into their health future in a way that few others have been able to do. Use of the technology also enabled diagnoses to be made with a greater degree of accuracy and gave parents the option of testing a fetus at risk to determine whether it had inherited the familial condition. However, these new opportunities were accompanied by new ethical challenges in health care. Was it acceptable to offer testing when there was no means of preventing or curing the disease? Could prior knowledge of a person's fate have a detrimental effect on their lives? How could the best interests of the patient be served?

Predictive testing for adult-onset neurological conditions has been the focus of much discussion and research. This chapter focuses on the counseling and testing for Huntington disease, but the principles discussed are equally pertinent to testing for a range of adult-onset genetic conditions, including other long-term neurological conditions and familial cancer.

Huntington Disease: A Description of the Condition

Huntington disease (HD) is an autosomal dominant genetic condition that has a profound impact on the life and health of affected individuals and their families. The gene mutation that is associated with HD has an effect on the functioning of the brain as it causes atrophy of the basal ganglia and cerebral cortex (NCBI 2007). The difficulties that arise for the affected individual fall into three main categories: movement disorder, depression, and dementia (Melone, Jori, and Peluso 2005).

The onset of symptoms of the disease can occur at any age, including childhood or adolescence, but most commonly occurs during middle age. In adults, the first signs may be forgetfulness, clumsiness, and difficulty in performing certain intellectual functions. However, as the disease progresses over the ensuing 15–20 years, involuntary choreic movements (uncoordinated, spastic jerking) and dementia usually become increasingly debilitating (Skirton and Glendinning 1997). Major causes of death are pneumonia (due to immobility and aspiration) or cardiovascular disease. However, because of changes in both physical and cognitive functioning, death may be accidental or due to suicide (Sorenson and Fenger 1992).

The huntingtin (scientific name) gene is located on chromosome 4. Each person has two copies of the gene, one inherited from each parent. An expansion of one copy of this gene will result in the person developing the disease, and the size of the expansion loosely correlates with the age of onset. That is to say that if one copy of the gene, if it is the abnormal version, will have a greater number of repeats of the three nucleotide base sequence, "CAG," and thus result in the appearance of the disease. The normal number of repeats in the huntingtin gene is 11–29, while the number of repeats in the abnormal version will range from 40 to 80 (from the website of the National Institutes of Health, National Human Genome Research Institute, http://www.genome.gov/10001215). In population terms, the larger the expansion, the earlier the onset. However, it is not possible to accurately predict the age of onset of the disease in individual cases.

The offspring of a person with one expanded gene will have a 50% chance of inheriting the gene mutation, and therefore of developing HD (NCBI 2007). As the age of onset is commonly in middle age, many affected persons have children before they develop signs and symptoms. Those children are often involved in the care of the affected parent and are very familiar with the physical, psychological, and social impact of the disease on the family.

Genetic Counseling for Families at Risk of Huntington Disease

Since George Huntington published the first paper on HD (Huntington, 1872), the heritability of HD has been understood and risk assessments for family members have been based on the autosomal dominant inheritance pattern (one copy of the gene from one parent is sufficient to cause manifestation of the associated health condition). Prior to discovery of the gene locus associated with HD, counseling a person who had a parent with the condition was a matter of conveying the information that the individual was born with a 50% chance of inheriting the disease. As the at-risk person grew older, the chances could be modified according to age-related tables. Thus, based on empirical evidence, a person born at 50% risk was said to have a chance of about 30% of having inherited the condition if they reached the age of 50 without developing any signs or symptoms (Harper, Walker, Tyler, Newcombe, and Davies 1979). Couples who were considering pregnancy had the option of not having a biological child or taking the risk that the child would be affected in the future. Some were advised by healthcare professionals not to have children in order to stamp out the disease.

However, with the advent of recombinant DNA technology, opportunities for genetic testing became a reality. The site of the gene on chromosome 4 was located in 1983 (Gusella, Wexler, Conneally, Naylor, Anderson, Tanzi, et al. 1983), enabling genetic testing to be performed by linkage analysis, tracking the faulty gene through the family using markers that were closely associated with (near) the gene. This necessitated using DNA samples from a number of family members, both affected and unaffected. In these circumstances, it was virtually impossible to maintain confidentiality of the person being tested, since he or she was compelled to ask relatives to donate a blood sample for DNA extraction and testing. In addition to the ethical aspects, in practical terms it was not possible to test those who had no living affected relatives or whose family genetic structure was uninformative (for example, there might be missing information about the condition of family members, or there might not be family members who manifested signs or symptoms of HD).

However, in 1993 the expansion in the huntingtin gene associated with HD was identified, and testing was simplified (Huntington's Disease Collaborative Research Group 1993). Once HD had been confirmed as the correct diagnosis in the family, each individual's sample could be tested without the need to involve other family members.

Research Basis for Predictive Testing

Initially, predictive genetic testing was performed under the auspices of clinical research projects. Naturally, there were concerns about possible adverse effects of testing for a serious condition for which there was no effective treatment. Candidates for testing underwent a number of psychometric tests (e.g., measuring levels of depression and anxiety), as well as a mandatory three sessions of pre-test counseling and post-test follow-up. However, as the research indicated that few adverse events were reported following testing (such as serious mental health problems), clinical services began to offer predictive testing on a widespread basis, using the research protocol as a model for preparation and follow-up care (Craufurd and Tyler 1992).

For some years these stringent protocols were observed, but gradually the need for patient autonomy, variation in the support needs of different families, and the lack of evidence of substantial harm (e.g., suicide attempts or serious mental health problems) from testing were acknowledged. Currently, many centers adhere to the guidelines published by the International Huntington Association (2005) but are willing to adopt a flexible approach to take the needs and preferences of individuals and families into account.

Demand for Testing

Prior to the introduction of predictive testing for HD, the majority of persons at risk reported an interest in testing and the intention to utilise the test personally (Evers-Kiebooms, Cassiman, and van den Berghe 1987; Kessler, Field, Worth, and Mosbarger 1987). However, following availability of the test, the uptake (actually having the test) was considerably less than predicted, with a maximum of 16% of at-risk individuals proceeding with the test (Maat-Kievit, Vegter-van der Vlis, Zoeteweij, Losekoot, van Haeringen, and Roos 2000).

Earlier, the number of patients being tested was affected by the need to also obtain samples from family members. However, this cannot entirely explain the discrepancy between intention and behaviour, because it was observed that the uptake did not change dramatically after the direct mutation tests became available. Following an initial surge in the number of tests after the direct test was introduced (possibly due to those people who were previously unwilling or unable to involve their families presenting for testing), the numbers of persons undergoing testing decreased. Currently, approximately 18%–24% of those eligible seek predictive testing (Maat-Kievit et al. 2000; Harper, Lim, and Craufurd 2000). It may be that respondents to the early studies agreed with predictive testing in principle, rather than as a personal option. It is also possible that for patients who were faced with the reality of the certainty of the results of mutational analysis rather than a risk estimate, living with the risk was preferable.

Ethical Issues in Predictive Testing

The predictive testing protocol is designed to ensure that the tests are offered ethically, with the best interests of the patient at the forefront of any service. Three principles help ensure this: autonomy, confidentiality, and non-maleficence.

Autonomy

The principle of autonomy dictates that an individual considering predictive testing is helped to make the decision based on his or her own best interests. The role of the professional is not to decide whether the individual should be offered testing, but to facilitate exploration of the direct and indirect implications of testing for the individual and help him or her to prepare to live with the result. Discussions between the health professional and the patient should include the impact of the test result on family members and support persons, and reproductive plans for the future (Burson and Markey 2001). Of those who seek a referral to genetic services for predictive testing, a minority actually proceed to testing (Cannella, Simonelli, D'Alessio, Pierelli, Ruggieri, and Squiteri 2001).

Within families, there may be some coercive behaviour that influences a person to request a test. For example, others in the family may find it difficult to live with the uncertainty of a relative's status. There may also be perceived pressure from other external sources, such as employers and insurance companies. In the genetic counseling setting, skilled exploration of the underlying reasons for requesting a test is appropriate. It is also important to identify the attitudes of the at-risk person toward their HD status. These areas of discussion are required to ensure that the person is able to make an autonomous choice. This approach can be described as nondirective counseling.

Nondirectiveness has been one of the salient principles of genetic counseling since the inception of genetic health care. It was based on the client-centered approach developed by Rogers (1951) as part of the psychotherapeutic technique, designed to empower the client in the interaction between client and professional. Some practitioners have interpreted nondirectiveness as neutrality, resulting in an unhelpful lack of engagement between themselves and the client (Wolff and Jung 1995). However, Kessler (1997) strongly refutes this notion of nondirectiveness, referring to a definition of nondirectiveness as an approach without coercion, deception, or threat. Both Kessler (1997) and Wolff and Jung (1995) maintain that skilled counseling rather than a stance of neutrality is required to truly empower clients to make the decisions that are personally appropriate. It would appear that it is therefore not ethical to practice in this context in genetic health care without prior training in counseling skills (Skirton, Patch, and Williams 2005).

Predictive testing for adult-onset diseases is not generally offered to children, because of the need for the individual to be able to make an autonomous choice and to provide informed consent . There are additional ethical issues around confidentiality, as due to the age and the dependence of the minor on parents or guardians, the results are more likely to be known by parents or others supporting the child. However, while professional guidance in this area is against testing, making children aware of their risk at an appropriate age is considered desirable (Dickenson 1999). In a qualitative study of communication of risk status to children, Skirton (1998) found that all adults interviewed who were at risk or affected by HD believed that children had a right to know their status. Opinions varied as to age at which children should be told of their risk. "When they are old enough to understand" was the most common response. Some of those studied reflected that they had been aware of "something different" in the family for a long time before they were told, and had felt that knowing about the condition would have explained the unusual or difficult behaviour of family members. While it is not the responsibility of healthcare professionals to disclose information to children in a family, it is often helpful to offer support to adults or children in the family following disclosure.

Confidentiality

The principle of patient confidentiality underpins all health care; however, it is often difficult to conceal the health status of a person because of the obvious nature of the condition. Within a genetic service context, discussion and testing may center around the future health of the individual, rather than on existing conditions. Furthermore, the information may have an impact on the individual's relationships, employment, and financial status. Ethically, the person's at-risk status cannot be divulged to another person or organisation without their express consent.

In some families, there are difficulties around disclosure of genetic information to others whom it concerns (Forrest, Simpson, Wilson, Van Teijlingen, McKee, Haites, et al. 2003). This can be exceptionally challenging when others in the family are unaware of their own risk and may benefit from such knowledge (Hakimiam 2000). In the situation where a person does not wish relatives to be told of the familial risk, the health professional must usually respect that wish while ensuring that the patient is aware of the potential impact of this decision on others. Understanding the familial patterns of communication and the response of the tested person to their own situation can enhance the practitioner's ability to facilitate communication between relatives (Forrest et al. 2003). In the United States, anonymous testing, which involves the use of pseudonyms so that the person's true identity is concealed in any records, has been practiced in some centers. However, disquiet about this has been expressed by health professionals (Visintainer Matthias-Hagen, Nance, and the U.S. Huntington Disease Genetic Testing Group 2001). Ongoing supportive care of patients can be very limited in these circumstances.

Non-Maleficence

Ethical guidelines for healthcare practice demand that whenever possible, causing harm is avoided. The greatest concern about the introduction of genetic predictive testing was the potential for harm among those who were tested. For this reason, psychological assessment of candidates for testing is considered an essential part of the pre-test counseling protocol. This involves counseling sessions with an experienced professional (such as a nurse, doctor, or psychologist) in which relevant issues are discussed, such as how the client has coped with stressful situations in the past, how they have prepared mentally for the test, and how they are able to access support from others. This type of clinical assessment may be augmented by the administration of psychometric questionnaires such as the State Trait anxiety inventory (Spielberger 1970) to identify those at increased risk of harm.

It is usual to discuss with the patient their motives and timing for being tested. Because of the use of psychological questionnaires and the stringent criteria for testing under research conditions, patients may perceive that they need to "pass" scrutiny in order to have a test. However, guidelines for testing support the view that it is the patient's autonomous right to be tested if they wish (International Huntington Association 2005). It is therefore more ethically sound to use exploratory questioning and counseling techniques to explore the patient's decision rather than interrogate the patient as to their motives. Tassicker (2005) identified the potential for fears of abandonment in persons who have had an affected parent to surface during pre-text counseling; this highlights the need for skilled and experienced counsellors to be involved in the predictive testing process. In a review of studies on predictive testing outcomes, Broadstock, Michie, and Marteau (2000) concluded that there was no evidence to suggest that such testing resulted in adverse psychological outcomes for patients, but strongly advocated studies on the relationship between the type and amount of test counseling and patient outcomes.

It may be necessary to discuss deferring testing in those patients who are suffering from depression or other mental illness, or who are currently experiencing difficult life events, as depression is associated with an increased chance of an adverse event (such as self-harm) after the results are given (Lawson, Wiggins, Green, Adam, Bloch, and Hayden 1996). Post-test supportive counseling for all those tested should be offered routinely, as studies have shown that those who have negative results ("good news") are equally at risk of adverse psychological sequelae after testing as those who receive positive mutation test results. However, the timing of the adverse events differs, with adverse events being more common in the immediate aftermath of the result (within 10 days) for those with positive results. We have found that adverse events in those having a negative test results are more likely to occur six months after the test or later (Lawson et al. 1996). Williams, Schutte, Evers, and Holkup (2000) studied the post-test psychological impact of predictive testing for neurological disease and concluded that a period of "redefinition" of self was necessary for those who had received good news results. The authors suggested that the adjustment period takes up to six months and it may therefore be that offering support for that period should be a component of care after testing.

Considerations Related to Other Members of the Family

Predictive Testing for Those at 25% Risk

An ethical conflict may arise if an individual at 25% risk of inheriting the condition (a grandchild of an affected person) wishes to be tested, while a parent at 50% risk does not wish to know their status. A positive test result for the affected person's grandchild will in effect provide information that the parent will also be affected in the future. In this situation, the autonomous choice of one person directly conflicts with that of the relative. In practical terms, discussion of the impact of testing on both parties can help to resolve the situation by enabling negotiation between family members. However, in cases where the person at 25% risk wishes to be tested, it is often felt that the most ethical course of action lies in acceding to their wishes, even though this may be to the detriment of another family member. A report by Benjamin and Lashwood (2000) indicated that over a five-year period (1994–1998) 161 such tests were performed in the United Kingdom. In four cases it was reported that the candidate for testing had agreed not to disclose the results to the at-risk parent, but in three out of four cases family members had subsequently been told of the negative test result.

Impact of Test Results on Other Family Members

The protocol for predictive testing requires that if possible a support person attend preparatory, result, and post-test counseling sessions with the person being tested. However, such support persons may have little preparation for the role and may themselves have support needs. Williams, Schutte, Holkup, Evers, and Muilenburg (2000) recommended that the needs of the support persons be assessed and met as far as practicable as part of the testing process. There is particular concern that the experience may be detrimental to support persons who are themselves at risk of HD.

Unsurprisingly, predictive testing has also been shown to have an effect on family function, over half the families studied by Sobel and Cowan (2000). They found changes in relationships, intrafamilial communication, and concerns about providing care in the future. Partners of those who were found to carry the mutation were under as much stress as the carriers five years after testing (Decruyenaere et al 2005), but the partner's stress was less well recognised by others. Richards (2004), in contrast, found that couples reported few adverse effects on their relationship from testing of one partner, although living with the risk of HD was said to result in breakdown of the relationship in some couples. These results confirm the need for healthcare professionals to address the needs of the family, rather than one individual, during the process of predictive testing.

Diagnostic Testing

In situations where a person has signs or symptoms of Huntington disease, as well as a family history of the condition, the need for pre-test counseling may not pertain in the same way as it does for predictive testing. However, even when the condition is suspected, the individual may need support to adjust to the result, which may also have powerful implications for other family members. Due to the cognitive changes that are part of the effect of HD, the person may genuinely not be aware of the signs and symptoms. In these situations, careful preparation for testing should be undertaken.

Prenatal Testing

In any family with a genetic condition where the disease-causing mutation has been detected, prenatal diagnostic testing can usually be offered. In families at risk for HD, only 2% of couples whose fetus is at risk opt for prenatal diagnostic testing (Maat-Kievet et al. 2000). This low uptake is typical for adult-onset conditions, and families often have faith that a cure or effective treatment will have been discovered for the condition before the child is old enough to develop the disease. There is no difference in the number of post-test pregnancies in families where a mutation has been found in one parent compared to individuals who have had a negative predictive test result (Richards and Rea 2005). Parents have the right to make an autonomous choice and to be fully supported in that choice by health professionals. However, where the parents would not wish to have a termination of pregnancy if the fetus were shown to be affected, prenatal diagnosis is not usually indicated, as this would result in the parents knowing the child's status, regardless of the child's eventual choice about predictive testing. This situation again highlights the potential for conflict between ethical principles of autonomy and confidentiality.

Implications for Healthcare Practice

The changing face of genetic health care and the increasing opportunities for predictive and prenatal genetic testing have raised ethical issues that may not have previously arisen in health care, and the impact of genomics will mean more patients, families, and professionals will be faced with similar dilemmas in health care. While Parker and Lucassen (2002) suggest that specific additional training in ethics for health professionals will enable them to deal with the concerns raised in this setting, others (Taylor 2004) believe that there is a potential conflict between the personal vulnerability that testing can expose and the drive to enforce individual responsibility in society today. Taylor argues therefore that the issues involved need to be approached from a broader societal base.

It is clear that to practice ethically, efforts to prepare both the person presenting for testing and their support persons is required. The need for support will vary from family to family, and an individual approach rather than rigid adherence to protocols is probably indicated. However, guidelines suggesting the minimum acceptable standards for service may be useful, especially for less experienced practitioners.

Ethical professional practice in this context depends on development of skills necessary to facilitate exploration of the individual's preferences and motivations for testing, to ensure that they are able to make an autonomous choice. The ability to effectively communicate the factual information required as a basis for decision making is also required, as is respect for individual privacy.

Conclusion

Genetic technology has enabled individuals and families to make choices about accessing knowledge to inform the future. There are potential benefits and disadvantages to undertaking predictive or prenatal tests for adult-onset neurological conditions. Preparation for safe and ethical practice enables professionals to support individuals and families through this process in a way that minimises risk and enhances individual autonomy.

References

Benjamin, C. M., and A. Lashwood. 2000. United Kingdom experience with presymptomatic testing of individuals at 25% risk for Huntington's disease. *Clinical Genetics* 58 (1): 41–49.

Broadstock, M., S. Michie, and T. Marteau. 2000. Psychological consequences of predictive genetic testing: A systematic review. *European Journal of Human Genetics* 8 (10): 731–738.

Burson, C. M., and K. R. Markey. 2001. Genetic counseling issues in predictive genetic testing for familial adult-onset neurologic diseases. *Seminars in Pediatric Neurology* 8 (3): 177–186.

Cannella, M., M. Simonelli, C. D'Alessio, F. Pierelli, S. Ruggieri, and F. Squitieri. 2001. Presymptomatic tests in Huntington's disease and dominant ataxias. *Neurological Sciences* 22 (1): 55–56.

Craufurd, D., and A. Tyler. 1992. Predictive testing for Huntington's disease: Protocol of the UK Huntington's Prediction Consortium. *Journal of Medical Genetics* 29 (12): 915–918.

Decruyenaere, M., G. Evers-Kiebooms, A. Boogaerts, K. Demyttenaere, R. Dom and J. P. Fryns. 2005. Partners of mutation-carriers for Huntington's disease: Forgotten persons? *European Journal of Human Genetics* [Epub ahead of print, July 6].

Dickenson, D. L. 1999. Can children and young people consent to be tested for adult onset genetic disorders? *British Medical Journal* 318: 1063–1066.

Evers-Kiebooms, G., J. J. Cassiman and van den Berghe, H. 1987. Attitudes towards predictive testing in Huntington's disease: A recent survey in Belgium. *Journal of Medical Genetics* 24 (5): 275–279.

Forrest, K., S. Simpson, B. Wilson, E. Van Teijlingen, L. McKee, N. Haites and E. Matthews. 2003. To tell or not to tell: Barriers and facilitators in family communications about genetic risk. *Clinical Genetics* 64 (4): 317–326.

Gusella, J. F., N. S. Wexler, P. M. Conneally, S. L. Naylor, M. A. Anderson, R. E. Tanzi, P. C. Watkins, K. Ottina, M. R. Wallace, A. Y. Sakaguchi, et al. 1983. A polymorphic DNA marker genetically linked to Huntington's disease. *Nature* 306 (5940): 234–238.

Hakimian, R. 2000. Disclosure of Huntington's disease to family members: The dilemma of known but unknowing parties. *Genetic Testing* 4 (4): 359–364.

Harper, P. S., D. A. Walker, A. Tyler, R. G. Newcombe, and K. Davies. 1979. Huntington's chorea: The basis for long-term prevention. *Lancet* 2: 346–349.

Harper, P. S., C. Lim and D. Craufurd. 2000. Ten years of presymptomatic testing for Huntington's disease: the experience of the UK Huntington's Disease Prediction Consortium. *Journal of Medical Genetics* 37 (8): 567–71.

Huntington, G. 1872. On chorea. *The Medical and Surgical Reporter of Philadelphia* 26 (15): 317–321.

Huntington's Disease Collaborative Research Group. 1993. A novel gene containing a trinucleotide repeat that is expanded and unstable on Huntington's disease chromosomes. *Cell* 72 (6): 971–983.

International Huntington Association. 2005. http://www.huntington-assoc.com/ (accessed October 8, 2008).

Kessler, S., T. Field, L. Worth, and H. Mosbarger. 1987. Attitudes of persons at risk for Huntington disease toward predictive testing. *American Journal of Medical Genetics* 26 (2): 259–270.

Kessler, S. 1997. Psychological aspects of genetic counseling. XI. Nondirectiveness revisited. *American Journal of Medical Genetics* 72: 164–171.

Lawson, K., S. Wiggins, T. Green, S. Adam, M. Bloch, and M. R. Hayden. 1996. Adverse psychological events occurring in the first year after predictive testing for Huntington's disease. The Canadian Collaborative Study Predictive Testing. *Journal of Medical Genetics* 33 (10): 856–862.

Maat-Kievit, A., M. Vegter-van der Vlis, M. Zoeteweij, M. Losekoot, A. van Haeringen, and R. Roos. 2000. Paradox of a better test for Huntington's disease. *Journal of Neurology, Neurosurgery, & Psychiatry* 69 (5), 579–583.

Melone, M. A., F. P. Jori and G. Peluso. 2005. Huntington's disease: New frontiers for molecular and cell therapy. *Current Drug Targets* 6 (1): 43–56.

National Center for Biotechnology Information (NCBI). 2007. *Online Mendelian inheritance in man.* http://www.ncbi.nlm.nih.gov/sites/entrez?db=OMIM (accessed October 8, 2008).

Parker, M., and A. Lucassen. 2002. Working towards ethical management of genetic testing. *Lancet* 360 (9346): 1685–1688.

Richards, F. 2004. Couples' experiences of predictive testing and living with the risk or reality of Huntington disease: A qualitative study. *American Journal of Medical Genetics* A 15 126 (2): 170–182.

Richards, F. H, and G. Rea. 2005. Reproductive decision making before and after predictive testing for Huntington's disease: An Australian perspective. *Clinical Genetics* 67 (5): 404–411.

Rogers, C. R. 1951. *Client-centered therapy: Its current practice, implications and theory.* Boston: Houghton Mifflin.

Skirton, H. 1998. Telling the children. In *The genetic testing of children,* ed. Angus Clarke. Oxford, England: Bios Scientific Publishers.

Skirton, H., and N. Glendinning. 1997. Using research to develop care for patients with Huntington's disease. *British Journal of Nursing* 6 (2): 83–90.

Skirton, H., C. Patch, and J. K. Williams. 2005. *Applied genetics in healthcare.* Abingdon, England: Taylor and Francis.

Sobel, S. K., and D. B. Cowan. 2000. Impact of genetic testing for Huntington disease on the family system. *American Journal of Medical Genetics* 90 (1): 49–59.

Sorensen S. A., and K. Fenger. 1992. Causes of death in patients with Huntington's disease and in unaffected first degree relatives. *Journal of Medical Genetics* 29 (12): 911–914.

Spielberger, C. D., R. L. Gorsuch and Lushene, R. E. 1970. *Manual for the state-trait anxiety inventory (self-evaluation questionnaire).* Palo Alto, CA: Consulting Psychologists Press.

Tassicker, R. J. 2005. Psychodynamic theory and counseling in predictive testing for Huntington's disease. *Journal of Genetic Counseling* 14 (2): 99–107.

Taylor, S. D. 2004. Predictive genetic test decisions for Huntington's disease: Context, appraisal and new moral imperatives. *Social Science and Medicine* 58 (1): 137–149.

Visintainer, C. L., V. Matthias-Hagen, M. A. Nance, and the U.S. Huntington Disease Genetic Testing Group. 2001. Anonymous predictive testing for Huntington's disease in the United States. *Genetic Testing* 5 (3): 213–218.

Williams, J. K, D. L. Schutte, P. A. Holkup, C. Evers and A. Muilenburg. 2000. Psychosocial impact of predictive testing for Huntington disease on support persons. *American Journal of Medical Genetics* 96 (3): 353–359.

Williams, J. K., D. L. Schutte, C. Evers, and P. A. Holkup. 2000. Redefinition: Coping with normal results from predictive gene testing for neurodegenerative disorders. *Research in Nursing and Health* 23 (4): 260–269.

Wolff, G., and C. Jung. 1995. Nondirectiveness and genetic counseling. *Journal of Genetic Counseling* 4 (1): 3–25.

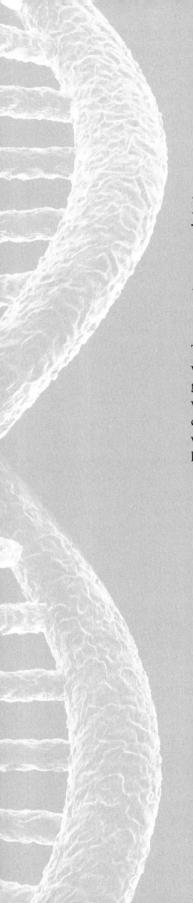

PART 4

Case Studies in Genetics and Ethics

This concluding part presents a variety of case studies illustrating what families face, in specific circumstances, in terms of genetics, genetic testing, and the care of family members who are affected with a genetic condition. Through each of these five studies, we can catch at least an accurate glimpse of the burdens associated with such gene mutations as may spread through families and have the potential to affect many future generations.

PART 4 CONTENTS

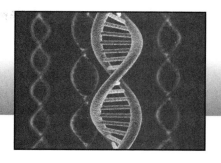

CHAPTER 23

Prenatal Case Study

Dale Halsey Lea, MPH, RN, CGC, APNG, FAAN

Background

A pediatric neurologist referred a couple, Mr. and Mrs. R., whose two year-old identical twin girls had recently been diagnosed with the rare neurodegenerative condition metachromatic leukodystropy (MLD), to our Medical Center Division of Genetics. The couple sought more information about "how this had happened to them," and what the chances were that they would have more children with the same condition. The twins, at the time of referral, had developed seizures and had lost their ability to walk.

Patient and Family Profile

Pregnancy History: Mrs. R.'s pregnancy with her twin girls was uncomplicated. She delivered them at 38 weeks via cesarean section. Both girls were assessed as healthy at birth. They were in the newborn nursery for three days before being discharged home.

Developmental History: Both girls developed normally until they were 15 months. Both began to develop gait disturbances and loss of fine motor abilities such as feeding themselves. One of the girls had a seizure at 16 months. They were referred to the pediatric neurologist at that point.

Diagnosis: Evaluation of the twins included a physical examination, which revealed that they both had developmental deterioration and diminished deep tendon reflexes. The following diagnostic studies were conducted for further evaluation:

- Brain MRI (magnetic resonance imaging): Both were abnormal, with white matter lesions and atrophy, characteristic of MLD.

- Leukocyte (white blood cells) cultures for arylsulfatase A enzyme activity—severely depressed activity of arylsulfatase A in leukocytes in both girls. This is generally considered diagnostic, leaving little doubt about the nature of the condition.

Based on these results, a diagnosis of MLD was made. The neurologist explained to Mr. and Mrs. R. that MLD is rare (1 in 40,000 individuals), and that there are several types. The type present in their daughters is the late infantile form in which symptoms appear at 4 years or younger. Typically, these children experience gait disturbances, loss of motor developmental milestones (normally expected neuromuscular function), optic atrophy, and diminished deep tendon reflexes. Progressive loss of both motor and cognitive functions is usually rapid and the children die usually within 5 years after the onset of clinical symptoms.

At the time of their diagnosis (2000), there was no effective treatment available to reverse the deterioration and loss of function. Bone marrow transplantation was available to stabilize neurocognitive function, but symptoms of motor function loss frequently progress even with this intervention. Gene therapy was under development as a possible solution, but at that time was still under investigation and not ready for clinical trials (Moore 2006; United Leukodystrophy Foundation 2008). Supportive care could be provided as needed for feeding difficulties, seizure disorder, and constipation.

Family History: A three-generation family history was taken on both Mrs. R. and Mr. R. (see pedigree in Figure 23–1). In the review of family history, Mr. and Mrs. R. noted the following issues of significance:

- Mrs. R. is one of three siblings. All are in good health. Her younger brother had a son who was born with a congenital heart defect (ventriculoseptal defect, VSD). He is in good health.

- Mrs. R.'s mother has a history of heart disease. She is 62 years old.

350

FIGURE 23–1
R Family Pedigree

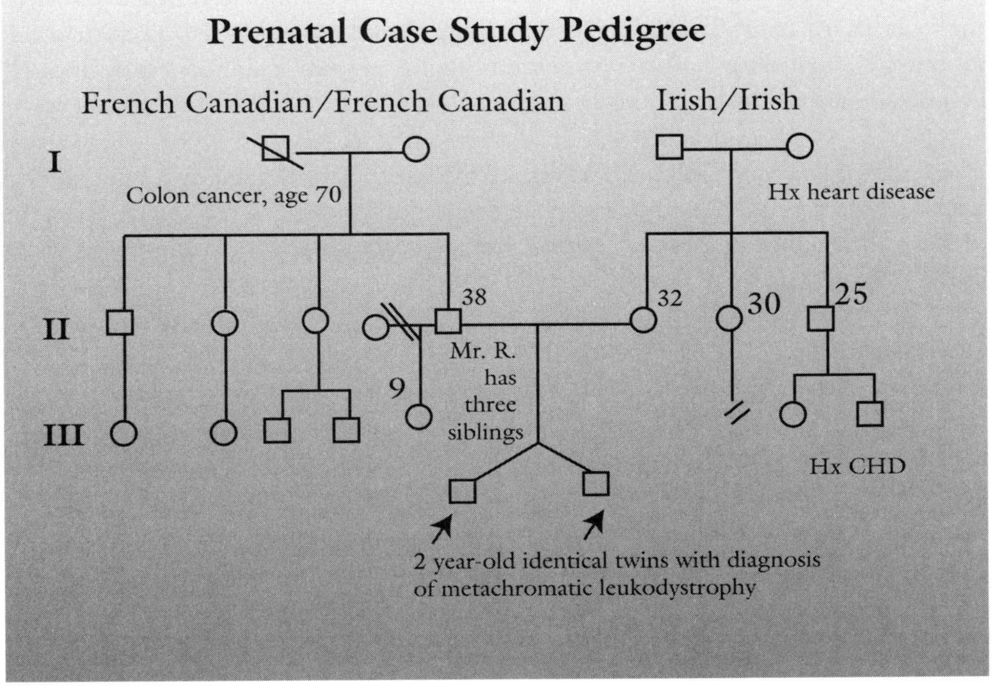

Prenatal Case Study Pedigree

2 year-old identical twins with diagnosis of metachromatic leukodystrophy

- Mr. R. is one of three siblings. All are in good health as are their children.
- Mr. R. has a nine-year-old daughter from a previous relationship. She is in good health.
- Mr. R.'s father died from complications related to colon cancer at the age of 71.
- Mrs. R. is of Irish ancestry and Mr. R. is of French Canadian ancestry. There is no history of consanguinity (biological relatedness).

Objective

Mr. and Mrs. R. came for their genetic counseling appointment and brought their twin girls with them. At the time that we provided genetic counseling, the girls had lost any speech that they had. They had recently undergone an ophthalmology evaluation that showed the beginnings of optic atrophy in both girls. Mr. and Mrs. R. explained that they were "still reeling from the diagnosis three months ago." Mrs.

R. stated, "I had such a healthy pregnancy, and our families are so healthy, I just can't believe that this is happening to us." The couple had many questions about the cause of MLD and the chance for having another child with MLD. Mr. R. said "We so want to have more children, especially since our girls will not be with us for very long. But is it possible to have a healthy child together?" At this time, the focus of the couple's concern was on the cause of MLD and recurrence. Therefore, the focus of the consultation was on explaining the inheritance of MLD, recurrence in future children and available prenatal testing. A physical examination of the girls was not indicated.

Laboratory/Diagnostic Results: Copies of the diagnostic evaluation (MRI, blood studies, and Pediatric Neurology consultation report) were faxed to us, with consent of Mr. and Mrs. R., before the consultation as verification of the diagnosis of MLD in the twin girls.

Family and Social Profile

Mrs. R. is a 32-year-old Caucasian female who is currently in good health. Mr. R. is a 38-year-old Caucasian male who is also in good health. Mr. R. has a nine-year-old daughter from a previous marriage who is in good health. She currently lives with her biological mother. Mr. and Mrs. R. live in a small town outside of a large city. Mr. R. teaches history at a local high school. Mrs. R. is a nurse who was practicing pediatrics in a physician's office before she gave birth to the twins. Mr. and Mrs. R.'s families live six hours away.

Medical Diagnosis and Plan

Pediatric Diagnosis: Late infantile Metachromatic Leukodystrophy (MLD)

Plan:

- Provide genetic counseling for Mr. and Mrs. R. (assessment, communicating information about MLD and risk of recurrence, decision-making support, coping enhancement, hope, follow-up support).
- Consider prenatal diagnosis. The Arylsulfatase A-deficient forms of MLD can be diagnosed prenatally using cells obtained by either amniocentesis or chorionic villi sampling. Prenatal diagnosis is normally only considered for couples who have had a child with MLD, or if the disease has occurred in a close relative.

- Consider gene mutation analysis in the girls for trying to identify a specific gene that could then be used for prenatal diagnosis in a future pregnancy.
- Offer support services.
- Follow up with the couple after counseling.

Genetic Assessment and Counseling with Mr. and Mrs. R.

Issue 1: The Disease Process

Mr. and Mrs. R. had many questions about the cause of MLD and whether the fact that they lived near a power plant might have caused exposures that "damaged our genes." Mrs. R. said, "My husband and I went on the Internet but the information we found was frightening and confusing to us. Please help us understand this condition in our girls in a way that we can understand."

Assessment: Lack of understanding about the cause of MLD.

Nursing Diagnosis: Knowledge deficit of the disease process

Nursing Outcome: Enhanced knowledge

Nursing Interventions and Nursing Actions:

- Ensure privacy and confidentiality. I assured the couple that all information discussed during the genetic counseling session and documentation of the consultation in their medical records was kept private and confidential. The genetic information would be shared only with their written permission and consent. Mr. and Mrs. R. asked that the summary letter be sent to them only at this time.
- Provide information about the inheritance of MLD. I explained that MLD is a rare autosomal recessive inherited condition ranging between 1 in 40,000 to 1 in 100,000, which would place the carrier frequency at 1 in 100–150. In response to Mr. and Mrs. R.'s concerns about exposure to the power plant and whether that might have caused damage to their genes, I explained that each of us is born with seven or so autosomal recessive gene changes, which when paired with a similar gene in a partner can cause an autosomal recessive condition to occur. I reassured Mr. and Mrs. R. that there is no evidence to date showing that living near a power plant causes gene changes that can lead to being a carrier of MLD. I provided written and visual information about autosomal recessive inheritance using graphics in an area Genetic Counseling Center booklet.

Issue 2: Risk of Recurrence

Mr. and Mrs. R. asked for information about future pregnancies. "Can we have a healthy pregnancy? Is there any testing that we can have that will tell us ahead of time that we are having another baby with this MLD?"

Assessment: Concern about the impact of their daughters' diagnoses of MLD on future reproduction and recurrence risks

Nursing Diagnosis: Knowledge deficit

Nursing Outcome: Enhanced knowledge; risk detection and health-seeking behavior

Nursing Interventions and Nursing Actions:

- Provide an estimate of the risk of recurrence based on the diagnosis of MLD. I explained that since MLD is an autosomal recessive condition, the chance for them to have another child with MLD is 25%. The chance for them to have a healthy child who does not inherit a gene for MLD is 25%, and the chance for them to have a child who is a carrier is 50%. This means that together, they have a 75% chance to have a child who is not affected with MLD.

- Discuss prenatal diagnosis options. I explained that the Arylsulfatase A-deficient forms of MLD can be diagnosed prenatally using cells obtained either by amniocentesis or chorionic villi sampling. Prenatal diagnosis is offered to couples, such as Mr. and Mrs. R. who have had a child with MLD. Enzymatic analysis using synthetic substrates is usually adequate, if it can be established that the pseudodeficiency gene is not present. I also discussed the possibility of gene mutation analysis in the girls for the purpose of trying to identify a specific gene that could then be used for prenatal diagnosis in a future pregnancy. The structure of the Arylsulfatase A gene, which is located near the end of the long arm of chromosome 22, is relatively short and consists of 8 exons. Between 50 and 100 variations in the reference gene structure have so far been noted. Disease-related mutations have tentatively been separated into two groups. One (0-type) results in the complete lack of any active gene product, while the other (R-type) provides a low level of functional enzyme. Two copies of 0-type mutations result in the late-infantile form of MLD, which is what Mr. and Mrs. R.'s daughters have.

- Monitor the response when the couple learns of their genetic risks. Mr. and Mrs. R. expressed relief when they learned that the risk of recurrence in a future pregnancy was 25%, stating "we thought the chance was 100%. We need to think about whether we want the girls to have genetic testing to see if there is a gene because they have already been through so much."

Plan: I offered to meet with Mr. and Mrs. R. again in follow-up for further discussion and, if they chose to have their daughters tested, to coordinate the blood drawing.

Issue 3: Prenatal Diagnosis

Mr. and Mrs. R. said that they needed to talk together when they got home about persuing prenatal diagnosis because they had never talked "about what we would do if the test shows that we are having another baby with MLD. We love our girls so, and it would be heartbreaking to consider ending a pregnancy when a baby has the same disease."

Assessment: Difficulty choosing between alternatives

Nursing Diagnosis: Decisional conflict

Nursing Outcome: Participation in healthcare decisions

Nursing Interventions and Nursing Actions:

Provide decision-making support. I reviewed the options available to Mr. and Mrs. R.—to pursue gene mutation testing of the girls for the purpose of prenatal diagnosis; to pursue another pregnancy with or without prenatal diagnosis. I explained that in their situation there are no right or wrong choices: each couple makes the choice that is right for them based on their personal values and beliefs. I supported their decision to take time and talk together. I explored with the couple whether they had any family members or friends they could talk with. Mr. and Mrs. R. said that they did not think they could talk with their families. They said that they had a very good friend who is a pastor in a nearby church and they thought they could talk with him, as they had already talked with him about the future for their daughters. I provided them with our 800 number and encouraged them to call me with any questions or if they needed support.

Plan: Mr. and Mrs. R. said that they planned to return for follow-up counseling if they decided to pursue gene mutation testing of their daughters and prenatal diagnosis. I told them that I would follow up with them in a month to see how they were doing.

Issue 4: Information and Support

Near the end of the counseling session, Mrs. R. said, " I am a nurse, so I am aware of some of the resources that are out there for families who have children with a chronic disease, but I want to get more information about MLD—like is there any research going on or any cures? I want to see if there are other families out there who have been through this and can give us help to get through these times with our daughters."

Assessment: Concern about the future health of her daughters and need for information; concern about Mr. and Mrs. R.'s emotional well-being and psychological adjustment to their daughters' prognosis

Nursing Diagnosis: Knowledge deficit; ability to manage stressors

Nursing Outcome: Enhanced knowledge; risk detection and health-seeking behavior

Acceptance: Health status; coping and hope

Nursing Interventions and Nursing Actions:

- Provide referral to a large, world-renowned neurogenetic center. I provided the couple with the name of a neurologist specializing in neurodegenerative disorders. I also gave them the web site for a listing of current clinical trials maintained by the National Institutes of Health, www.ClinicalTrials.gov.
- Provide referral for community, local, and national resources including support resources. I provided information to the couple about the United Leukodystrophy Foundation (http://www.ulf.org/), the National Organization for Rare Disorders (http://www.rarediseases.org/), and the Genetic Alliance (www.geneticalliance.org).
- I offered referral to a local support organization the Matthew Fund, a group that provides support to families who have a child with a terminal illness.

Plan: I told Mr. and Mrs. R. that I would be glad to help coordinate a referral to the neurogenetic center with the girls' pediatric neurologist if they desired. I also offered to contact the Matthew Fund. Mr. and Mrs. R. expressed gratitude and said that they wanted me to make these contacts.

Genetic Assessment and Counseling with Mr. and Mrs. R. in Follow-up

I remained in contact with Mr. and Mrs. R. on a regular basis over the next three months. Mr. and Mrs. R. decided that they wanted to return for follow-up counseling to discuss their options for prenatal diagnosis.

Assessment: Decision-making and choosing between alternatives

Nursing Outcome: Decision-making; participation; healthcare decisions

Nursing Interventions and Nursing Actions:

- Provide decision-making support. I reviewed with Mr. and Mrs. R. the inheritance, the prenatal diagnostic options (chorionic villus sampling and amniocentesis), and gene mutation analysis of the girls to determine whether a specific mutation could be identified for prenatal diagnosis. Mr. and Mrs. R. said that they had talked together intensively and with their friend who was a pastor. They said that they had come to the decision to go forward with another pregnancy and to have prenatal diagnosis. They had decided not to pursue gene mutation testing of the girls because "they have been through so much already." I supported their decision and gave them referral information about the high-risk maternal/fetal medicine center in the city where they would have additional counseling and prenatal diagnosis.

- Monitor the response when the patient learns of genetic risks. Mr. and Mrs. R. said that they felt hopeful about their decision to pursue another pregnancy. "We still don't know what we will do if the test shows that our baby has MLD, but at least we will know one way or the other."

Follow-up Nursing Outcome Evaluation: Health Seeking Behaviors and Hope

Six months after our follow-up appointment, I received a call from Mrs. R. She was tearful and elated to inform me that she was currently 14 weeks pregnant. She had had early amniocentesis and results of the prenatal diagnostic testing for MLD showed that her baby did not have the condition. She had also had a chromosome analysis that showed she was having a boy, and the chromosomes were normal (46, XY). "We are just so thankful." Mrs. R. also told us that her daughters now required full-time nursing care, and had feeding tubes. She had been working with a regional community resource for ongoing support. Mrs. R. later delivered a healthy boy, and sent us a picture of the family together with her two daughters.

References

Moore, T. 2006. *Metachromatic leukodystrophy*. www.emedicine.com/ped/topic2893.htm (accessed October 9, 2008).

National Institute of Neurological Disorders and Stroke. NINDS Metachromatic Leukodystrophy Page. www.ninds.nih.gov (accessed October 9, 2008).

OMIM—Online Mendelian Inheritance in Man. Metachromatic Leukodystrophy. http://www.ncbi.nlm.nih.gov/sites/entrez?db=omim (accessed October 9, 2008).

United Leukodystrophy Foundation. 2008. *Mission statement*. http://www.ulf.org/whoweare/mission.html (accessed October 9, 2008).

CHAPTER 24

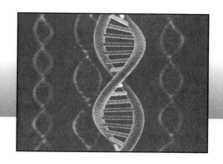

Sickle Cell Disease Case Study

Victoria Odesina, MS, APRN-BC, CCRP, APGN

Sickle Cell Disease

Sickle cell disease (SCD) is an inherited anemia that follows the autosomal recessive (AR) pattern of inheritance requiring two copies of the sickle genetic mutation (one from each parent). A child who inherits the two copies of the sickle mutation will be diagnosed as having sickle cell anemia (with hemoglobinSS, also designated as Hgb SS). One who inherits a copy of a sickle hemoglobin gene mutation from one parent and a normal hemoglobin gene from the other parent will have HgbAS, which renders the child a carrier of the sickle cell trait. It is also possible that a parent may carry a normal copy of the hemoglobin gene and one of the other hemoglobin variants, resulting in the child's hemoglobin being designated as HgbAC, AD, or AE.

Both parents who carry a normal hemoglobin gene and the sickle cell hemoglobin are usually healthy carriers (heterozygotes) of the sickle trait (HgbAS); they will have inherited this trait, and it is a condition that under normal circumstances will not make them sick. However, under certain conditions (for instance, low oxygen tension at very high altitudes), having the sickle trait can lead to health problems such as hematuria (blood in the urine), pain, splenic sequestration (blood entrapment or pooling of blood in the spleen), and sudden death. Parents who are heterozygote carriers with one copy of the sickle cell gene may have one copy of the variant hemoglobin genes and may or may not have health problems associated with their carrier status.

Athletes with sickle cell trait (heterozygote carriers of one copy of the sickle cell gene mutation) have been known to develop red blood cell sickling as a result of rhabdomyolosis (destruction of muscle tissue associated with trauma, strenuous exercise, or related events) during uncontrolled training exercises, a condition which could be fatal. According to the 2007 Consensus Statement by the National Athletic Trainer's Association, nine young athletes have died from exertional sickling during team sports training.

Identification of trait status, prevention, early recognition, and prompt treatment of exertional sickling will reduce mortality. If both parents carry the sickle trait (Hgb AS), each of their offspring has a 25% chance of receiving two copies of the sickle cell mutation (HgbSS) and having sickle cell anemia, a 50% chance of receiving only one copy and being a carrier of the trait (HgbAS), and a 25% chance of receiving the normal gene and having normal hemoglobin (HgbAA).

The majority of forms of SCD involve a missense mutation in the gene for beta globin, a component of the HgbSS molecule resulting in sickle- or crescent-shaped red blood cells that cannot traverse fine capillaries and deliver oxygen to body cells as normal red blood cells do. These sickle-shaped red blood cells clog up the fine circulation in bones and internal organs, leading to pain and damage especially in the spleen, heart, lungs, and kidneys as well as large blood vessels, as may be seen in cerebrovascular accidents associated with strokes (Gelehrter, Collins, and Ginsberg 1998). This sickling phenomenon and the occlusion in blood vessels that results in the above complications can lead to renal insufficiencies (poor kidney function), leg ulcers, and for women with HgbSS, preterm delivery. Additionally, red cell dehydration, endothelial damage, inflammatory response, and erythrocytes damage can lead to avascular necrosis (severe deterioration of body tissue) and even death (Yale, Nagib, and Guthrie 2000; Buchanan, DeBaun, Quinn, and Steinberg 2004).

The lifespan of the sickle-shaped red blood cell (HgbSS) is only between 10 and 20 days compared to120 days for the normal HgbAA. Because of constant red blood cell hemolysis (destruction), SCD is associated with chronic anemia, and leads to joint pain, leg ulcers, pneumonia, infections, acute chest syndrome (a potential life threatening pneumonia-like phenomenon which may require respiratory support; National Heart, Lung, and Blood Institute 2003), and pulmonary hypertension.

Sickle cell anemia (Hgb SS) is the most common of the sickle cell syndromes or diseases; other types include Hgb SC, Hgb SD, and Hgb SBthal. Hemoglobin electrophoresis, a diagnostic test, is the preferred approach for family testing before a confirmatory diagnosis is made. This test may identify some of the other hemoglobin variants that may be present and can modify the diagnosis, course of illness, and management of the patient and other family members, as well as genetic counseling and community support services that are needed.

Today, with preventive care such as prophylactic penicillin until age five (to protect from infections), and lifelong follow-up, persons with SCD can live into their 50s and some have lived into their 60s and 70s. New approaches such as hydroxyurea to increase the somewhat healthier fetal hemoglobin and minimize pain episodes have been very successful in the treatment of some adults and children (Buchanan, DeBaun, Quinn, and Steinberg 2004). Other treatments involving stem cell transplants (Chandler 2006) and other therapies are being investigated today to improve the health and quality of life of those affected.

The incidence of SCD in African Americans is 1 in 600 live births and 1 in 1,000–4,000 live births among Hispanic Americans, affecting about 72,000 persons in the United States. SCD is commonly found in peoples from sub-Saharan Africa, the Mediterranean, the Middle East, and India. About 2 million Americans (about 1 in 12 African Americans) are heterozygote carriers with the sickle trait (National Heart, Lung, and Blood Institute 2003). Newborn screening in most states in the United States, Puerto Rico, and the Virgin Islands detects infants who are affected with SCD (for early identification and management) or who are carriers of the sickle trait.

At present, there is no nationwide, uniform policy with regard to genetic counseling for those with HgbAS, who have a chance of transmitting one copy of the sickle cell gene mutation to their offspring. There are, however, a number of healthcare centers which specialize in the treatment of those with sickle cell anemia and other conditions that involve variations in the hemoglobin molecule. Some helpful websites that provide more information include: the American Sickle Cell Anemia Association, www.ascaa.org, the National Heart, Lung, and Blood Institute, www.nhlbi.nih.gov/health/dci/Diseases/Sca/SCA_Causes.html; the National Coalition for Health Professional Education in Genetics, www.nchpeg.org; and the National Human Genome Research Institute, www.genome.gov.

Narrative of the Orca Family's Care
(names changed to protect confidentiality)

Case History

Mr. Orca, a Caucasian with Caribbean heritage, just moved to this area from Canada with his wife, two daughters (Kala and Dana, ages 10, 7), and one son (Benji, age 4, diagnosed with SCD in infancy). (See Figure 24–1, pg. 366.) They had been referred to a Sickle Cell Center in a neighboring community after Benji was seen at the urgent care about three months ago with swollen hands and feet. The pain has not been responding to warm compress and Tylenol at home. The boy had been unable to put on his shoes or walk for about two days. The Sickle Cell Center team provided care for Benji, including management of his SCD and approaches to ease his recurrent pain.

Mr. Orca states that their first son, Ricky, had HgbAS and died suddenly at 16 years of age three years ago from a swollen abdomen and severe pain, after a skiing trip in the Canadian Rockies. This trip was taken soon after the family arrived in Canada and before the family realized that skiing would be a significant health risk to the boy. When he was transported to a hospital for emergency care, the family refused a blood transfusion because of their religion. The hospital staff tried without success to save his life.

Mr. Orca said that his wife should be giving the children the traditional herbs from his own family cultural practices on a regular basis. He seemed concerned that not enough was being done to help their children. Mrs. Orca said that she felt that modern medical care would be better for their children.

The Orcas said that Kala, their ten-year-old daughter, had pain in her joints during cold weather when she was younger but had "outgrown it." Apart from being a girl who loves video games and reading rather than exercise, Mr. Orca said Kala only gets occasional pains in other parts of her body and the whites of her eyes turn yellow at times. Kala was diagnosed with SCD (Hgb SS), and 7-year-old Dana with sickle cell trait (HgbAS) during infancy.

Mrs. Orca (34), a Caucasian with Mediterranean heritage, is six months pregnant with her fifth child. She has two brothers (30 and 24) with no children and one 28-year-old sister with two daughters (6 and 2). Mrs. Orca's parents are alive. Her mother, the youngest of four children, is 58 years old and has diabetes. Her father is 60 years old and has knee pain. Her mother is the only woman alive on her side of the family. Mrs. Orca's one maternal aunt and two uncles died very young. There has been very little discussion in Mrs. Orca's family of these illnesses or why the aunt and uncles died in childhood.

Mr. Orca's parents emigrated from Puerto Rico and left behind a healthy sister and two healthy brothers who are in their 60s. His 58-year-old father and 56-year-old mother are both healthy. Mr. Orca's paternal aunt has two adult male children who have been diagnosed with SCD and have both been hospitalized for severe pain and pneumonia. Mr. Orca's mother was an only child. Nobody talks about the family illnesses because of fear of stigmatization. Mr. Orca (34) has one brother, 37 years old with one child (14), and a 20-year-old sister who is, as yet, unmarried. The couple denied consanguinity (reproduction between two blood relatives) in the family.

Issues for Discussion

Diagnosis: Mrs. Orca and Mr. Orca both have HgbAS (establishing their status as heterozygous carriers of the sickle cell trait) confirmed on hemoglobin electrophoresis.

Education: The nurse discussed the details of sickle cell trait, SCD, risk factors for future illnesses, pain management in the immediate future and long term, necessary preparation for elective procedures if any come up, prevention of complications of SCD, and healthy lifestyle modifications for all the family members.

Medical: The family will be encouraged to continue with the Sickle Cell Center healthcare team to assure appropriate care for the two children with SCD and to provide support services to other family members; consultation with the hematologist and pediatrician will continue. The children affected with SCD will continue their care with providers who specialize in SCD and care of youth and adults. The family was given instructions and contacts for emergency care, especially for the two children with SCD, who will need expert management in the event of sickle cell pain episodes and other health problems that might need emergency attention.

Genetic counseling: The nurse provided two sessions of counseling explaining the genetics of SCD, the inheritance patterns seen in the family history, and possible transmission of SCD and sickle traits to offspring. Because Mrs. Orca was 6 months pregnant with a male fetus identified on ultrasound, there was a discussion of possible testing options (including amniocentesis) and possible decisions that would be necessary pending the test results (therapy options). Mr. and Mrs. Orca decided not to have prenatal testing and said that they felt that they could accept whatever God had sent them with the current pregnancy.

The nurse recommended additional testing, genetic counseling, and support counseling, if desired, for Mr. and Mrs. Orca's siblings and other family members. Support group resources and information about the local sickle cell advocacy agency, the American Sickle Cell Anemia Association (online at http//www.ascaa.org), and the Genetic Alliance, an organization that serves patients and families with or at risk for genetic diseases (online at http://www.geneticalliance.org/), were provided.

Psychosocial issues: The nurse recognized the complex feelings of guilt, shame, and confusion as Mr. and Mrs. Orca described their family history and the many losses in the past. The death of an older son (and its relationship to the sickling process with probable splenic sequestration) was ever fresh in their minds and had left them with sadness that would last for many years. They worried about more emergencies that might affect their older girl, Kala, and their young son, Benji. The nurse explored their feelings about the sudden loss of Ricky and how that may affect the other children. In addition, the nurse acknowledged the use of traditional herbs and the need to discuss their use with health providers for safety (including possible drug interactions) as well as with the psychologist or community elder to resolve Mrs. Orca's blame for Ricky's death. The nurse offered a referral to a psychologist to further discuss their feelings and related issues.

Pregnancy: Mrs. Orca's current pregnancy and the discussions of autosomal recessive inheritance brought new questions about the health of the expected baby. These parents expressed hopes for his healthy future, and appeared to be supportive of each other as they described their fears. The nurse asked about the possibility of disclosure of this genetic information to family members, to the other children, and to friends. The Orca's were hesitant about this topic and said that they would talk about it at home before proceeding to inform others in their family. The nurse offered to provide assistance if the time came that these concerns would be discussed. There were still issues of stigma and uncertainty surrounding the initial two sessions of counseling, and the nurse urged the Orcas to use coping measures, support services, and possibly their pastor for assistance. The nurse was aware of the complex cultural and religious pressures on Mr. and Mrs. Orca and offered to discuss these further if they wished.

School: The nurse made plans with the family to consult with the children's schools for individual healthcare plans (IHCP) and individual educational plans (IEP) as appropriate for the affected children. Mr. and Mrs. Orca were appreciative of this assistance with the school system and had not yet had a chance to speak with the school personnel about their two children with SCD.

Prophylaxis and health maintenance: Future management of SCD in the two Orca children was explored in detail by the Orca parents and the nurse. Additional concerns for pain management and prevention of complications associated with SCD were outlined, and appointments were set for follow-up care at the Sickle Cell Center. The Orcas said that they would continue with a local family primary care provider for their usual care and keep this person up to date with the care the children were receiving at the Sickle Cell Center.

Support group: The nurse invited the Orcas to join the Sickle Cell Center or the local sickle cell community-based agency's Family Support Group that met on a regular basis and held family fun events, a summer camp program, and year-round social gatherings in the community. The Orcas were receptive to this invitation and thanked the nurse for the counseling and information they received.

Follow-up: About a year later, the nurse met again with the Orcas. The new baby, now nearly 10 months old, was healthy (HgbAA) and developing along expected milestones. Kala and Benji were progressing well in school and had not been hospitalized in the interim. Dana was also healthy and excelling in her schoolwork. The Orcas had not yet broached the subject of SCD with their families, but had received quite a bit of support at their church and had helped with the summer camp program at the Sickle Cell Center coordinated by the community-based sickle cell agency. They said that Mr. Orca's sister was planning a visit in several weeks, and they hoped to talk things over with her during this time. They had not been to the psychologist but instead had discussed with Mr. Orca's parents and community elders the use of traditional herbs.

The Orcas and the nurse agreed that the young infant's hemoglobin status might be an issue in later years as he and the family begin to discuss the presence of sickle cell disease and traits. Because he might ask questions about these conditions in view of his own normal hemoglobin, the nurse urged the Orcas to be receptive to his thoughts and to seek additional counseling and support as they feel appropriate.

Comments

We can see the influence of family, cultural, and religious influences on how this couple reacted to a life-threatening illness in their children and the risk for others in this kindred to be affected or to be carriers of the sickle trait. In the early period of contact, the nurse could not ask Mr. and Mrs. Orca to discuss the risks with their siblings who might have the trait, whose children might have inherited the trait, and

FIGURE 24–1
Sickle Cell Family Pedigree

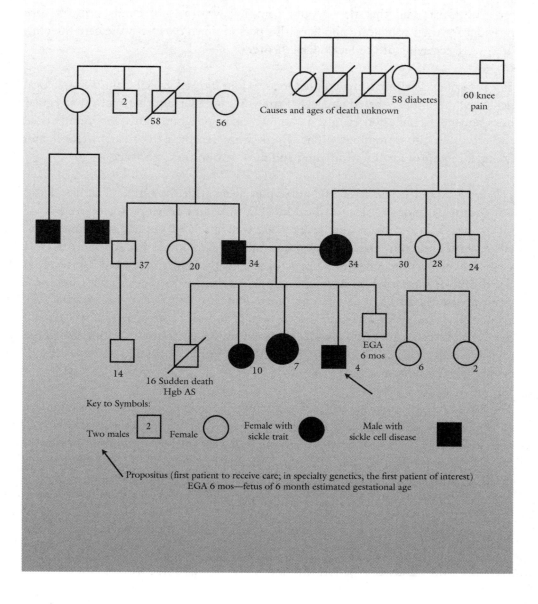

Causes and ages of death unknown

58 diabetes

60 knee pain

EGA 6 mos

16 Sudden death Hgb AS

Key to Symbols:

Two males | 2 | Female ⬤ | Female with sickle trait ⬤ | Male with sickle cell disease ◼

Propositus (first patient to receive care; in specialty genetics, the first patient of interest)
EGA 6 mos—fetus of 6 month estimated gestational age

who might be in a position to have children affected with SCD. The possibility of identification of SCD in a fetus early in pregnancy also presents difficult decisions regarding early termination, carrying an affected pregnancy to term, and preparation for appropriate treatment of the child during the first years of life and beyond. The nurse found it best to allow the Orcas to adjust to the issues among their own children and to approach the issues with extended family members later. She felt confident that in their own time, the Orcas would be ready to discuss the health risks in this family and that they could resolve their feelings with the resources they had at hand. The possibility of other family members requesting information was welcomed and the nurse assured them of continuing future assistance.

References

Buchanan, G. R., DeBaun, M. R., Quinn, C. T., and Steinberg, M. H. (2004). Sickle cell disease. *Hematology*, 2004: 35–47.

Chandler, K. 2006. Stem cells show promise in treating sickle cell. *The Westside Gazette.* http://news.pacificnews.org/news/view_article.html?article_id=1d9acb720a23fbf70ded6bde6c39651b (accessed October 9, 2008).

Gelehrter, T.D., Collins, F.S., and Ginsburg, D. 1998. *Principles of medical genetics* (2nd ed.). Baltimore, MD: Williams & Wilkins.

National Heart, Lung, and Blood Institute. 2003. *What is sickle cell anemia?* http://www.nhlbi.nih.gov/health/dci/Diseases/Sca/SCA_WhatIs.html (accessed October 9, 2008).

Yale, S. H., Nagib, N., and Guthrie, T. 2000. Approach to the vaso-occlusive crisis in adults with sickle cell disease. *American Family Physician*, 61: 1349–1356. http://www.aafp.org/afp/20000301/1349.html (accessed October 9, 2008).

CHAPTER 25

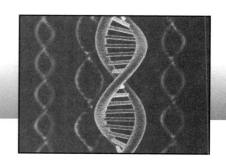

Case Study in Hereditary Breast and Ovarian Cancer

Susan Miller-Samuel, MSN, RN, APNG

Hereditary Breast Cancer

An estimated 5%–10% of all breast cancers are believed to have a hereditary component. Most forms of hereditary breast cancer are thought to be part of hereditary breast ovarian cancer syndrome (HBOCS), an autosomal dominant cancer predisposition syndrome in which germline gene mutations in the BRCA1 or BRCA2 gene have a 50–50 chance of being passed from generation to generation. Fewer hereditary breast cancers are believed to be associated with mutations in the TP53, and STK11/LKB1 genes (Mincey 2003).

Additional rarer mutations are seen in the ERBB2 (also called HER2/neu) and the PTEN genes. According to summaries available at the Genetics Home Reference (National Library of Medicine 2008) the ERBB2 (or HER2/neu) and PTEN genes play an important role in cell growth, function, adhesion to neighboring tissue, and movement. Mutations in the ERBB2 (or HER2/neu) gene can lead to unregulated growth and establishment of tumors (25% of all breast cancers and tumors in several other areas of the body have a mutation in this gene). The PTEN gene is a tumor suppressor gene that normally occurs in many cells all over the body and functions to control cell growth and death cycles (apoptosis is the process of cell decay and death). Mutations in the PTEN gene can mean the absence of these controls and the appearance of cancerous and abnormal non-cancerous cells (uncontrolled cell growth and proliferation). The gene known as p53 is a tumor suppressor with oncogenic properties. Mutations in the p53 gene are thought to occur in over 50% of all human cancers.

The BRCA1 and BRCA2 genes follow the autosomal dominant pattern of inheritance, are present in the germline line (cellular material in ova or sperm that is inherited and can be transmitted to offspring) and play a role in DNA repair mechanisms, cell cycle regulation, and the integrity of the genome (Yarden and Papa 2006). A number of researchers have estimated the risk of development of breast cancer among those with the BRCA1 mutation at 59%–87% and the BRCA2 mutation at 38%–80% (Mincey 2003). Moreover, the risk of ovarian cancer among carriers of the BRCA1 gene ranges from 28% to 44% and that for carriers of the BRCA2 gene ranges from 16% to 27% (Mincey 2003). Those with hereditary cancer, including those who carry the BRCA1 or BRCA2 genes, often demonstrate the onset of disease before the age of 50 (some sources say 45). Other cancers associated with germline mutations in the BRCA1 and BRCA2 genes include pancreatic, early-onset prostate, and laryngeal. It remains unclear whether colon cancer risk is absolutely increased in families who carry BRCA1 or BRCA2 mutations, although mutation carriers are given screening guidelines that manage them at increased risk of colorectal cancer.

Families who demonstrate increased rates of cancer, especially first-degree relatives (parents, children, and siblings), are candidates for further surveillance and possible study of genetic material. An accurate family history covering at least three generations with as much information as possible about ages at onset of illness, medical diagnoses, relevant co-morbidities, causes of death, and related issues is an essential part of health services delivery. A number of models (for example BRCAPRO and Myriad) have been used by specialists in cancer risk assessment to determine the likelihood of the presence of a mutation in the BRCA1 or BRCA2 genes in an individual. These models take into account such variables as the patient's age and history of breast or ovarian cancer diagnosis, family history of breast cancer, family history of ovarian cancer, family history of men with breast cancer, and ethnic background. While these models help guide clinicians and families in decision making for genetic testing, they are but one type of tool used in making decisions.

Recurring themes in the cancer genetics literature dealing with management of risk assessment include the essential ingredients of genetic counseling, accuracy of cancer diagnoses, and completeness of family and medical histories, when available. Careful and sensitive handling of preparation for genetic testing, informed consent, and disclosure of genetic testing findings by professionals with training in genetics (including physicians, nurses, and genetic counselors) are paramount. Appropriate referral of patients to specialists is essential. An essential component of genetic risk assessment and counseling includes patients knowing that their genetics providers are there to respond to concerns and support them long after results have been disclosed.

Ms. Crandall's Opening Assessment

We met Ms. Crandall for the first genetic consultation related to a strong family history of cancer. (See Figure 25–1 on page 381.) Ms. Crandall was diagnosed several months prior to our first visit with a breast cancer at age 38. Surgery was performed with subsequent pathology reports citing a left-sided 2.3 cm infiltrating ductal nuclear grade III, histological grade 2, ER/PR/HER2-negative tumor. Five of 12 axillary nodes were positive for metastasis. The patient was treated with bilateral mastectomy without reconstruction, preferring to wait one year until after completing chemotherapy treatment. Based on information provided to me, I believed that Ms. Crandall (at her relatively young age of cancer onset, still during reproductive years) could be at increased risk of a hereditary cancer syndrome such as Hereditary Breast Ovarian Cancer Syndrome (HBOCS).

Ethnic background: Italian (maternal and paternal)

Contributory Family History:

Sister: Thyroid cancer, not otherwise specified (NOS, meaning that a specific cell type or more detailed description of pathology was not given or available) at age 39

Mother: Ovarian vs. endometrial cancer at age 55, died at age 65

Maternal grandfather: Stomach v. Colon cancer, NOS, died at age 60

Maternal aunt: Breast cancer age 36, died at age 37

The patient and I discussed the information regarding hereditary breast cancer and associated conditions. We reviewed the risks, benefits, and limitations of gene testing, and cancer screening recommendations for Ms. Crandall and her at-risk family members. The patient appeared to have an appropriate understanding of the reviewed information and asked appropriate questions throughout the genetic consultation. Based on the current literature, Ms. Crandall's probability of having a

BRCA1 or BRCA2 mutation was estimated to be 42.2% (Myriad Genetics 2006). This estimation took into account Ms. Crandall's personal and family history of breast or ovarian cancer, and her non-Ashkenazi Jewish heritage (the Ashkenazi Jewish population is an ethnic group with increased risks for having BRCA1 and BRCA2 genetic mutations). Based on this estimate, we discussed the option of testing for mutations in the BRCA1 or BRCA2 genes. We also discussed the fact that risk probability models do not outweigh the patient's personal and family history.

The patient and I reviewed other background information: the BRCA1 and BRCA2 genes are important cancer tumor suppressor genes, and mutations in these genes account for a significant proportion of hereditary breast and ovarian cancer. Cancer-predisposing mutations have been identified throughout the BRCA1 and BRCA2 genes. The current technology for BRCA1 and BRCA2 testing may miss up to 10%–12% of mutations thought to exist within these genes. Therefore, a negative gene test result in a family with a striking family history must be interpreted with caution.

We discussed that there are, most likely, other breast or ovarian cancer syndrome-related genes which exist, but we do not yet have solid research that identifies other genes to test in any given individual or family. Often, variable penetrance factors (conditions that affect the appearance of a disease in persons who posses a given genetic mutation) are at play that are not completely understood now. Also, if we did have additional mutational analysis to offer, this might give Ms. Crandall and her family useful risk information at some future time.

General Genetic Information

We discussed that everyone is born with two copies of each gene, one from the mother, the other from the father. With tumor suppressor genes and mismatch repair genes, because each person inherits two copies of each gene, it takes two "injuries" to completely disable a gene by disabling both copies. We described that a person who inherits a mutation in a tumor suppressor gene such as BRCA1 or BRCA2 or PTEN is born with one copy of the gene already damaged. Injury to the second copy can greatly increase the risk of cancer. This also explains why hereditary cancer often develops at a younger age than non-hereditary or sporadic cancer. Individuals who are born with inherited risk (a damaged copy) have only one working copy of the gene, which if damaged may set the stage for cancer to develop. In contrast, sporadic cancers tend to develop later in life because both normal, working copies of a gene must become disabled by random mutations. We reviewed the fact that in true hereditary cancers, the inherited mutation is present in every cell in the body, which is why blood testing can identify the majority of such mutations.

We discussed that males and females have an equal chance of both carrying and transmitting these particular mutations. We also discussed that not everyone who carries a mutation in the genes we discussed develops cancer. Just as we cannot predict if a person with a genetic mutation will develop cancer, we cannot predict what type of cancer that person may develop, if in fact they do. A person who carries a mutation but never develops the disease may still transmit the mutation to their children. We also discussed the significance of finding a BRCA1, BRCA2, or other gene mutation in Ms. Crandall and the possibility of testing for her other family members if desired later.

Cancer Risks for BRCA1 and BRCA2 Carriers

We reviewed cancer risks associated with BRCA1 and BRCA2 mutations in detail. If a mutation in either gene is found, the person's lifetime risk to develop breast cancer is 50%–87%. There is a 20% risk of a second primary breast cancer within five years diagnosis of the first for BRCA1 gene carriers and up to a 60% risk for a second primary breast cancer by age 70 (a similar risk has been estimated for BRCA2 carriers). The associated risk for ovarian cancer is 20%–44% for BRCA1 and 10%–27% for BRCA2 compared to the lifetime risk of 1.4% for the general population. In general, if a mutation were found in Ms. Crandall, she would have a significantly increased risk for ovarian cancer as well as an increased risk of developing a second breast cancer. Although rare, males who carry a BRCA1 or BRCA2 mutation are also at increased risk for developing breast cancer, although the risk is higher in families where a BRCA2 mutation is identified. The estimate for male breast cancer is 6% by the age of 70 years, as compared to the average population risk of about 0.5%. We also discussed that there are increased risks for colon, pancreatic, and prostate cancers associated with BRCA1 families, and increased risks for prostate, laryngeal, and pancreatic cancer in BRCA2 families.

Risks, Benefits, and Limitations of Genetic Testing

We reviewed that genetic testing for cancer susceptibility is not a screening test intended for the general population; it is meant for individuals and their families thought to be at high risk for developing certain cancers based on their family or personal cancer history. We also discussed that gene testing has both risks and benefits and should always be a choice made by the individual after being fully informed, since testing results can often affect family members as well as the person being tested. Gene testing should be done only after carefully considering why an individual and family wants the information, as well as what they will do with it. Individuals should carefully plan for how and when to tell other family members of their gene testing results before it is done.

We reviewed potential benefits of gene testing, including helping to clarify the risk of developing cancer, to enhance early detection and prevention of cancer through increased surveillance, and to determine whether children or other family members may carry a mutation. Some of the cancer detection and risk-reduction strategies include lifestyle changes, increased screening, chemoprevention such as tamoxifen therapy, and risk-reduction surgery.

We discussed that genetic testing is not for everyone, and reviewed the risks and limitations. These include: psychological distress (anxiety, guilt, decreased self esteem, stigmatization, grief, and changes in family dynamics); loss of privacy; discrimination by insurers; and false sense of security for individuals who test negative for a mutation. Technical limitations of gene testing include: not all mutations are detectable; there may be uncertain significance of some mutations; and a negative result is fully informative only if a mutation has actually been identified in the family. Most gene testing results can indicate only a probability, not a certainty, of developing certain types of cancer.

Should Ms. Crandall opt for genetic testing, we discussed the fact that she would need to come back to our center to receive her genetic testing results in person. It is a policy of the center that all results be disclosed to patients in person. No genetic testing results will be given to patients or physicians over the phone. Results cannot be released to the patient's physician unless the patient gives written permission to the center to do so.

Final recommendations are always deferred until genetic testing results are disclosed. At the disclosure session, a follow-up management plan is provided. In the event that genetic testing results are negative, I would still recommend that Ms. Crandall follow the high-risk cancer screening guidelines listed below. If genetic testing results are indeterminate, or of uncertain significance, these results would be specifically addressed at the time of results disclosure.

All of the patient's questions were answered. The patient was asked to contact us should any questions arise. I told the patient I would contact her when I received her test results in approximately four to five weeks.

Genetic Consultation Summary: Results Disclosure

Results of Gene Testing

Genetic testing was performed at Myriad Genetic Laboratory in Salt Lake City. Analysis consists of sequencing all translated exons and immediately adjacent intronic regions of the BRCA1 and BRCA2 genes and a test for five specific BRCA1 rearrangements. Results of testing did find the Y130X (BRCA1) deleterious mutation in Ms. Crandall's blood sample. Results of this analysis are consistent with the germline mutation Y130X, resulting in a premature truncation of the BRCA1 protein at amino acid position 130. At-risk blood relatives are encouraged to be tested for this single-site mutation by the time they reach their mid-20s so appropriate screening guidelines can be firmly settled. Until that time, aggressive screening recommendations should be followed, some beginning at age 18. At-risk blood relatives are managed as though they carry the germline genetic mutation until genetic testing proves otherwise.

Summary of the Results Disclosure

Cancer risks associated with BRCA1 mutations were reviewed with Ms. Crandall in detail:

- In known mutation carriers, the person's lifetime risk to develop breast cancer is estimated to be 50%–87% with a 20% risk for a second primary breast cancer within five years of diagnosis of the first breast cancer (Verhoog, Brekelmans, Seynaeve, van den Bosch, Dahmen, van Geel, et al. 1998).

- The associated risk for ovarian cancer would be tenfold over that of the average population risk of 1.4% (Frank, Manley, Olopade, Cummings, Garber, Bernhardt, et al. 1998).

- Studies suggest that the chance to develop breast cancer approaches 50% by age 50 in BRCA mutation carriers. In the general population, the lifetime risk to develop breast cancer by age 80 is about 13%.

- Although rare, males who carry a BRCA1 mutation are also at increased risk for developing breast cancer; the risk is higher for men who carry a BRCA2 mutation (Ford, Easton, Stratton, Narod, Goldgar, Devilee, et al. 1998). The estimate for male breast cancer in mutation carriers is 6% by the age of 70, compared to the average population where the risk is approximately 0.5%–1.0%. BRCA1 mutations are thought to confer a somewhat lower risk for male breast cancer than those related to BRCA2 mutations, but still greater than that of the general population.

We also discussed that there are increased relative risks for prostate and pancreas cancers associated with BRCA1 families. It remains unclear whether an association exists between colon cancer and BRCA mutations. We reviewed the fact that female and male children of BRCA mutation carriers also have a 50–50 chance to inherit the BRCA1 mutation. If inherited, these children have a 50–50 chance to pass the mutation to each of their children.

Risk Reduction and General Information

Screening

We recommend that Ms. Crandall follow high-risk screening recommendations.

High-risk Breast Cancer Screening

- Monthly breast/chest-wall self-examinations.
- Clinical breast/chest wall examinations by a qualified clinician, preferably a breast surgeon, every 6 months.
- Studies have shown that BRCA1-related breast cancers can present with an unusually aggressive phenotype; therefore, bilateral breast MRI is recommended every 3–6 months along with mammography. Breast ultrasound may be considered as an adjunct to MRI.

High-risk Ovarian Cancer Screening

- Consultation with a gynecologic oncologist is strongly encouraged to clinically assess ovarian cancer risk via twice-yearly bi-manual rectovaginal pelvic examination, transvaginal ultrasound with color Doppler flow and CA-125 levels.
- The gynecologic oncology consultation can help answer questions regarding risks and benefits of prophylactic oophorectomy.

Prophylactic oophorectomy be thought to mainly reduce ovarian, but not breast cancer risk, since the majority of breast cancers related to BRCA1 mutations are "triple negative": Estrogen Receptor negative/Progesterone Receptor negative/HER2 negative. This particular tumor type has become associated with an unfavorable prognosis and aggressive phenotype. Studies have shown a relationship between BRCA1-related breast cancers and this triple-negative phenotype (Seewaldt and Scott 2007; Kaas, Kroger, Peterse, Hart, and Muller 2006; Turner and Reis-Filho 2006).

However, BRCA1-positivity does not rule out a future ER-positive breast cancer. (The patient's prior breast cancer was ER-negative). It was noted that the patient's mother was diagnosed with ovarian vs. endometrial cancer at age 52 years.

Colonoscopy

- The relationship between colon cancer and BRCA mutation carriers remains unclear. However, we recommend that starting now, Ms. Crandall have colonoscopy every 3–5 years. Depending on clinical symptoms and pathology results if specimens are taken, this recommendation could increase in frequency.
- At-risk blood relatives should be managed as though they are gene mutation-positive until genetic testing proves otherwise.

High-risk Screening

- Monthly breast self-examinations beginning at age 18.
- Baseline bilateral breast MRI and mammogram by age 28 (10 years earlier than the age at which the proband was diagnosed with breast cancer) and every six months thereafter.
- Clinical breast examinations by a qualified healthcare professional, preferably a breast surgeon, every year starting at age 18.
- Consultation with a gynecologic oncologist to clinically assess ovarian cancer risk via annual bimanual rectovaginal pelvic examination, transvaginal ultrasound with color Doppler flow and CA-125 levels; baseline at age 18.
- Colonoscopy may be indicated; however, the relationship between colon cancer and BRCA mutation carriers remains unclear. We do recommend that all at-risk blood relatives have baseline colonoscopy by age 40, 10 years earlier than the age suggested for the general population.

Recommendations for Men

These may at some time be applicable to a member of Ms. Crandall's family.

- Prostate cancer screening via digital rectal exam (DRE) and prostate specific antigen (PSA) every year beginning at age 35.
- Monthly breast self-exam beginning at age 18.
- Annual clinical breast exam by a breast surgeon beginning at age 25.
- Baseline bilateral mammogram and bilateral breast MRI by age 28.
- Monthly testicular exam beginning at age 18.
- Colonoscopy: Baseline at age 40.

The above recommendations could change if family members test negative for the known familial BRCA mutation.

Preventive Risk-Reduction Surgery

These risk-reduction options carry significant physical and psychological risks, along with the potential risk-reduction benefits they offer.

Prophylactic mastectomy (removal of the breasts) with or without reconstruction is an option for high-risk family members to further discuss with a board certified breast surgeon and breast reconstructive surgeon. Prophylactic mastectomy significantly reduces the risk to develop breast cancer, but does not reduce the risk to zero since every breast cell cannot be removed. Those women at significant risk to develop breast cancer, such as those who carry a deleterious genetic mutation, should carefully weigh prophylactic mastectomy in terms of their own lives, their perceptions of risk, and personal decision making.

Prophylactic oophorectomy (removal of the ovaries) is an option for high-risk women to further discuss with a board-certified gynecologist or gynecologic oncologist. Removal of the ovaries causes immediate surgical menopause. In pre-menopausal women, removal of the ovaries can also reduce the risk for breast cancer because the primary endogenous source of estrogen is removed. However, this lack of estrogen can significantly increase a woman's risk to develop osteoporosis, which can increase the risk for bone fractures. Bone density should be evaluated via bone densitometry (DEXA scan) prior to prophylactic oophorectomy and every 2–3 years thereafter. Pre-menopausal prophylactic oophorectomy may deleteriously affect cardiovascular health. Even in women who have had their ovaries removed, a type of ovarian cancer can still occur. This cancer is called primary peritoneal carcinoma (PPC) and is managed as ovarian cancer when it occurs. For this and other general health reasons, meticulous gynecological follow-up is essential.

Lifestyle Risk Reduction Strategies

Alcohol

A byproduct of alcohol metabolism is estrodial, a most potent form of estrogen. Women at increased risk for breast cancer are generally advised to limit their alcohol consumption to 1–2 drinks per week (5 ounces of wine, 12 ounces of beer, or 1.5 ounces of hard liquor).

Diet

A diet based on the American Cancer Society (ACS) guidelines encourages a variety of vitamins, minerals, antioxidants, and fiber. This recommendation has sound evidence, and we support a diet of this type for most people with out special issues such as diabetes. The role of phytoestrogens (plant estrogens), or soy products remains somewhat controversial. Some experts feel that plant estrogens or soy may increase breast cancer risk since they are in fact a source of estrogen. Others feel the exposure to the "weaker" soy products which compete for endogenous estrogen receptors may help to reduce breast cancer risk. More research is needed. Studies have shown that high-fiber diets can help reduce the risk of colorectal cancer. It was noted that individuals should always check with their personal healthcare provider before starting or altering any diet.

Exercise

Studies have shown that a moderate amount of aerobic exercise (4–5 times per week for 20–30 minutes each time) can help lower breast cancer risk. Studies have shown that weight-training or resistance training (lifting free weights, using resistance bands, using gym-style weight machines, push-ups, pull-ups, and squats) can help prevent, stabilize, or moderately reverse osteoporosis. It was noted that individuals should always check with their personal healthcare provider before beginning or altering any exercise regimen.

Body Weight

Weight gain, especially postmenopausal weight gain, is associated with an increased risk for breast cancer. Fat tissue secretes estrogen; estrogen exposure is associated with increased risk for breast cancer.

Smoking

Tobacco is associated not just with lung cancer but with cervical, bladder, and other cancers. Tobacco cessation programs are available at our center and other community facilities.

UVA/UVB Exposure

It is unclear whether certain skin cancers may be associated with BRCA mutations. Risk-reduction measures for all people include using an SPF of 45 of greater when out of doors and reapplying liberally after becoming wet, not using tanning booths, wearing long sleeves and long pants when out of doors for prolonged periods, and wearing wide-brimmed hats instead of baseball-style caps.

Talc

Studies have shown an association between regular talc exposure in the perineal area and ovarian cancer occurrence. This may be due to the fact that over 20 years ago, asbestos was an ingredient found in talc. We are unsure whether the relatively recent removal of asbestos from talc products now renders these products safe for use in the perineal area. Therefore, we recommend against it.

Chemoprevention Risk Reduction Options

Tamoxifen

Tamoxifen is the only drug FDA-approved to reduce breast cancer risk in pre- and post-menopausal women at increased risk for, but never diagnosed with, breast cancer. Tamoxifen may reduce breast cancer risk in certain individuals by up to 50%. Tamoxifen is also known to reduce the risk for breast cancer recurrence in women with estrogen receptor-positive breast tumors. However, it can have potentially serious side effects including increased risk for uterine cancer, including uterine sarcoma, and increased risk for blood clots. Smokers should not use Tamoxifen due to the increase risk for blood clots. A history of blood clot or phlebitis is considered a contraindication for Tamoxifen therapy. Concominent hormone therapy is contraindicated with Tamoxifen therapy.

Raloxifene (Evista)

In September 2007, Raloxifene was FDA-approved for breast cancer risk reduction in post-menopausal women at increased risk for the disease. Research findings from the STAR trial (a large national study on cancer risk reduction medications) indicate that Raloxifene may be as effective as Tamoxifen in reducing certain breast cancer risks (Vogel, Costantino, Wickerham, Cronin, Cecchini, Atkins, et al. 2006) and carries a less serious side effect profile. At this time, Raloxifene is NOT approved for pre-menopausal women. Raloxifene carries a less serious risk for blood clots than Tamoxifen; however, the risk is still substantial, therefore, smokers should not use Raloxifene. A history of blood clots or phlebitis is considered a contraindication for Tamoxifen and Raloxifene therapy. Concominent hormone therapy is contraindicated with Raloxifene therapy.

Aromatase Inhibitors

Femara and Arimidex are being evaluated to see if they may give the same, or better, risk reduction benefits as Tamoxifen, with less serious potential side effects. At

FIGURE 25-1
The Crandall Pedigree

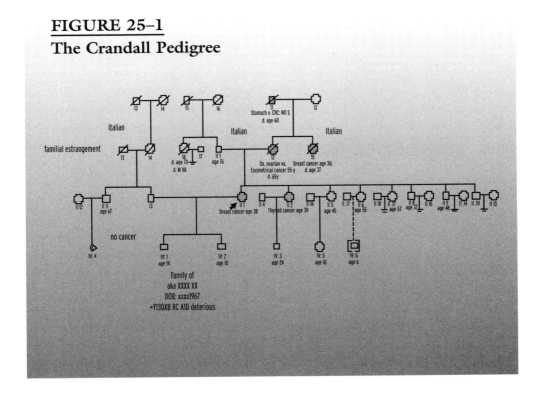

this time, aromatase inhibitors are only approved for postmenopausal women who have been diagnosed with breast cancer.

Oral Contraceptives

Studies have shown that oral contraceptives (birth control pills) are associated with a decreased risk for ovarian cancer, seemingly because ovulation stops, thus reducing the "activity" of the ovaries with less chance for a DNA transcription error to occur. However, oral contraceptives contain estrogen, which may increase the risk for breast cancer. Alternatives to oral contraceptives include barrier methods such as a diaphragm, or tubal ligation (having the Fallopian tubes tied). Studies have shown that tubal ligation also reduces the risk for ovarian cancer.

Closing Discussion

After summarizing all of this information, I reassured Ms. Crandall that I always remain available to answer questions or make referrals for issues such as reproductive genetic testing if they arise. In addition, given Ms. Crandall's relatively young age and the possibility that she or another family member might somehow become concerned about pregnancy, I included information about the www.fertilehope.org website. She or another relative might become interested in preimplantation genetic testing (testing of embryonic cells within the first weeks of pregnancy). Ms. Crandall was referred to the Women's Center for a gynecologic oncology consultation. I stressed that until Ms. Crandall's at-risk relatives are genetically tested, they should follow high-risk screening and moderate cancer risk-reduction measures.

In conclusion, I believe that Ms. Crandall had time to have all of her questions answered. As with all of my patients, I asked her to contact me at least once per year to update her family history.

References

Ford, D., D. F. Easton, M. Stratton, S. Narod, D. Goldgar, P. Devilee, D. T. Bishop, B. Weber, G. Lenoir, J. Chang-Claude, et al. 1998. Genetic heterogeneity and penetrance analysis of the BRCA1 and BRCA2 genes in breast cancer families. *American Journal of Human Genetics* 62 (3): 676–89.

Frank, T. S., S. A. Manley, O. I. Olopade, S. Cummings, J. E. Garber, B. Bernhardt, K. Antman, D. Russo, M. E. Wood, L. Mullineau, et al. 1998. Sequence analysis of BRCA1 and BRCA2: correlation of mutations with family history and ovarian cancer risk. *Journal of Clinical Oncology* 16 (7): 2417–2425.

Kaas, R., Kroger, R., Peterse, J. L., Hart, A. A., and Muller, S. H. 2006. The correlation of mammographic-and histologic patterns of breast cancers in BRCA1 gene mutation carriers, compared to age-matched sporadic controls. *European Radiology* 16: 2842–2848.

Mincey, B. A. 2003. Genetics and the management of women at high risk for breast cancer. *The Oncologist* 8: 466–473.

Myriad Genetics Inc. 2006. *BRCA Mutation prevalence tables.* http://www.myriadtests.com/provider/brca-mutation-prevalence.htm (accessed September 16, 2008).

National Library of Medicine. 2008. *Genetics home reference.* http://ghr.nlm.nih.gov (accessed September 16, 2008).

Seewaldt, V. L., and Scott. V. (2007). Images in clinical medicine: Rapid progression of basal-type breast cancer. *New England Journal of Medicine* 356 (13): e12.

Turner, N. C., and Reis-Filho, J. S. 2006. Basal-like breast cancer and the BRCA1 phenotype. *Oncogene* 25 (43): 5846–5853.

Verhoog, L.C., C. T. Brekelmans, C. Seynaeve, L. M. van den Bosch, G. Dahmen, A. N. van Geel, M. M. Tilanus-Linthorst, C. C. Bartels, A. Wagner, A. A. van den Ouweland, et al. 1998. Survival and tumour characteristics of breast-cancer patients with germline mutations of BRCA1. *Lancet* 351 (9112): 1359–1360.

Vogel, V. G., J. P. Costantino, D. L. Wickerham, W. M. Cronin, R. S. Cecchini, J. N. Atkins, T. B. Bevers, L. Fehrenbacher, E. R. Pajon, J. L. Wade, et al. 2006. Effects of tamoxifen vs. raloxifene on the risk of developing invasive breast cancer and other disease outcomes: the NSABP study of tamoxifen and raloxifene (STAR) P-2 trial. *Journal of the American Medical Association* 295: 2727–2741.

Yarden, R. I., and M. Z. Papa. 2006. BRCA1 at the crossroad of multiple cellular pathways: approaches for therapeutic interventions. *Molecular Cancer Therapeutics* 5: 1396–1404.

CHAPTER 26

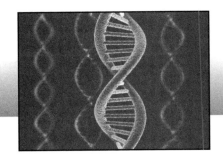

Lynch Syndrome (Hereditary Nonpolyposis Colon Cancer): A Case Study of Ethical Implications

Deborah J. MacDonald, PhD, RN, APNG

Most cancer occurs as a result of acquired genetic changes in a specific cell type. However, 5%–10% of some cancers occur because of a germline mutation (abnormality) in a single gene. These mutations are passed on to subsequent generations via the egg or sperm, generally in an autosomal dominant manner. In autosomal dominant inheritance, each child of a carrier of a cancer-associated gene mutation has a 50% (1:2) chance of inheriting the mutation. Individuals who inherit a cancer-associated gene mutation are at high risk for early-onset cancers, when screening or risk-reducing strategies are typically not in place. Genetic testing to identify these individuals is increasingly being incorporated into clinical practice and is now standard medical management for some heritable malignancies (American Society of Clinical Oncology 2003; Weitzel 2003). Although the technology enables implementing strategies to reduce cancer risk and help find cancer at an earlier stage, genetic testing for cancer predisposition has complex ethical, legal, and social implications (ELSI) not only for the person undergoing testing but also their family.

The International Society of Nurses in Genetics (ISONG) and the Oncology Nursing Society (ONS) have published position statements about the role of the nurse in genetic risk assessment, counseling, and testing (ISONG 2000, 2001, 2002, 2003; Oncology Nursing Society 2000a, 2000b). Counseling based on cancer predisposition testing must be more directive than traditional non-directive genetic counseling because persons desiring test results expect to be given recommendations for prevention or early detection of cancer. Nurses knowledgeable about the ELSI issues in hereditary cancer can provide anticipatory guidance, education, advocacy, psychological support, and appropriate referrals for individuals and their families (ANA 2007; MacDonald 1997; Dimond, Calzone, Davis, and Jenkins 1998; Lea, Jenkins and Francomano 1998; Tranin, Masny and Jenkins 2003; Lashley 1998; Loescher 1999; Flach and Jennings-Dozier 2000).

The following case composite depicts some ELSI issues confronted in the course of genetic cancer risk assessment (GCRA) for a family with Lynch syndrome. All names have been changed to maintain patient confidentiality, and details have been altered to protect anonymity while maintaining an accurate portrayal of ethical dilemmas. The case is presented from the viewpoint of the nurse on the cancer genetics team. The role of the nurse in facilitating positive outcomes for a family faced with ELSI issues is discussed.

Lynch Syndrome Case (Hereditary Nonpolyposis Colon Cancer)

Jane is a 47-year-old woman who had a colonoscopy at age 44 for evaluation of rectal bleeding, anemia, and unexplained weight loss. She was found to have an adenocarcinoma of the transverse colon with lymph node involvement, for which she had a segmental resection and chemotherapy. Her oncologist referred her for GCRA because her mother, brother, and maternal grandmother had also been diagnosed with colon cancer.

Cancer Risks in Lynch Syndrome

In Lynch syndrome, colon cancer typically occurs in the mid-40s, with few polyps, and a predominance of right-sided colon cancer. Colonoscopy (vs. sigmoidoscopy) is the appropriate screening tool. The distinguishing features of Lynch syndrome are early onset cancers as well as multiple primary tumors in affected individuals. This syndrome is most often caused by an abnormality in one of several mismatch DNA repair pathway genes (most often *MLH1* or *MSH2*; occasionally *MSH6*, or more rarely, *PMS2*).

The risk for colon cancer in Lynch syndrome is about 80%. Women who have a mutation in one of the syndrome's associated genes also have about a 35%–40% risk of endometrial cancer and up to a 10% risk of ovarian cancer. Persons with this syndrome also have a very high risk (>50%) for additional primary colorectal cancers and a small risk for upper GI cancers, transitional cell carcinomas of the renal pelvis, and cancers of the pancreato-biliary tract. The strictest diagnosis of Lynch syndrome is based on the "Amsterdam 3–2–1" criteria of having three affected family members with colon cancer, at least two generations affected, one case diagnosed before age 50, and one affected being a first-degree relative of the other two. Each child or sibling of a person with a mutation in one of the Lynch syndrome genes has a 50% (1:2) chance of inheriting the mutation.

Family History

Figure 27–1 depicts the family history in the form of a pedigree. Jane and her husband have a 16-year-old daughter, Kim, and two sons, John, age 23 and Steven, age 20. Jane has a 43-year-old sister, Anne, who does not have children. Jane and Anne's only brother, Tom, died of colon cancer nearly six years ago, shortly after being diagnosed with the disease at age 45. Tom has a 31-year-old son, Scott, who does not have children. Jane's 77-year old mother was treated for colon cancer in her cecum at age 65. The mother also had a hysterectomy and removal of both ovaries at age 50 for uterine fibroids, as did Jane's only maternal female cousin, Linda, at age 45. Linda does not have children, neither does her 44-year-old brother, but their 49-year-old brother has two daughters, ages 18 and 20. Linda's mother, age 75, had uterine cancer at age 49. Jane's other maternal aunt died at age 29 in an automobile accident. The only maternal uncle, age 74, has not had cancer. The maternal grandmother had stomach cancer at age 55 and died of disease at age 56. She had one sibling, a brother who died at age 78 of heart disease. The maternal grandfather died at age 28 of leukemia. Jane had no further knowledge of his side of the family. There are no cancers in the paternal lineage other than a lung cancer at age 85 in the paternal grandfather.

Genetic Cancer Risk Assessment (GCRA)

At each counseling session the family was offered the support of the cancer center's social worker and psychologist. Jane presented to clinic with her husband, expressing that her major motivation for the genetic consultation was to learn about her daughter's risk for colon cancer. Jane states that she is not concerned about her sons having colon cancer, because they resemble her husband's side of the family physically and in their personalities, in contrast to her daughter who is the "spitting image of me." Jane also believes that her cousin Linda is not at risk for colon cancer since Linda's mother, Jane's maternal aunt, has not had the disease.

Jane and her husband received extensive counseling from the GCRA multidisciplinary team regarding Lynch syndrome and its implications for Jane's health care as well as for their children and other relatives. The couple decided that trying to identify the cause of the colon cancers was something they wanted to pursue. After discussing this with their family, they returned to the clinic anxious to proceed with genetic testing.

Jane and her husband said they understood the information discussed in the counseling sessions. Jane desired to proceed with genetic testing, and gave written consent and a blood sample for analysis. When results were ready the couple returned to the clinic with Jane's mother. The test result revealed that Jane had a cancer-associated mutation in the *MLH1* gene. The genetics team again reviewed the recommendations for persons with Lynch syndrome, including the rationale for colonoscopy every 1–2 years generally beginning between the ages of 20 and 25, and for women, annual transvaginal ultrasound or endometrial aspirate generally beginning at ages 25–35 and consideration of hysterectomy and removal of both fallopian tubes and ovaries by age 35–40 or after completion of childbearing (Hendriks, de Jong, Morreau, Tops, Vasen, Wijnen, et al. 2006; Hadley, Jenkins, Dimond, de Carvalho, Kirsch, and Palmer 2004; National Comprehensive Cancer Network 2007). They also reiterated the importance of sharing this information with other relatives (ASCO 2003). Jane stated that she intended to share the test result with her family and would suggest that her at-risk adult family members seek genetic counseling. She understood that genetic testing would determine whether these relatives had inherited the mutated or normal working copy of the *MLH1* gene, which would have significant implications for her relatives' and their children's health care.

To help guide her mother's health care and confirm what appeared to be maternal inheritance of the mutated gene, Jane's mother proceeded with genetic testing. As expected, she was found to carry the *MLH1* gene mutation.

Ethical Dilemmas

Testing of Minors

Jane and her husband discussed Lynch syndrome with their children after expressing how surprised they were to learn that each of their sons had the same chance (1:2) of inheriting the mutated *MLH1* gene as did their daughter. Although the couple understood that testing their 16-year-old daughter was not warranted, upon learning Jane's test result they insisted that all their children be tested for the gene mutation. Jane stated that if their daughter did not have this testing now, she would worry too much about her daughter's risk for cancer.

Non-Paternity

A few days after Jane learned her test result, she called the cancer genetics team nurse, quite distressed because her nephew Scott had told her he had scheduled a colonoscopy for the following month. As the nurse explored Jane's concerns, Jane revealed that shortly before his death her brother Tom had told her that Scott was not his biological child. Scott had been raised to believe Tom was his biological father, and no one in the family knew otherwise. Jane had promised her brother that she would not divulge this information.

Jane was seeking advice about how to handle this situation because she knew that Scott did not need a colonoscopy before age 50 and that the procedure had a risk, albeit very small, for colon perforation. She insisted, however, that she intended to uphold her deceased brother's wishes and would not inform Scott that her brother was not his biological father. She pleaded with the nurse to keep this information confidential.

Scott and his wife thought that Scott had a 50% chance of inheriting the *MLH1* gene mutation, because they assumed that Tom, who died of colon cancer, had the same genetic abnormality responsible for Jane's colon cancer. Therefore, Scott thought that he was being proactive by following Lynch syndrome colonoscopy guidelines. He and his wife recognized the value of genetic testing, but decided not to have this testing because Scott mistakenly thought that his group health insurance would be dropped if he were found to have "the gene."

Family Coercion or Disagreement

Jane's maternal aunt and her three adult children were aware of Jane's test result. The children tried to convince their mother to have genetic testing to determine if she had inherited the mutated *MLH1* gene.

The aunt had previously had uterine cancer, which is the most common extra-colonic cancer in women with Lynch syndrome. The optimal means to determine if the aunt's children were at risk for the cancers associated with this syndrome was for their mother to undergo genetic testing of the known mutation. If she had it, then each of her three children had a 50% chance of inheriting it. Although each of her children could individually pursue testing, if the mother did not have the mutated gene, testing of her children would be unnecessary. Conversely, if one of the children had testing and was found to have the mutation, then by default the mother's genetic status would be identified, as she would need to have the mutation for her children to inherit it. Jane informed the genetics team that her aunt did not want to have this testing because her aunt's husband, whom her aunt relies on to make healthcare decisions as is customary in his culture, did not want her to have the test.

Applying the Nursing Code of Ethics

Earlier this monograph discussed how *Code of Ethics for Nurses with Interpretive Statements* provides a framework for nurses regarding their professional and ethical obligations and duties (American Nurses Association 2001), and how *Genetics and Genomics Nursing: Scope and Standards of Practice* may be used to guide ethical nursing care related to genetic conditions (ANA 2007). This section describes how the nurse helped the family work through their ethical dilemmas.

Testing of Minors

The primary consideration in genetic testing of minors is the welfare of the child (American Society of Human Genetics/American College of Medical Genetics 1995). Although parents generally have the authority to decide medical care for their minor children, in the case of genetic testing for Lynch syndrome, testing minors is not ethically justified (ASCO 2003; ASHG/ACMG 1995).

Jane and her husband discussed with the nurse why Jane wanted their 16-year-old daughter to be tested for an adult-onset condition. The nurse explored Jane's concerns, which revealed that Jane mistakenly thought that because her daughter was "as physically and mentally mature as any 30-year-old" she was more likely to develop cancer in her teens. The nurse explained that in Lynch syndrome chronological age, not physical appearance or mental capacity, was an important factor in the onset of cancer. The nurse reviewed the age of cancer onset and care recommendations, and the reasons why genetic testing of children is not deemed ethical:

- Because Lynch syndrome is an adult-onset cancer syndrome, testing of minors is not warranted because minors are not at risk for the cancers in this syndrome.
- There are no interventions for minors that can prevent or lower the chances for these cancers.

- Testing of a minor takes away the minor's chance to make an autonomous and informed decision when they are adults whether they want to pursue this testing (ASCO 2003; ASHG/ACMG 1995; MacDonald and Lessick 2000).

At the end of the session Jane stated that although she would like to know her daughter's genetic status, she better understood why leaving this decision up to her daughter to consider when she was at least age 18 was "the right thing to do."

Non-Paternity

An ethical principle in health care is the just and fair use of healthcare resources. The nurse knew, as Jane did, that colonoscopy and genetic testing was not needed for 31-year-old Scott, because he was not Jane's biological nephew. Yet, to prevent the misuse of healthcare resources and the minor but real chance of physical harm from a colonoscopy, Scott would need to know that he was not at risk for Lynch syndrome and why this was so, which would breach the confidentiality Jane requested, cause psychological distress for Scott and the family, and could seriously and irreparably disrupt family dynamics and their trust in the nurse and genetics team.

Without identifying the family, the nurse consulted genetic, ethical, and legal experts to determine the most ethically prudent way to handle this situation. The ethical principles of self-determinism, nonmaleficence, beneficence, and justice were taken into consideration in determining if there was a way for Jane to inform Scott that colonoscopy and genetic testing was not needed, while maintaining the family secret. Also of concern was whether there was any legal obligation to inform Scott or his doctor that colonoscopy was not indicated and to let Scott know that he was not at risk for Lynch syndrome.

The nurse was well aware of the ethical and legal duty to uphold patient confidentiality except in rare, extreme circumstances of imminent serious danger that could not otherwise be avoided. The risks and benefits of alternative approaches that might respect Jane's wishes, not cause harm, promote the welfare of the family, and use healthcare resources appropriately were weighed. Legal liability and obligation to warn relatives was taken into account, noting that the federal Health Insurance Portability and Accountability Act (HIPAA) precludes warning family members of genetic risk and that the American Society of Clinical Oncologists and American Medical Association believe that the duty to warn, if any, is fulfilled by encouraging persons having genetic testing to communicate this information to their relatives (ASCO 2003; U.S. Congress 1996; Offit, Groeger, Turner, Wadsworth, and Weiser 2004).

Although in this situation the issue pertained to informing Scott or his doctor of the lack of genetic risk rather than potential risk, Scott was not in any life-threatening danger that warranted breaching patient confidentiality. Thus the nurse concluded that the primary duty was to the patient, Jane. Although the nurse was privy to information that went against the fair use of resources and had a small potential to cause harm, the ethical principles of confidentiality and self-determinism prevailed, supporting Jane's right to not disclose the non-paternity. The nurse and genetics team, backed up by professional guidelines and a legal expert, concurred that there was no ethical or legal obligation to disclose information to Scott or his doctor.

The nurse assured Jane that the non-biological relationship would be kept private. She advised Jane to share with Scott the written information she had been given about state and federal anti-discrimination. She reminded Jane that the HIPAA law prohibits using genetic test results as pre-existing conditions in the absence of disease and denying insurance obtained through group health plans.

Jane was greatly relieved. She stated that she would urge Scott to come in for a genetics consultation right away so that he could have the testing done, which she would offer to pay for. Jane expected that Scott would then cancel the colonoscopy since his test result would show that he did not have the familial mutation, and reiterated her relief that her secret would not be disclosed.

Family Coercion and Cultural Differences

Nurses have a professional responsibility to ensure that their clients have accurate and adequate information to enable them to make fully informed decisions about genetic testing. Consent for genetic testing should be freely given, without undue coercion from others, including healthcare professionals and family members. Although the nurse agreed that the most efficient strategy in this situation was for the aunt to undergo genetic testing, she recognized her ethical obligation to put aside her personal opinion. Doing so preserved her professional integrity, allowed patient autonomy, and enabled her to provide unbiased and supportive care. Additionally, while the nurse values individuals' right to act freely on their own behalf, she also recognizes that in some cultures the accepted norm is that healthcare decisions are made by others in the family. Therefore the nurse has an ethical duty to support the aunt's preference to defer the genetic testing decision to her husband.

FIGURE 26–1
Lynch Syndrome
(Hereditary Nonpolyposis Colon Cancer)

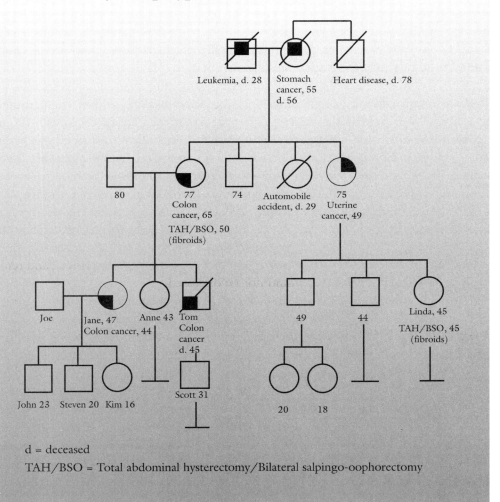

Leukemia, d. 28   Stomach cancer, 55 d. 56   Heart disease, d. 78

80   77 Colon cancer, 65 TAH/BSO, 50 (fibroids)   74   Automobile accident, d. 29   75 Uterine cancer, 49

Joe   Jane, 47 Colon cancer, 44   Anne 43   Tom Colon cancer d. 45   49   44   Linda, 45 TAH/BSO, 45 (fibroids)

John 23   Steven 20   Kim 16   Scott 31   20   18

d = deceased

TAH/BSO = Total abdominal hysterectomy/Bilateral salpingo-oophorectomy

393

The nurse discussed the situation with Jane and her mother, maintaining a neutral stance while acknowledging that their concerns were understandable. The nurse ensured that they understood that genetic counseling is always available to the aunt and her husband and their children, if desired, and proposed that Jane or her mother could provide written information about Lynch syndrome to relatives who are amenable to receiving such information. The nurse also discussed that although Jane and her mother believe "testing is the right thing to do," not everyone will have the same opinion and that it may take time for family members to adjust to new genetic information that may affect their health care.

Regarding Jane's inquiry about genetic testing for her cousins, who were interested in learning their genetic status, the nurse stated that the cousins could call for an appointment to be seen for genetic counseling or testing individually or as a group if they preferred. The cousins presented together for counseling and the genetics team urged them to consider how the family would be affected if one or more of them were found to carry the familial mutation. Role playing about receiving positive and negative test results was used to stimulate critical thinking of how the test results could influence personal and family relationships; this helped the cousins decide to defer testing until they had a chance to talk about this again with their parents. One of the cousins called a few weeks later to say that their parents were willing to come in for counseling. At the counseling visit, misconceptions regarding cancer risk factors, genetic testing, and Lynch syndrome were addressed with the family. Subsequently, the father decided that genetic testing would be of benefit to his family. Testing revealed that the aunt did not carry the gene mutation. Thus, none of their children were at increased risk for colon cancer, a great relief to the family.

Conclusion

This case illustrates how emerging genetic technology presents new ethical, legal, and social challenges to traditional healthcare practice. Although a family with Lynch syndrome (HNPCC) is depicted, the ELSI issues are germane to many situations that nurses may encounter. Each nurse's involvement with genetics will vary depending upon her focus and scope of practice. As genetics continues to influence the prevention, diagnosis, and treatment of various diseases and disorders, all nurses must be mindful of the ethical, legal, and social implications of utilizing genetic technology. Nurses are obliged to be cognizant of their personal feelings and beliefs, help families clarify their values, support autonomous fully informed decision making, and recognize that the manner in which information is presented and comprehended will affect how individuals and families cope. Multiple resources exist for nurses faced with ethical, legal, and social dilemmas.

References

American Nurses Association (ANA). 2001. *Code of ethics for nurses with interpretive statements.* Washington, DC: American Nurses Publishing.

———. 2007. *Genetics and genomics nursing: Scope & standards of practice.* Sliver Spring, MD: American Nurses Association.

American Society of Clinical Oncology (ASCO). 2003. American Society of Clinical Oncology policy statement update: Genetic testing for cancer susceptibility. *Journal of Clinical Oncology* 21 (12): 2397–2406.

American Society of Human Genetics (ASHG)/American College of Medical Genetics (ACMG). 1995. Points to consider: Ethical, legal, and psychosocial implications of genetic testing in children and adolescents. *American Journal of Human Genetics* 57: 1233–1241.

Dimond, E., K. Calzone, J. Davis, and J. Jenkins. 1998. The role of the nurse in cancer genetics. *Cancer Nursing* 21: 57–70.

Flach, J., and K. M. Jennings-Dozier. 2000. Bioethical considerations in cancer prevention and early detection practice and research. *Oncology Nursing Forum* 27 (9 Suppl.): 37–45.

Hadley, D. W., J. F. Jenkins, E. Dimond, M. de Carvalho, I. Kirsch, and C. G. S. Palmer. 2004. Colon cancer screening practices after genetic counseling and testing for hereditary nonpolyposis colorectal cancer. *Journal of Clinical Oncology* 22 (1): 39–44.

Hendriks, Y. M., A. E. de Jong, H. Morreau, C. M. J. Tops, H. F. Vasen, J. Th. Wijnen, M. H. Breuning, and A. H. J. T. Bröcker-Vriends. 2006. Diagnostic approach and management of Lynch syndrome (hereditary nonpolyposis colorectal carcinoma): A guide for clinicians. *CA: A Cancer Journal for Clinicians* 56 (4): 213–225.

International Society of Nurses in Genetics (ISONG). 2000. *Informed decision-making and consent: The role of nursing.* http://www.isong.org/about/ps_consent.cfm (accessed September 16, 2008).

———. 2001. *Privacy and confidentiality of genetic information: The role of the nurse.* http://www.isong.org/about/ps_privacy.cfm (accessed September 16, 2008).

———. 2002. *Genetic counseling for vulnerable populations: The role of nursing.* http://www.isong.org/about/ps_vulnerable.cfm (accessed September 16, 2008).

———. 2003. *Access to genomic healthcare: The role of the nurse.* http://www.isong.org/about/ps_genomic.cfm (accessed September 16, 2008).

Lashley, F. R. 1998. *Clinical genetics in nursing practice.* 2nd ed. New York: Springer Publishing.

Lea, D. H., J. Jenkins, and C. A. Francomano. 1998. *Genetics in clinical practice: New directions for nursing and health care.* Sudbury, MA: Jones and Bartlett.

Loescher, L. J. 1999. Genetics and ethics: The family history component of cancer genetic risk counseling. *Cancer Nursing* 22: 96–102.

MacDonald, D. J. 1997. The oncology nurse's role in cancer risk assessment and counseling. *Seminars in Oncology Nursing* 13: 123–128.

MacDonald, D. J., and M. Lessick. 2000. Hereditary cancers in children and ethical and psychosocial implications. *Journal of Pediatric Nursing* 15 (4): 217–225.

National Comprehensive Cancer Network (NCCN). 2003. Colorectal cancer screening: Clinical practice guidelines in oncology. *Journal of the National Comprehensive Cancer Network* 1 (1): 72 .

Offit, K., E. Groeger, S. Turner, E. A. Wadsworth, and M. A. Weiser. 2004. The "duty to warn" a patient's family members about hereditary disease risks. *Journal of the American Medical Association* 292 (12): 1469–1473.

Oncology Nursing Society. 2000a. Cancer predisposition: Genetic testing and risk assessment counseling. *Oncology Nursing Forum* 27: 1349.

Oncology Nursing Society. 2000b. The role of the oncology nurse in cancer: Genetic counseling. *Oncology Nursing Forum* 27: 1348.

Tranin, A., A. Masny and J. Jenkins. 2003. *Genetics in oncology practice: Cancer risk assessment.* Pittsburgh, PA: Oncology Nursing Society.

U.S. Congress. 1996. *Health Insurance Portability and Accountability Act of 1996.* 104th Cong., Public Law No. 104–191.

Weitzel, J. N. 2003. Screening and genetic counseling for the patient with cancer. In *Clinical hematology and oncology: Presentation, diagnosis, and treatment,* eds. B. Furie, P. Cassileth, M. B. Atkins, and R. J. Mayer, 1193–1208. Philadelphia: Churchill Livingstone.

The author acknowledges Sharon Sand, CCRP, for her careful review of this manuscript.

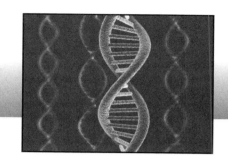

CHAPTER 27

The P Family, At Risk for Alzheimer's Disease

Rita Black Monsen, DSN, MPH, RN, FAAN

Overview of Alzheimer's Disease

Alzheimer's disease affects 4.5 million Americans, double those affected in 1980, and this figure is expected to grow to as many as 16 million by the year 2050 (Alzheimer's Association 2006a). It accounts for the majority of dementias and is characterized by neuron loss in the brain, especially in the cortex and hippocampus, leading to progressive memory loss, degradation in cognition, and deterioration in language (Nussbaum and Ellis 2004). Generally, early onset of Alzheimer's disease, prior to age 65 is rare, with the more prevalent late-onset form appearing on average at age 80 (Helmer, Joly, Letenneur, Commenges, and Dartigues 2001).

The early-onset forms of the disease that follow autosomal dominant inheritance are associated with one of three genes discovered in family linkage studies (studies of genes and markers that are located close to each other on chromosomes and tend to be transmitted through family lines), and DNA sequencing analysis (identification of base pairs in specific areas of DNA, often performed in persons affected with a given health condition) (NHGRI n.d). These three genes are presinilin1 (PSEN1 on chromosome14), presenilin2 (PSEN2 on chromosome 1), and the gene associate with beta-amyloid precursor protein on chromosome 21 (Nussbaum and Ellis 2004). PSEN1 was found in over half of patients from affected families in a community study of early-onset Alzheimer's Disease in France (Campion, Dumanchin, Hannequin, Dubois, Belliard, Puel, et al. 1999).

The vast majority of affected individuals are thought to have a combination of genetic and environmental factors (known as multifactorial inheritance) that causes the appearance of Alzheimer's disease late in life. There have been some reports of attempts to detect Alzheimer's disease before the affected person becomes incapacitated, and testing for mild cognitive impairment (MCI) has shown some promise because it separates those who have a greater likelihood of developing "clinically probable" Alzheimer's from those with expected cognitive loss in normal aging (Petersen, Doody, Kurz, Mohs, Morris, Rabins, et al. 2001). Petersen and his colleagues describe Alzheimer's disease as "clinically probable" because, at the present time, confirmation of the diagnosis requires autopsy examination of the brain for "plaques" and "tangles," the hallmark abnormal structures associated with this condition (Alzheimer's Association 2006b)

Perhaps as great a sadness for families who have a member affected with Alzheimer's disease is the burden accepted by their caregivers. Over two-thirds of those affected live at home and the majority of these are cared for by family members (Alzheimer's Association 2006a). The Alzheimer's Association (http://www.alz.org) offers resources, education, and support for families and friends. The many community agencies who serve the elderly provide information about therapies, respite care, and counseling to assist in coping with the stresses of living with an affected person.

The P. Family

Mr. and Ms. P. (a fictional family) came to our Genetic Services Center requesting information and possible genetic testing for Alzheimer's disease. Ms. P. was more worried than her husband and had been referred by a neurologist in the local community who suggested genetic counseling, especially for the couple's children.

Mr. and Ms. P. related the history of their family (see Figure 27–1) on our first visit. Ms. P. and her husband (who is adopted and has no information about his family background) have 18-year-old twins, a boy and a girl, both healthy. Ms. P. is age 41, has no health problems, is a non-smoker, and works as an elementary school teacher.

FIGURE 27–1
P Family Pedigree

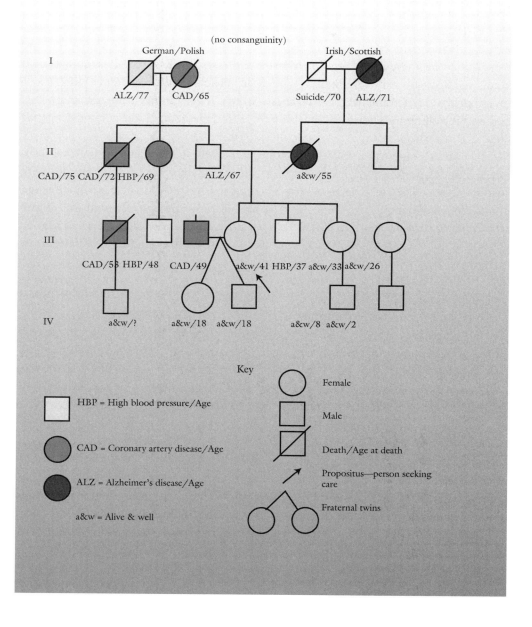

Her husband is age 49 and was diagnosed with coronary artery disease in the last two months. He takes medication and exercises regularly, but occasionally smokes cigars. Mr. P. is the pastor of a large congregation in a local Protestant church. The P.'s refrain from alcohol and eat a "heart-healthy" diet.

Ms. P. has a younger brother, age 37, who was diagnosed two years ago with high blood pressure and takes medication. This younger brother has no children and works as an accountant in another city not far from the P.'s. Ms. P. has a younger sister, age 33, who is healthy and lives with her husband and eight-year-old son in a neighboring community. Ms. P.'s younger sister works with her husband in a family business installing aluminum siding.

Ms. P.'s father is age 69 and has high blood pressure. He lives nearby in a "golf-centered" condominium complex. He has an older brother, who died at age 75 with coronary artery disease. This uncle has a son, now 53 years old with coronary artery disease and living in another state. The family has only rare contact with this cousin and believes that he has one son who is healthy. No other information is known about this cousin and his son. Ms. P.'s father also has an older sister age 72 who has been diagnosed with probable Alzheimer's disease. She has a 48-year-old son with high blood pressure. This paternal aunt and her son live close to Ms. P.'s cousin in another state and are rarely contact the P. family.

Ms. P.'s paternal grandfather died at age 79 with probable Alzheimer's disease (onset after age 72, no autopsy confirmation) and her paternal grandmother died at age 65 with coronary artery disease. They are of German and Polish ethnicity, and there is no known consanguinity in the family background.

Ms. P.'s mother died at age 67 with Alzheimer's disease diagnosed at age 60 (confirmed on autopsy); she had no other health problems. Ms. P.'s mother had a sister (fraternal twin) who was diagnosed at age 61 and died at age 69 with Alzheimer's disease (also confirmed on autopsy). This twin never married and did not have children. These twins were close throughout their lives and close to their younger brother, Ms. P.'s uncle, who is age 60 and was recently found to have mild cognitive impairment (MCI). This uncle lives with his healthy 26-year-old daughter and a healthy two-year-old grandson. This side of the family lives in close proximity and sees each other several times a year.

Ms. P.'s maternal grandfather was described as a "heavy drinker" and thought to suffer bouts of depression. He committed suicide at age 70, a circumstance that profoundly saddened the entire family, particularly the twins, Ms. P.'s mother and her aunt. Ms. P.'s maternal grandmother died at age 71 with probable Alzheimer's disease (diagnosed approximately 8–10 years before her death and unconfirmed by autopsy) after several years at home being cared for by her husband and daughters, Ms. P.'s mother and aunt. They were of German and French ethnicity. There is also no known consanguinity on this side of the family.

Ms. P.'s mother and her twin sister were part of early family linkage studies conducted several years ago in a large academic research center near their home community about one year after being diagnosed with probable Alzheimer's disease. Because of the parameters of the research protocol, Ms. P.'s mother and aunt consented to participate as subjects and gave blood samples. The researchers specified that the results of the testing would not be revealed to them, but would contribute to a summary report of the findings among family members who qualified to participate in the research. Since that time and after the death of her mother and her aunt, Ms. P. and her relatives have not discussed this study and did not receive any further contact from the researchers.

Assessment and Genetic Counseling

The P. family pedigree suggests that early onset Alzheimer's disease appeared in Ms. P.'s maternal grandmother, her mother, and her aunt who were in their early 60s at the time of diagnosis and that MCI was diagnosed in her maternal uncle only recently at age 60. Ms. P.'s brother's diagnosis of high blood pressure is noted as well. There is a significant history of coronary artery disease in Ms. P.'s father's family, appearing in her paternal uncle, aunt, and paternal grandmother, as well as high blood pressure in her father and first cousin, son of her paternal aunt. The appearance of probable Alzheimer's disease in Ms. P.'s paternal grandfather in his 70s does not suggest the early-onset form of the disease.

Ms. P., her siblings, and her cousin may be at risk for early-onset Alzheimer's disease coming down to them from Ms. P.'s maternal grandmother. In view of the pattern of disease appearance in maternal grandmother, mother, and maternal aunt, as well as MCI in the maternal uncle, it may well be that there is a genetic mutation with an autosomal dominant (AD) mode of inheritance. Ms. P. asked about the possibility of learning the results of genetic testing done on her mother and aunt, both having been part of a family linkage study conducted in another center some time back. I acknowledged this request and noted that the circumstances of the study were such that the findings on specific individuals would have been sealed and unavailable for later review by family members.

It is possible that Ms. P. and her family, having French heritage, may have inherited the PSEN1 gene as reported by Campion and colleagues in 1999. PSEN1 is known to follow AD inheritance and there is a chance that this mutation was present in Ms. P's maternal grandmother. The offspring of individuals affected with conditions that follow AD inheritance have a 50% chance of inheriting the genetic mutation. The presence of the genetic mutation does not confer a 100% guarantee of having the illness, but does depend on the penetrance of the mutation—the likelihood that those with the mutation will have the illness. The form of Alzheimer's with AD inheritance has been found to have high penetrance (Campion, Dumanchin, Hannequin, Dubois, Belliard, Puel, et al. 1999), meaning that those with the mutation have a strong likelihood of developing the disease.

Offering genetic testing for conditions that have no possibility for prevention or treatment is not appropriate in view of the fact that knowledge of the presence of such a mutation could do more harm and even destroy the mental stability of a family. Definitive genetic testing for one or more genetic mutations associated with Alzheimer's disease would not be considered at the present time because there is no current available treatment. The young P. twins, now age 18 and able to give informed consents as adults, might at some future date be candidates for genetic testing. This testing is not likely to be recommended until there is firm evidence of efficacious treatment, and if available, preventive measures. Such testing would also have implications for the P. children as far as reproductive decision making.

The P. family was encouraged to stay in touch with the Genetic Services Center in the event that future developments promise prevention and treatment as well as genetic testing. In addition, I gave the P.s' information about the Alzheimer's Association, www.alz.org, and urged them to share this resource with other family members who would benefit from additional information and support.

I did provide the P. family with information about the risks for coronary artery disease and high blood pressure suggested by Ms. P.'s paternal side of the family. I urged early screening, healthy lifestyles, and contact with community support resources to possibly prevent or reduce the severity of these conditions in family members. I urged them to consider discussing these preventive measures with Ms. P.'s paternal aunt and cousins as the occasion arises.

Unfortunately, I did not have any information about Mr. P.'s family and could not offer any counseling that would be based on his family history. Someday the P.'s may discover information about Mr. P.'s parentage and the young twins may return with a more complete picture of health conditions with possible risks for inherited problems later in their adult years.

Evaluation of Outcomes

I heard from Ms. P. a few months after our genetic counseling session and was saddened to hear that her brother had reported bouts of depression. I noted that he would be a candidate for a professional mental health evaluation and treatment. I offered community resources, including the National Alliance on Mental Illness (NAMI), for her family to seek further assistance. In addition, I noted that depression is among the conditions that are currently being studied for genetic causation and that the presence of depression in her brother as well as suspected depression in her maternal grandfather could indicate that further genetic counseling might be appropriate for her family.

Ms. P. said that she suspected as much and noted that the pressures of realizing that Alzheimer's disease, and now depression, were part of their family heritage. She said, "we are a family that is going to go crazy some day and there isn't a darn thing we can do about it." I noted the distress in her voice and asked if there had been additional conversations among family members along these lines. She denied this, but was very receptive when I recommended that arrangements could be made for mental health counseling in cooperation with our Genetic Services Center. I assured her that such services might be very beneficial in helping her and other family members identify and discuss their fears and worries as well as make provision for preventive care. I also assured her that her husband and young children would benefit from supportive counseling. I had the impression that she was receptive to these recommendations and offered to make a referral for help. She expressed her appreciation and said that she hoped to do all in her power to give her children as many resources as possible to live healthy lives.

Conclusion

The P. family illustrates the suspicion, even knowledge, that one or more genetic mutations threaten their well being. Moreover, the present state of gene-based diagnostics and therapeutics in the area of Alzheimer's disease does not permit prevention or cure, or even amelioration in a practical, meaningful way. As well accepted testing for mental health conditions become more available, and as more efficacious prevention and treatment methods are developed, problems such as depression are likely to become more manageable.

In the last quarter of the twentieth century, family linkage studies were one of the few tools available to assist clinicians in understanding the presence of inherited illness and provide some estimate of risk for appearance in later generations. Families who participated in linkage analysis as part of research protocols gave generously of their blood, body tissue, and histories in hopes of contributing to larger databases that may contribute to our understanding of such conditions in the future. Today, more sophisticated and direct methods of searching for mutations that lead to conditions that affect mental health are commonplace, especially in highly specialized academic centers.

The P.'s inherit a family experience of serious mental illness (as well as cardiovascular disease) that bestows on them the dread of mental anguish in later life. Finding a way to accept this burden is difficult, and for some families in similar circumstances impossible. The memories of seeing parents care for grandparents and other family members with deteriorating mental health may cast a prophetic path for children, some of whom may abdicate. Yet one cannot escape the inevitable. Respite from caring for sick family members may provide a chance to forget, at least temporarily, about the difficult daily lives they have. Mental health therapies, counseling, and support services that help families build on their strengths are appropriate in most instances. As we learn more about genetic causes and discover new therapies that use molecular technologies for control of previously untreatable illnesses, we are able to offer hope to future generations.

References

Alzheimer's Association. 2006a. *Alzheimer's facts and figures.* http://www.alz.org/alzheimers_disease_facts_figures.asp (accessed September 16, 2008).

———. 2006b. *Risk factors.* http://www.alz.org/alzheimers_disease_causes_risk_factors.asp (accessed October 9, 2008).

Campion, D., C. Dumanchin, D. Hannequin, B. Dubois, S. Belliard, M. Puel, C. Thomas-Anterion, A. Michon, C. Martin, F. Charbonnier, et al. 1999. Early-onset autosomal dominant Alzheimer disease: Prevalence, genetic heterogeneity, and mutation spectrum. *American Journal of Human Genetics* 65 (3): 664–670.

Helmer, C., P. Joly, L. Letenneur, D. Commenges, and J. F. Dartigues. 2001. Mortality with dementia: Results from a French prospective community-based cohort. *American Journal of Epidemiology* 145: 642–648.

National Human Genome Research Institute (NHGRI). n.d. *Talking glossary.* http://www.genome.gov/glossary.cfm?key=linkage (accessed September 16, 2008).

Nussbaum, R. L., and C. E. Ellis. 2004. Alzheimer's disease and Parkinson's disease. In *Genomic medicine: Articles from the New England Journal of Medicine,* eds. A. E. Guttmacher, F. S. Collins, and J. M. Drazen, 93–105). Baltimore, MD: Johns Hopkins Press/Boston: The New England Journal of Medicine.

Petersen, R. C., R. Doody, A. Kurz, R. C. Mohs, J. C. Morris, P. V. Rabins, K. Ritchie, M. Rossor, L. Thal, and B. Winblad. 2001. Current concepts in mild cognitive impairment. *Archives of Neurology* 58: 1985–1992.

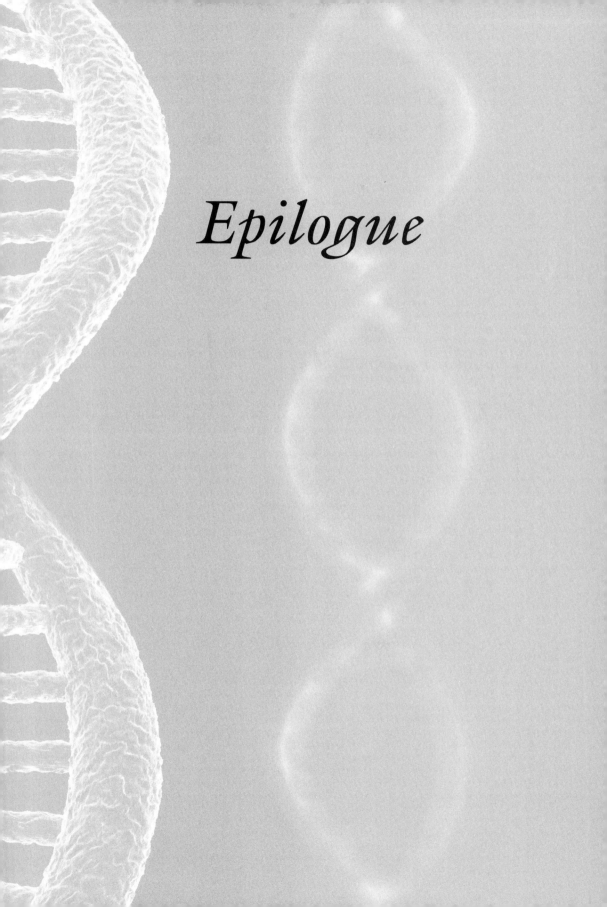

Epilogue

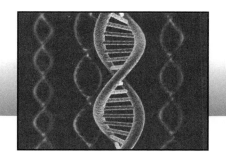

Genetics and Ethics in Health Care and Nursing: Epilogue and Future Directions

Rita Black Monsen, DSN, MPH, RN, FAAN

Epilogue: The Range of Allegiances and Commitments

This monograph has traced some of the major belief systems and cultural perspectives of the world's peoples, and it has brought forward a few major questions that we must ask today because of the advances of genetics and genomic technologies in health care. We can now appreciate that spiritual, religious, and cultural allegiances and commitments are integral to human life and population health. We can also witness the unprecedented revolution in diagnosis and treatment that will become possible with the application of genomics to healthcare services. These two great movements form a trajectory that is unprecedented in human history and call us to confront new questions about the meanings of person, family, and society. We can know a significant amount of information about our genetic makeup, the makeup of our families, and the genetic basis for human diversity on earth. We can project risks for health and illness as never before, yet we are still not able to provide cures for many major killers. We will not have to wait more than a few years for some of these cures, based upon genetic and genomic research and applications of gene-based therapeutics. As these new ways of thinking about health and illness unfold, we will see many changes in our cultural and religious values and practices.

Truth-Telling: A Basic Assumption About Relationships Among Nurses and Patients

Pellegrino (2001) notes that the ordering value of science is truth. We must listen to our patients and attend to the integrity of their lives as they place their trust in us. We must tell them the truth to the extent that we possibly can, and we must honor their desires and decisions without allowing harm to themselves or others.

We can strive to realize that culture is integral with family life as we encounter each new patient who seeks information and counseling about genetic concerns. We can inform ourselves about their values and traditional beliefs by being sensitive to cultural practices and patterns of behavior. Patients and families will tell us of their hopes for the future and for the coming generations of children as they confront decisions about gene-based testing and related therapeutics. Each family and kindred with whom we interact will signal how they accept the risk of illness and the risk of transmission of illness or the propensity for it to their offspring.

As advocates for better lives for patients and families, nurses stand for protection of personal interests and for development of public policies that promote healthful living. We should work to curb the use of genetic technologies to modify crops and animal products in agriculture without adequate establishment of safety to consumers and to the environment, indeed to the integrity of the cultural landscapes of entire populations. Nursing joins the many professions that work for recovery and preservation of safe environments because, ultimately, the quality of the air we breathe, the waters we drink and bathe in, and the earth from which our food comes determine the quality of our health as we live out our lives. We must advocate for environments that are free of toxins and safe for humans of all ages.

Worrisome developments in genetics and genomic research, particularly in areas where commercial exploitation of new technologies may generate short-term profits at the expense of population health and long-term public safety, have increased in recent decades. Testing in less than appropriate circumstances, such as laboratories that operate with few quality controls, undermines the credibility of test results and can dismantle trust between patients, families, and healthcare providers. New options for learning about inherited traits from widely advertised and easily accessible analyses of tissue (such as scrapings from the inner surface of the mouth) via direct marketing of genetic test kits to the public are becoming commonplace now. Health-care providers have serious concerns about such testing being conducted without adequate assessment of personal and family health histories, genetic counseling, and follow-up evaluation of testing outcomes.

Healthcare Genetics/Genomics and Nurses' Responsibilities in Caring for Families and Communities

Genetic information pervades our self-images and expectations for the future. Our understanding of health and well-being rests on our genetic makeup, and our lives are intertwined inextricably with those of our immediate family, especially those of our spouses and children. Our genetic makeup undergirds our ethnicity which, in turn, contributes to our understanding of ourselves and where our families and communities of origin come from and what future paths lay before us. Our spirituality and sense of goodness are integral to our cultural allegiances and govern our conduct and decisions along the way.

Nurses and the patients, families, and communities they serve are one and the same, yet nurses are obligated to understand the meanings of the lives of those they serve. They are obligated to inform themselves, to the greatest possible degree, of the parameters of risk, illness, and therapies their patients live with. And they are obligated to watch for the signposts on the horizon that lead to wellness or further suffering. Genetic information, while evolving at an unprecedented rate in today's technology-focused society, stands as a clear set of signposts for patients and families and for their progeny. Nurses need genetic information and need to appreciate its many implications for all those they serve.

Nursing, as the preeminent healthcare profession, should therefore continue to lead its members to ever-evolving education coupled with recognition of the ethical obligations attendant on new knowledges and technologies. A precept such as this is timeless, no matter what social and economic pressures present themselves in healthcare delivery. The American Nurses Association has consistently led all the nurses in our nation over the past century, as our professional organization, by its dissemination of standards of care, scopes of practice, and Code of Ethics. As genomic healthcare becomes more and more commonplace in the next decades, nursing will be obligated to keep its professionals ready and well prepared to serve. Certainly, this obligation supersedes any other in nursing's agenda for our nation and across the world.

Future Directions: The Full Measure of a Post-Genomic World

The success of the Human Genome Project has equipped us with the knowledge, methods, and tools to understand how genes are expressed, to some extent, and how they work in concert to produce various states of health and illness. Genomics, the study of all of the genetic activity in an organism, has been extended into the field of proteomics, the study of all of the proteins and their activities in a biological organism (Bowler, Ellison, and Reisdorph 2006). The field of proteomics has engendered discoveries in several specialized areas of protein metabolism that are now being used to capture and understand the behaviors of protein molecules in a number of clinical areas (for example, oncology, nephrology, immunology, infectious diseases, pulmonology, and cardiology).

Also, as an adjunct to the Human Genome Project, work has progressed over the past two decades in the study of epigenetics, the developmental processes that are associated with gene expression level over the course of a lifetime and result in phenotypic features (body and behavioral characteristics) (Gallon-Kabani and Junien 2005). Epigenetics encompasses methylation and related biochemical activities of DNA in cells, the essential processes that govern cell growth, regulation of gene and chromosome activities, and responses to environmental influences (Novik, Nimmrich, Gene, et al. 2002). Indeed, epigenomic studies that exploit rapidly emerging computational and biological technologies to capture genome-wide phenomena in cells are leading to the establishment of the Human Epigenome Project. The field of epigenomics is providing greater understanding of the mechanisms that contribute to cancer (Plass 2002), diabetes (Gallon-Kabani and Junien 2005), and cardiovascular disease (Fornage and Doris 2006), as well as the role of nutrition in disease development (Milner 2007).

Indeed, the *post-genomic era* is upon us with emerging technologies that pinpoint genomic and metabolic phenomena as well as how proteins interact in groups and in tandem with environmental influences, allowing us to understand and predict disease progression and the responses of individuals to pharmacologic, nutritional, and other interventions (Cho 2007; Iguchi, Watanabe, and Katsu 2006; Polotsky and O'Donnell 2007). These advances will become more commonplace as they identify which molecular processes signal illness, how illness can be expected to worsen or improve, and how therapeutic approaches can reverse or ameliorate disease courses.

As for the greater fabric of developments in health care, we can be sure that increasing successes will be sought for understanding our genetic makeup, for manipulating our genes and genomes to enhance our capacities for longer and more comfortable lives. I suspect that those of us interested in the human experience will continue to ask about the boundaries of a meaningful, fulfilling life, about the access and appropriateness of care for all peoples, about respect for cultural and religious allegiances and traditions, and about the ultimate center of control of the human experience—the individual in the context of family and community. We will see advances in technology transfer from the laboratory bench to the healthcare setting as long as society supports excellence in scientific scholarship (and scholarship in all areas of human inquiry), human and material resource deployment for genomic testing and treatment, and proliferation of adequately prepared nursing professionals and other providers of direct care services.

I fully expect that there will continue to be exploitation of vulnerable populations: we haven't really learned a great deal from history (as is seen is many of the discussions in this text) and are likely to repeat some of our mistakes. To the extent that we permit inquiry into ethical practices and engage in conversations that call for truth telling (most importantly to ourselves), we can hope to realize greater benefits from our discoveries and hope to ease the suffering of all those who wish for help.

This book was intended to highlight some of the new questions facing us now, and questions that will appear on the horizon in the next decade. It is likely that our culture and our values regarding health and illness will change as these new possibilities emerge. Nurses, other healthcare professionals, and scholars in the sciences and humanities must join together to consider the immense impact of genomic developments on our civilization. This book is one early step in that direction.

Rita Black Monsen, DSN, MPH, RN, FAAN
Hot Springs, Arkansas

References

Bowler, R. P., M. C. Ellison, and N. Reisdorph. 2006. Proteomics in pulmonary medicine. *Chest* 130: 567–574.

Cho, W. C. 2007. Contribution of oncoproteomics to cancer biomarker discovery. *Molecular Cancer* 6: 25.

Fornage, M., and P. A. Doris. 2006. Genomics and epigenomics of hypertension. *Current Opinion in Molecular Therapy* 8: 206–214.

Gallon-Kabani, C, and C. Junien. 2005. Nutritional epigenomics of metabolic syndrome: New perspective against the epidemic. *Diabetes* 54: 1899–1906.

Iguchi, T., H. Watanabe, and Y. Katsu. 2006. Application of ecotoxicogenomics for studying endocrine disruption in vertebrates and invertebrates. *Environmental Health Perspectives* 114 (Supplement 1): 101–105.

Milner, J. A. 2007. Nutrition in the "omics" era. *Forum of Nutrition* 60: 1–24.

Novik, K. L., I. Nimmrich, B. Gene, S. Maier, C. Piepenbrock, A. Olek, and S. Beck. 2002. Epigenomics: genome-wide study of methylation phenomena. *Current Issues in Molecular Biology* 4: 111–128.

Pellegrino, E. D. 2001. *Physician and philosopher.* Charlottesville, VA: Carden Jennings.

Plass, C. 2002. Cancer epigenomics. *Human Molecular Genetics* 11: 2479–2488.

Polotsky, V. Y., and C. P. O'Donnell. 2007. Genomics of sleep-disordered breathing. *Proceedings of the American Thoracic Society* 4: 121–126.

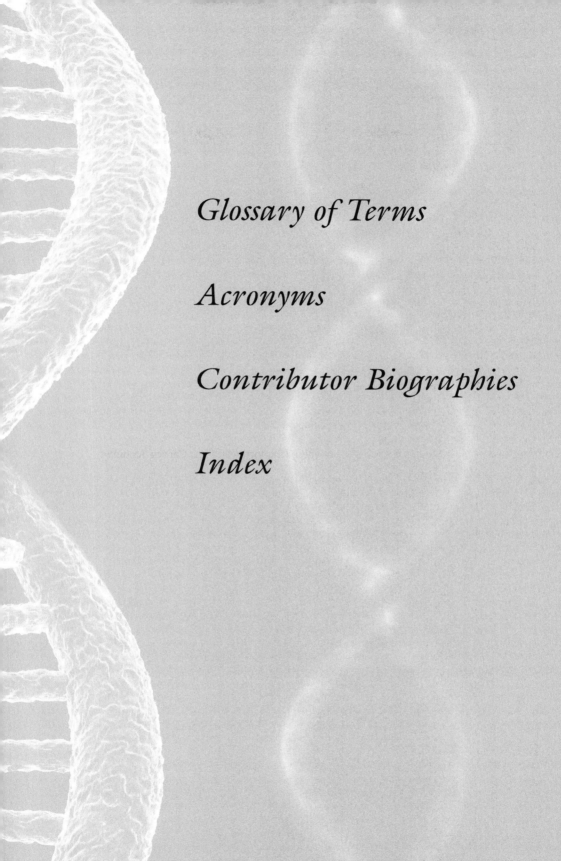

Glossary of Terms

Acronyms

Contributor Biographies

Index

GLOSSARY OF TERMS

The list of acronyms begins on page 423.

(* A term adapted from a glossary of the National Human Genome Research Institute: http://www.genome.gov/glossary.cfm accessed October 22, 2008.)

allele
A variation of a particular gene at a particular location on a specific chromosome, associated with inherited characteristics that vary such as eye color, skin pigmentation, and certain bodily functions; may be dominant (usually manifested) or recessive (less likely to be expressed unless there are two copies of the same allele present).

assent
To agree with, the act of understanding and agreeing; often associated with consent, usually by a minor.

AD inheritance
Autosomal dominant inheritance; one copy of the gene from one parent is sufficient to cause manifestation of the associated health condition; each child of a person who has a gene mutation that follows AD inheritance has a 50% chance of inheriting the mutation (half of offspring will inherit the abnormal genetic material); offspring without the mutation will not have the abnormality, nor can they pass it to their own offspring

AR inheritance
Autosomal recessive inheritance; two copies of the gene (one copy from each parent) are required to cause manifestation of the associated health condition. There is a 25% chance for offspring to inherit both copies of the mutation from parents who are carriers of a genetic mutation that follows AR inheritance, resulting in the appearance of the condition. There is a 50% chance for offspring to inherit one copy of the mutation from parents who are carriers of a genetic mutation that follows AR inheritance, making them a carrier of the mutation like their parents. Lastly, there is 25% chance for offspring from carrier parents to inherit neither copy of the mutation, meaning that these children do not have any copies of the mutation and will neither manifest the condition nor pass the mutation to their offspring.

autosomes
Chromosomes other than the sex chromosomes, X and Y.

cascade effect
An ancillary benefit of carrier testing where family members can be alerted to their risk for carrying a mutation and may seek genetic testing.

congenital
Present at birth

consanguinity
Reproduction between two blood relatives.

consent
To agree with or comply with what is desired or recommended.

consultand
Person who seeks and receives counseling and/or additional services from one or several professional providers.

chromosome
Strands of tightly coiled DNA; the normal human has 46 chromosomes, of these 44 are autosomes and 2 are sex chromosomes.

de novo mutation
A change in a gene (a change in the base pairs in a part of an organism's DNA), not inherited from parents.

DEXA scan
An examination of bone density (densitometry).

disclosure
Genetic counseling session aimed at revelation of results of genetic testing; entails sensitive discussion of the results of analysis(es) of genetic material in body tissue (frequently blood or cells from mucosa such as that from the inside of the mouth).

DNA
Deoxyribonucleic acid, strands of nucleotide base pairs that compose strands forming a double helix inside the cell nucleus providing the instructions for proteins and related substances essential to life.*

DNA sequencing analysis
Identification of base pairs in specific areas of DNA in persons affected with a given health condition.*

exon
Coding regions of a gene.

expressivity
The signs and symptoms caused by one or more genes in an individual organism or person who possesses that gene or combination of genes. For example, a gene may be described as having full expressivity, meaning that all of its associated signs and symptoms appear in the affected person. Also, a gene may be spoken of as having variable expression, meaning that not all of its associated signs and symptoms appear in the affected person

family linkage studies
Studies of genes and markers that are located in close to each other on chromosomes and tend to be transmitted through family lines.*

gene
Group of nucleotides that direct the assembly of proteins and related cell materials leading to bodily structure and function; genetic material is arranged in specific sequences associated with the formation of amino acids in living cells, often referred to as "spelling" such as TTT in DNA. In an example of protein synthesis, TTT in an active coding area of DNA is translated in messenger RNA (mRNA) to AAA, which is then transcribed into one of the amino acids, lysine.

genetic counseling
Short-term, educational counseling process for individuals and families who have a genetic disease or who are at risk for such a disease. Genetic counseling includes a family health history, construction of as complete a pedigree as possible (graphical drawing of the members of a family or kindred arranged to show relationships across generations), and discussion of risk of the appearance of health conditions in family members. In genetic counseling, professionals with training in genetics inform patients about their condition and help them make informed decisions about their plans in life (such as plans for reproduction).*

genetic screening
The process of testing a population or group for the presence and/or risk of having or passing on a specific genetic condition.*

genetic testing

The process of testing an individual for the presence and/or risk of having or passing on a specific genetic condition; often involving identification of one or more specific mutations.*

geneticization of health

Understanding or description of health as derived from a person's or a group's genetic make-up.

genome

All of the genetic material in an organism.

genotype

The genetic material in an organism that determines bodily characteristics.

genomic healthcare

Diagnostic and/or therapeutic procedures that consider a combination of genetic and environmental factors and their manifestation(s) in the body.

germline

Cellular material in ova and/or sperm that is inherited and can be transmitted to offspring.*

heritability

The ability of a gene or combination of genes to be inherited by offspring; often refers to the pattern of inheritance of genetic material in a family, kindred, or population.

inheritance

The presence of genetic material in offspring from biological parents.

kindred

Extended family, includes blood relatives from several generations

mtDNA

Mitochondrial DNA (genetic material contained in the mitochondria of cells).

multifactorial inheritance

A combination of genetic and environmental factors known or suspected of causing a health condition; a significant majority of commonly occurring conditions that appear to "run in families" are associated with multifactorial inheritance, examples include certain forms of cardiovascular disease, cancer, diabetes, and hypertension.

mutation
Gene associated with illness or risk for illness; mutations may entail redundant base pair repeats, mistakes in "spelling" (erroneous deletion or substitution of nucleotides), or rearrangement of one or several base pairs.

pedigree
A graphical diagram of the relationship of the members of a family or kindred that includes more than one generation, often several generations.

penetrance
The appearance signs and symptoms caused by one or more genes in a population that possesses that gene or combination of genes, often expressed as a percent. For example, a gene may be described as 80% penetrant, meaning that 80% of the population with that gene will show signs or symptoms of its affect(s).

pharmacogenomics
The study of variation associated with an individual's genes that influence the metabolism of pharmaceutical products.

phenotype
The bodily characteristics of an organism determined, in part, by the genetic material one possesses.

polymorphism
A common variation in the sequence of DNA among individuals.*

proband
The first person in a family to be identified with or at risk for a condition (also referred to as propositus in some instances where this is the first person in a family who seeks care).

proteomics
A field of biotechnology in which molecular biological, genetic, and biochemical analysis focuses on the development and behavior of proteins expressed by genes, often with implications for diagnosis and treatment of health conditions.

risk
The chance of inheritance of genetic material; also may refer to the chance that a health condition may appear in a person with one or a combination of causative genes.

workup

A series of diagnostic procedures that assist in determining the nature and cause(s) of a health condition and might indicate the presence of a specific health problem.

x-linked dominant inheritance

One copy of the gene located on an X chromosome in a male or a female is sufficient to cause manifestation of the associated health condition.

x-linked recessive inheritance

One copy of the gene located on the X chromosome in a male is sufficient to cause manifestation of the associated health condition (because males with one X and one Y chromosome possess only one copy of the genes on the X chromosome, conditions associated with these genes are likely to be manifested); females with two X chromosomes (one from each parent, and only one of these X chromosomes has the mutated gene) will not manifest the condition.

ACRONYMS

ACMG	American College of Medical Geneticists
ACOG	American College of Obstetricians and Gynecologists
AIS	artificial insemination
ANA	American Nurses Association
APC	adenomatous polyposis coli gene mutation
APRN	Advanced Practice Registered Nurse (occasionally APN, Advanced Practice Nurse); a nurse with advanced education and preparation, capable of independent specialized clinical management of clients: patients, families, and communities). There are four types of APRN: Nurse Practitioner, Clinical Nurse Specialist, Certified Nurse Midwife, and Certified Registered Nurse Anesthetist.
ASCO	American Society of Clinical Oncology
ASHG	American Society of Human Genetics
ATM	ataxia telangiectasia mutation
BCC	basal cell carcinoma
BCE	before the Christian or common era (generally used in dating historical events, periods, and objects)
BCP	birth control pills
BRCA	gene mutation for certain forms of inherited breast cancer; BRCA1 and BRCA2 are two mutations that are associated with inherited breast cancer
CABG	coronary artery by-pass graft
CBAVD	congenital bilateral absence of the vas deferens
CD	Cowden disease or Cowden syndrome
CDC	Centers for Disease Control and Prevention in Atlanta, GA, a division of the U.S. Department of Health and Human Services

CF	cystic fibrosis
CFF	Cystic Fibrosis Foundation
CFRD	Cystic Fibrosis-Related Diabetes Mellitus
CFTR	cystic fibrosis transmembrane regulator
CIA	census of India
CLIA	Clinical Laboratory Improvement Amendments, a mechanism for assurance of quality in laboratory testing; regulated by the Centers for Medicare and Medicaid Services (http://www.cms.hhs.gov/clia accessed 22 October 2008)
CMS	Centers for Medicare and Medicaid Service, a division of DHHS
COBRA	Consolidated Omnibus Budget Reconciliation Act
CRC	colorectal cancer
CYP genes	genes associated with isoenzymes that play a role in the metabolism of drugs and other chemicals
DHHS	U.S. Department of Health and Human Services
DNA	deoxyribonucleic acid, consists of four types of nucleotides (thymine, guanine, adenine, and cytosine, often written briefly by capitalized initials, T, G, A, C) arranged in pairs, known as base pairs. There are approximately 3 billion base pairs in all of the genetic material in humans, comprising an estimated 30–40,000 genes. About 5% of human DNA is thought to be biologically active (coding for specific bodily functions). As yet, the activities of the rest of human genetic material are not well understood. Additional information about DNA, genes, and inheritance can be obtained at the websites of the National Human Genome Research Institute (www.genome.gov) and the National Coalition for Health Professional Education in Genetics (www.nchpeg.org)
DNR	do not resuscitate (an order prohibiting lifesaving procedures for a selected patient)
DOE	U.S. Department of Energy
DTC	direct-to-consumer, refers to advertising of genetic and genomic technological applications to the public

ECIB	Education and Community Involvement Branch of the NHGRI
EGAPP	Evaluation of Genomic Application in Practice and Prevention Project, a model program established at the CDC for guiding the transfer of genetic and genomic technologies to clinical application (more information available online at http://www.cdc.gov/genomics/gtesting/EGAPP/docs/egappInfo.htm, accessed October 7, 2008)
ELSI	Ethical, Legal, and Social Implications of genetic conditions and associated health care; there is an ELSI Division of the National Human Genome Research Institute at the National Institutes of Health in Bethesda, MD.
EMT	emergency medical technician
ERBB2 (HER-2/neu)	gene approved symbol for *v-erb-b2 erythroblastic leukemia viral oncogene homolog 2, neuro/glioblastoma derived oncogene homolog (avian)*. Also referred to as HER-2/neu by some clinicians, this gene is one of a family of genes that provide instructions for producing growth factor receptors. (From the Genetics Home Reference http://ghr.nlm.nih.gov/gene=erbb2; accessed October 22, 2008.)
FAP	familial adenomatous polyposis
FDA	U.S. Food and Drug Administration
FTC	U.S. Federal Trade Commission
GCRA	genetic cancer risk assessment
GINA	Genetic Information Nondiscrimination Act of 2008; U.S. legislation to protect Americans against any discrimination based on their genetic information in employment and health insurance.
GOVA	ANA's Governmental Affairs Department
HBOC	hereditary breast ovarian cancer
HCP	health care providers
HD	Huntington disease
HER2	human epidermal growth factor receptor-2; see also ERBB2 above
HGP	Human Genome Project

HIPAA	Health Insurance Portability and Accountability Act, U.S. legislation enacted in 1996
HIV/AIDS	human immunodeficiency virus/acquired immunodeficiency syndrome
HNPCC	hereditary nonpolyposis colon cancer
HRQOL	health-related quality of life
HRSA	Health Resources and Services Administration, a division of DHHS
HRT	hormone replacement therapy
ICN	International Council of Nurses
IEP	individual education plan
IECP	individual emergency care plan
IHCP	individual health care plan
IOM	Institute of Medicine, part of the U.S. National Academy of Science, an advisory group serving the United States in matters of science, engineering, and medicine (http://www.iom.edu)
ISONG	International Society of Nurses in Genetics
ITR	immunoreactive trypsinogen (associated with cystic fibrosis, a genetic disease
IVF	in vitro fertilization
LPS	lipopolysaccharide
MCI	mild cognitive impairment
MEN2a	multiple endocrine neoplasia, type 2a
MLD	metachromatic leukodystropy
MRI	magnetic resonance imaging
MSI	microsatellite instability (distinctive patterns of repetitive stretches of short sequences of DNA used as genetic markers to track inheritance in families)*
NCHPEG	National Coalition for Health Professional Education in Genetics (http://www.nchpeg.org)
NBS	newborn screening

NCEMNA	National Coalition Ethnic Minority Nurse Association
NF2	neurofibromatosis, type 2
NHGRI	National Human Genome Research Institute (part of NIH)
NIH	National Institutes of Health, a division of the DHHS
NOS	Not otherwise specified (in some instances this may refer to a general disease description, meaning that a specific cell type or more detailed description of pathology was not given or available)
NPD	nasal potential difference
NSAIDS	nonsteroidal antiinflammatory drugs
NSGC	National Society of Genetic Counselors
NSRV	New Standard Revised Version (edition of the Bible)
OMIM	Online Mendelian Inheritance in Man, http://www.omim.org, an online listing and description of genetic conditions that follow Mendelian inheritance patterns.
ONS	Oncology Nursing Society
PGD	pre-implantation genetic diagnosis
PHAD	pre-hospital advanced directives
PHI	protected health information
PKU	phenylketonurea
PPC	primary peritoneal carcinoma
PSDA	Patient Self-Determination Act voted into law by the U.S. Congress in 1991
PTEN	approved symbol for *phosphatase and tensin homolog* (mutated in multiple advanced cancers; (from the Genetics Home Reference, http://ghr.nlm.nih.gov/gene=pten accessed October 22, 2008)
RN	Registered Nurse; registered nursing is characterized by its initial educational paths of a bachelor's degree, an associate degree, or a diploma from an approved nursing program.
RNA	ribonucleic acid, similar to one strand of DNA except that uracil (U) substitutes for thymine (T); RNA participates in cell physiology by bringing the DNA directions for assembly of proteins to cell cytoplasm.*

SACGHS	U.S. Department of Health and Human Services Secretary's Advisory Committee on Genetics, Health, and Society
SACGT	U.S. Department of Health and Human Services Secretary's Advisory Committee on Genetic Testing
SCD	sickle cell disease
SERMS	selective estrogen receptor modulators
SNP	single nucleotide polymorphism, a "spelling" variation in one base pair, may or may not be associated with illness or risk for illness
STAR	Study of Tamoxifen and Raloxifene (a specialized protocol for the prevention of certain forms of breast cancer)
TAH/BSO	total abdominal hysterectomy/bilateral salpingo-oophorectomy
VSD	ventriculoseptal defect, a congenital defect in the heart

Margaret Abbott, MPH, BS, RN

Margaret Abbott is a pioneering clinician who served the major portion of her career with the Johns Hopkins University and Medical Center in the Division of Medical Genetics. She practiced with Victor McKusick, MD, the "Father of Medical Genetics," and a multidisciplinary team of professionals who led efforts in laying the twentieth-century groundwork for the diagnosis and management of patients and families with genetic conditions and gene-based illness. She has worked with a diverse group of trainees in medical genetics at Hopkins from all parts of the world.

Imam Johari Abdul-Malik, MS

Dar Al-Hijrah Islamic Center, and Bioethicist and
Genetics Counselor, Washington, DC

Imam Abdul-Malik received his medical training at Howard University, earning a bachelor's of Science degree in chemistry and a master's degree in genetics and human genetics. After 30 years of dedication to medical research, genetics counseling, health education, and advocacy, he now serves as the Executive Director of Faces of Our Children-Sickle Cell Foundation. His clinical bioethics training at Georgetown University's Kennedy Center for Ethics and his service as a Health Care Reform Commissioner for Washington, DC, uniquely qualify him to present this material. He has co-authored more than 30 scientific articles and developed the first survey to assess the health status of Muslims in the United States.

Franklin R. Ampy, PhD

Professor and Acting Chairman, Department of Biology,
Howard University

Dr. Ampy is a member of the Genetics Society of America, American Society of Cell Biologists, American Institute of Biological Sciences, Association of Southeastern Biologists, and Sigma Xi, The International Research Society. A biostatistician, he teaches and consults with graduate students from most of the life sciences departments at Howard University.

Laurie Badzek, JD, MSN, RN, LLM, NAP
Professor, West Virginia University School of Nursing, Director
Dr. Badzek, a nurse attorney, scholar, and researcher, is Director for the ANA Center of Ethics and Human Rights (2003 to present, 1998–1999) and a tenured professor at West Virginia University School of Nursing, where she teaches nursing, ethics, law, and health policy. In her ANA work she has been instrumental in developing both the current Code of Ethics for Nurses and the 2007 genetic and genomic core competencies for nurses. In the latter initiative, Dr. Badzek led ANA's collaboration with the Genetic/Genomic Nursing Competency Initiative (GGNCI) and the AAN Genetic Health Expert Panel.

Lynne Taylor Bemis, PhD
Associate Professor of Medicine, University of Colorado (Denver).
In addition to her position at the University of Colorado, Dr Bemis is also a co-founder of Genetic Education for Native Americans (GENA), a team-taught genetics curriculum whose subject is cultural concerns about genetics. Dr. Bemis actively conducts research on genetic changes in cancer predicting response to therapy. Her current research includes projects on microRNA and the use of nanotechnology for cancer diagnostics.

Noureddine Berka, PhD, D(ABHI)
Clinical Director, Tissue Typing Laboratory, Calgary Laboratory Services, Calgary, AB, Canada
A board certified immunogeneticist, Dr. Berka is also Adjunct Assistant Professor, Department of Pathology and Laboratory Medicine, Faculty of Medicine, University of Calgary, Canada and a member of the Institute of Infection, Immunity, and Inflammation. He also serves with the Canadian Institute for Health Information for the redevelopment of MIS Standards for Clinical Laboratory Services.

Triptish Bhatia, PhD
Postdoctoral Fellow (Genetic Counseling and Genetic Epidemiology), University of Pittsburgh
Dr. Bhatia holds a PhD in Psychology from HP University India and the Gold Medal in MPhil. Her postdoctoral work focuses on a training program for psychiatric genetics in India (a Fogarty NIH-funded program). She has conducted research on the genetics of schizophrenia for the last 12 years, publishing a number of book chapters and more than 20 peer-reviewed research articles.

Linda Burhansstipanov, DrPH, MSPH, CHES
Director, Native American Cancer Initiatives, Inc.

Dr. Burhansstipanov (Cherokee Nation of Oklahoma) has worked in public health since 1971, primarily with Native American issues. With 18 years of experience as faculty for California State University Long Beach, she has authored over 90 peer-reviewed publications, the majority of which focus on health and wellness concerns of Native peoples. She developed and implemented the Native American Cancer Research Program at the National Cancer Institute from 1989 to1993. She serves on such national boards as the CDC Health Disparities Board, ICC Governing Board, and chairs the American Indian Alaska Native National Advisory Council of the Susan G. Komen for the Cure.

Bernice Coleman, PhD, ACNP
Heart Transplantation and Ventricular Assist Programs,
Cedars Sinai Medical Center

Dr. Coleman has 23 years of advanced practice nursing experience as a Clinical Nurse Specialist and as a board certified Acute Care Nurse Practitioner. She completed post-doctoral studies in the Histocompatibility Laboratory (HLA), Cedars Sinai Medical Center, and later attended the National Institute of Nursing Research (NINR) Summer Genetics Institute, a collaboration between the National Institute of Health's NINR and Georgetown University. Her research specializes in bench explorations of the clinical ethnic impact of cytokine gene polymorphisms on heart transplantation outcomes. She has presented and published on topics associated with care of cardiac surgical patients, ethnic immunogenetics of heart transplantation, and critical care nursing issues.

Rebecca B. Donohue, MSN, FNP-BC, AOCN, APNG
Cancer Genetic Counselor, Acadiana Medical Oncology

Currently pursuing a PhD in nursing research with an oncology focus through the University of Utah, Ms. Donohue is certified as a Family Nurse Practitioner, licensed by the state of Louisiana as an APRN with prescriptive authority, and certified as an Advanced Oncology Certified Nurse and as an Advanced Practice Nurse in Genetics. She has been employed as an oncology nurse practitioner and cancer genetic counselor with Acadiana Medical Oncology in Lafayette, Louisiana for 8 years, and has developed and implemented preventive health, supportive care, and disease management evidence-based practice tools. A national speaker on a variety of oncology topics, she has been published in a variety of media.

Robbie J. Dugas, DNS, APRN
Assistant Professor, Louisiana State University Alexandria

Dr. Dugas received a Doctorate of Nursing Science from Louisiana State University, Health Science Center in New Orleans. She is currently an Assistant Professor and Coordinator of the RN to BSN Program at Louisiana State University Alexandria. Dr. Dugas holds two advanced practice licensures as an Adult and Family Nurse Practitioner. Dr. Dugas has studied and researched the cultural factors related to the transjectory of Friedreich's Ataxia, a genetic disease within the Acadian population, and presented this research at local and international conferences. She has published an article related to genetic and ethics called "Nursing and Genetics: Applying the *American Nurses Association's Code of Ethics*" in a peer-reviewed journal. Dr. Dugas has attended the Genetic Program for Nursing Faculty at the Genetic Institute, Cincinnati Children's Hospital, and from this implemented genetic courses in two BSN programs.

Rabbi Michael L. Feshbach
Senior Rabbi of Temple Shalom

Rabbi Feshbach is the Senior Rabbi of Temple Shalom, a Reform synagogue in Chevy Chase, MD. He is the author of numerous columns and articles, including "Obedience to Which Commander: An Examination of a Jewish Soldier's Right to Disobey Immoral Orders," (with Peter Schaktman) in *Reform Jewish Ethics and the Halakha,* and "A Name for Ourselves: On Infertility, Meaning and Hope," in *A Guide to Infertility and Reproductive Technology* from the Union for Reform Judaism Department of Family Concerns, and on the Internet, "Faces in the Mirror," an America Online feature from 1996 to 2002. Rabbi Feshbach previously served congregations in Buffalo, New York; Erie, Pennsylvania; and Boca Raton, Florida.

Melissa H. Fries, MD, Colonel, USAF, MC
Clinical Mentor, Medical Genetics, Uniformed Services University of the Health Sciences

Dr. Fries received her undergraduate degree in Biology from California State University (Sacramento), a Master's of Science in Education from the University of Southern California (Los Angeles), and a Medical Doctoral degree from the Uniformed Services University of the Health Sciences. Her postgraduate education includes an obstetrics and gynecology residency, medical genetics and reproductive ultrasound fellowship, and APGO Solvay Education Fellowship. With interests in inherited breast and ovarian cancer and sonographic assessment of chromosomal anomalies, she has published numerous articles and book chapters.

Elizabeth Gettig, MS, CGC
Associate Professor and Co-Director of the Genetic Counselor Training Program, Graduate School of Public Health, University of Pittsburgh

A noted expert in the field of genetic counseling and education, Ms. Gettig recently received a career development award with the Office of Genetics and Disease Prevention at the Centers for Disease Control and Prevention. With clinical work including Huntington Disease, cancer genetics, and newborn screening, her research also extends to national genetic services. Such analysis provides information for policy development and establishment of uniform minimum criteria for genetic service delivery nationally. A board certified (ABMG/ABGC) genetic counselor who publishes and lectures frequently, Ms. Gettig is a past president of the National Society of Genetic Counselors and recipient of two national awards in genetic counseling.

Ellen Giarelli, EdD, RN, CRNP
Research Associate Professor, Biobehavioral Research Center, University of Pennsylvania School of Nursing

Dr. Giarelli is an advanced practice nurse certified as an adult nurse practitioner with two years post-doctoral training (2000–2002) in psychosocial oncology at the University of Pennsylvania School of Nursing. Her clinical experiences include bedside care for adult and pediatric patients in cardiothoracic surgical intensive care that has led to considerable knowledge of the experiences of informal caregivers (spouses and parents) of people with chronic disorders. She has extensive research experience in lifelong management of chronic illness and the experiences of parents and families caring for children with chronic genetic and non-genetic disorders.

Cathleen M. Goetsch, MSN, ARNP, AOCNP
Virginia Mason Medical Cancer Institute

Ms. Goetsch is a hereditary cancer risk consultant at Virginia Mason Medical Center Cancer Institute. She has been providing cancer genetic services since 1996. Experienced in cancer prevention clinical trials and adult hematology and oncology outpatient care, she also provides surveillance for women with increased breast cancer risk. She is a member of the International Society of Nurses in Genetics (ISONG) and the Cancer Genetics Special Interest Group of the Oncology Nursing Society (ONS).

Karen Greco, PhD, RN, ANP

Clinical Associate Professor, University of Arizona College of Nursing

Dr. Greco's clinical practice has been in cancer genetics for over 15 years; her research has studied breast and colorectal cancer screening decision-making in high-risk individuals and families. She is an adult nurse practitioner and holds a PhD (focusing on gerontology and genetics) and Master's in Nursing, both from Oregon Health & Science University. A longtime member of the International Society of Nurses in Genetics (ISONG), she received the 2005 ISONG President's Award for her leadership in writing and bringing to publication *Genetics and Genomics Nursing: Scope and Standards of Nursing,* one of several awards for her work in genomics nursing.

Chris Hackler, PhD

Professor and Director of the Division of Medical Humanities of the College of Medicine, University of Arkansas for Medical Sciences

Dr. Hackler received a PhD in philosophy from the University of North Carolina and has received awards from the Woodrow Wilson Foundation, the Fulbright Commission, and the National Endowment for the Humanities. He has served on the governing board of the Society for Health and Human Values, editing its newsletter from 1992 to 1998. He received the Society's Distinguished Service Award in 1996. Dr. Hackler was Sealy & Smith/NEH Visiting Scholar at the Institute for the Medical Humanities at the University of Texas Medical Branch in Galveston in 2001. He publishes primarily on end-of-life issues and heathcare policy. His current research is centered on ethical issues in public health and genetic interventions into the aging process.

Barbara W. Harrison, MS, CGC

Assistant Professor, Howard University College of Medicine

Mrs. Harrison is a Certified Genetics Counselor who received her degrees from University of Maryland and University of Pittsburgh. She is an Assistant Professor at Howard University and the Co-Director of the Howard University Genetics Counseling Program, where she teaches graduate and medical students, as well as residents in various specialties. In addition to her academic duties, she sees patients at Howard University Hospital in areas that include prenatal, pediatric, adult, and cancer genetics.

Verle Headings, MD, PhD

Professor in Pediatrics and Human Genetics, Howard University College of Medicine

Dr. Headings received an MD and PhD (Human Genetics) at the University of Michigan (Ann Arbor). He serves as Professor in Pediatrics and Human Genetics at Howard University and as Clinical Geneticist at Howard University Hospital. He is Director of Graduate Studies in Genetics and Human Genetics, as well as Director of the MD/PhD Program at Howard University.

Jean F. Jenkins, PhD, RN, FAAN

Senior Clinical Advisor, Office of the Director of the National Human Genome Research Institute (NHGRI), National Institutes of Health

In this NIH leadership role, Dr. Jenkins is committed to the preparation of others to become aware of, plan for, and integrate genetics and genomics concepts throughout healthcare practice. In 2005 she received the Michael J. Scotti Jr. award for National Coalition for Health Professional Education in Genetics (NCHPEG) efforts as content and instruction co-chair. She coordinated the development and consensus of the NCHPEG competencies and the 2007 publication, *Essential Nursing Competencies and Curricula Guidelines for Genetics and Genomics* and its 2008 update. She has co-authored three nursing texts, including *Nursing Care in the Genomic Era: A Case-Based Approach* with Dale Halsey Lea (2005).

Dale Halsey Lea, MPH, RN, CGC, APNG, FAAN

National Human Genome Research Institute, National Institutes of Health

A board certified genetic counselor with more than 20 years experience in clinical and educational genetics, Ms. Lea is the Health Educator with the Education and Community Involvement Branch and the Genomic Healthcare Branch, National Human Genome Research Institute (NHGRI). There she conducts research in and develops numerous consumer health education and community involvement programs and resources in genetics and genomics. Along with leadership roles with the International Society of Nurses in Genetics (ISONG), the National Society of Genetic Counselors, and the National Coalition for Health Professional Education in Genetics (NCHPEG), she has published widely on integrating genetics into nursing practice, particularly interdisciplinary partnerships in genetic-related health care.

Robin R. Leger, PhD, MS, RN, CCRP
University of Connecticut Health Center

A clinical nurse specialist working for over 17 years with children, adults, and families with chronic and disabling conditions, Dr. Leger has spent 16 years on the faculty of schools of nursing. Now a Research Facilitator in the Department of Orthopaedics and an Assistant Professor in Community Medicine and Health Care at University of Connecticut Health Center, she has produced numerous service demonstration publications. A board member of the Spina Bifida Association of Connecticut and Citizens for Quality Sickle Cell Care, Dr. Leger has been a member of the New England Regional Genetics Group for two decades, and chaired the North East Myelodysplasia Association for 10 years. A co-investigator on grant-funded projects focused on sickle cell disease education, community screening, and hemoglobinopathy counseling certification, she mentors students and collaborates with family leaders on genetic and disability issues.

Deborah J. MacDonald, PhD, RN, APNG
City of Hope Clinical Cancer Genetics Department

Assistant Professor in the Division of Population Sciences, and of the City of Hope Clinical Cancer Genetics Department *Cancer Screening & Prevention Program,* Dr. MacDonald was among the first nurses credentialed as an Advanced Practice Nurse in Genetics. She is a writing member of the National Comprehensive Cancer Network's panel to establish practice guidelines for breast cancer risk reduction. A past president of the International Society of Nurses in Genetics (ISONG), and recognized internationally for her cancer genetics presentations and publications, her research focuses on family communication of genetic cancer risk and risk reduction behaviors.

Agnes Masny, RN, MSN, MPH, CRNP
Fox Chase Cancer Center

Ms. Masny is a nurse practitioner and research assistant in the Division of Population Science at the Fox Chase Cancer Center. Her work is part of the Margaret Dyson Family Risk Assessment Program, which evaluates genetic and clinical approaches to reduce the risk of breast and ovarian cancer. Her research includes health professional education in cancer genetics and the integration of genetic and genomic technologies into community-based practice. She served on the Secretary of Health and Human Services' Advisory Committee on Genetics Health and Society from 2002 to 2006, and chaired the Genetic Discrimination Task Force. She was the 2002–2004 coordinator of the Oncology Nursing Society (ONS) Cancer Genetic Special Interest Group and was the 1997–2001 ONS representative to the National Coalition for Health Professional Education in Genetics (NCHPEG) and the ANA working group on Nursing Genetic and Genomic Competencies (2005).

Susan Miller-Samuel, MSN, RN, APNG
Thomas Jefferson University Hospital
Ms. Miller-Samuel is an Advanced Practice Nurse in Genetics at the Breast Care Center of Thomas Jefferson University Hospital in Philadelphia. Ms. Miller-Samuel's clinical genetic expertise centers on cancer genetics, with a specialization in hereditary breast and ovarian cancer. Her multidisciplinary practice includes genetic consultation, risk assessment, genetic testing, results disclosure, risk-reduction options, and long-term patient management. Educating the community and professional colleagues about breast and ovarian cancer risk, and comprehensive genetic consultation, are also key components of her work.

Rita Black Monsen, DSN, MPH, RN, FAAN
Dr. Monsen has been involved in clinical genetics and genetics in nursing education since the late 1970s. Now an independent consultant in the field, she was a faculty member and chairperson of the Department of Nursing at Henderson State University in Arkadelphia, AR. As well, she has served in founding, development, and leadership roles with the Arkansas Department of Health Genetics Advisory Board, the National Coalition for Health Professional Education in Genetics (NCHPG), the Genetic Nursing Credentialing Commission (GNCC), the International Society of Nurses in Genetics (ISONG), and the Arkansas Nurses Association. In addition to editing the first book on the use of professional portfolios in nursing, Dr. Monsen has published several articles on genetics in nursing and is an editor of the *Journal of Pediatric Nursing.*

Robert F. Murray, Jr., MD, MS
Chief, Division of Medical Genetics, Department of Pediatrics,
and Chairman of the Department of Genetics and Human Genetics,
Howard University College of Medicine
Dr. Murray is a graduate of Union College, Schenectady, New York, and received an MD degree from the University of Rochester School of Medicine and Dentistry. He earned a Master's of Science in Genetics from the University of Washington and also did a fellowship in Medical Genetics. He served three years in the U.S. Public Health Service while stationed at the National Institutes of Health doing medical research.

Isaac M. T. Mwase, PhD, MDiv, MBA
Associate Professor of Philosophy, Tuskegee University

Dr. Mwase is an Associate Professor of Philosophy with the Tuskegee University National Center for Bioethics in Research and Health Care. Having joined the Tuskegee faculty in 2004 as part of the Public Health and Bioethics Education and Training Core of Project EXPORT, he is a Bioethics Shared Resource investigator in the NCI U-54 Cancer Research Partnership between the Morehouse School of Medicine, Tuskegee University, and the University of Alabama (Birmingham). Serving a two-year term as a Governing Councilor for the American Public Health Association, Dr. Mwase was also recently selected as a Cancer Prevention Fellow with the NIH/NCI Cancer Prevention Fellowship Program. His research interests include epistemology, research ethics, genetics, neuro-ethics, business ethics, public health ethics, global health justice, and the role of religion in bioethics and public health.

Melinda Granger Oberleitner, DNSc, RN, APRN, CNS
Professor, Department Head, Associate Dean, Department of Nursing and Allied Health Professions, University of Louisiana at Lafayette

Dr. Oberleitner is a nurse educator and administrator and holds advanced practice licensure as an Oncology Clinical Nurse Specialist. She has over 30 years of oncology nursing experience. In 1996, she was named the Oncology Certified Nurse (OCN) of the Year by the Oncology Nursing Certification Corporation in recognition of her outstanding contributions to the specialty of oncology nursing. A long-standing member of the Editorial Review Board of the *Oncology Nursing Forum*, Dr. Oberleitner also serves on the Editorial Advisory Board of *The Oncology Nurse*. She spearheaded faculty efforts to successfully secure the prestigious National League for Nursing Center of Excellence in Nursing designation for the Department of Nursing at the University of Louisiana at Lafayette for 2005–2008.

Victoria Odesina, MS, APRN-BC, CCRP, APGN
Clinical Research Associate and Program Manager,
University of Connecticut Health Center

Ms. Odesina received her nursing and midwifery training in Nigeria, where she was a registered nurse/midwife before she obtaining her BA in Health Services Administration and MS in Community Health Education at Western Illinois University. Actively involved with sickle cell issues for more than 20 years, she has authored or co-authored several educational works and made numerous presentations on sickle cell disease (SCD) and sickle cell pain management for providers, patients, and their families. Two of her three children are living with sickle cell disease. Co-founder of an advocacy organization in New Britain, Connecticut called Citizens for Quality Sickle Cell Care, Inc., she received the 2000 Alan Crocker Award for her activities in genetics both at the consumer and professional levels.

Sharon J. Olsen, PhD(c), MS, RN, AOCN
Assistant Professor, Johns Hopkins University School of Nursing
Holding a joint appointment with the Department of Oncology of the School of Medicine at JHU, Dr. Olsen's research interests include clinical cancer genetics and cancer prevention and screening. In 2002 she was an NIH Fellow in the National Institute of Nursing Research Summer Genetics Institute. Her publications include edited books, book chapters, and peer-reviewed journal articles. She is active with the American Nurses Association, the Oncology Nursing Society (ONS), the International Society of Nurses in Genetics (ISONG), and the National Association of Clinical Nurse Specialists.

Carmen T. Paniagua, EdD, RN, CPC, ACNP-BC
University of Arkansas for Medical Science (UAMS) College of Nursing
Dr. Paniagua is the Adult Acute Care Nurse Practitioner Program Coordinator at UAMS, where she has also served as Chair of the Department of Nursing Practice, and a Clinical Assistant Professor. She also works with the UAMS Adult Cancer Genetic Clinic and Emergency Department Urgent Clinic. One of her active research interests is integrating genomics, cultural diversity, and healthcare disparities into the nursing curriculum. She has developed online cultural diversity modules, collaborated with multiple healthcare providers, served as a consultant for various hospitals, and presented at the local, state, national, and international level. She has also served as a Commissioner for the Arkansas Health Minority Commission and as a member of the Arkansas Governor Hispanic Advisory Committee. She has completed post-doctoral fellowships in molecular genetics at NIH and in interventional pain management at Georgetown University.

Daniel G. Petereit, MD
Rapid City Regional Hospital
A radiation oncologist at Rapid City Regional Hospital in Rapid City, South Dakota, Dr. Petereit is a nationally-respected expert in gynecological and other cancer treatments such as brachytherapy. He has special emphases in a NIH Clinical Disparities Research Grant for Native Americans and brachytherapy for gynecologic, prostate, lung, and breast cancer. Dr. Petereit has recently published articles and abstracts related to prostate studies and cancer health disparities research. Receiving his MD in 1989 from the University of South Dakota School of Medicine, he performed his residency in Radiation Oncology at the University of Wisconsin Hospital and Clinics from 1990 to1994. His hospital appointments are to the University of Wisconsin Hospital and Clinics and the Rapid City Regional Hospital, with academic appointments to the University of Wisconsin Medical School and the University of South Dakota Medical School.

Connie C. Price, PhD, MPS
Associate Professor of Philosophy, Tuskegee University
Dr. Price teaches philosophy at Tuskegee University. Her BA in philosophy is from William Jewell College, and her doctorate in philosophy is from Pennsylvania State University. Her Master of Professional Studies degree is in Interactive Telecommunications from New York University's Tisch School of the Arts. In addition to chairing Tuskegee's department of philosophy from 1988 to 1998, she has participated in major University grant programs (including membership of the proposal team for the Tuskegee Bioethics Center) and piloted courses and research in engineering and agricultural ethics. She has held offices in several national and international philosophical societies and has presented and published numerous papers and articles.

Diane Seibert, PhD, MS, WHCNP, ANP, CRNP
Uniformed Services University of the Health Sciences
Dr. Seibert received her undergraduate nursing degree in 1979 and has practiced as a Women's Health Nurse Practitioner for the past 14 years. She joined the faculty of the Uniformed Services University of the Health Sciences 11 years ago and is the Program Director for the Family Nurse Practitioner program. Dr. Seibert has published over 20 articles and book chapters on women's health, educational technology, and genetics, and has conducted research in improving learning outcomes. Her current research is in telehealth technology and developing genetic decision support tools for primary care providers. Her clinical practice includes genetic counseling and obstetrics and routine gynecologic care at the National Naval Medical Center.

Heather Skirton, PhD, MSc, RGN
University of Plymouth School of Nursing
Dr. Skirton has over 30 years of clinical experience in nursing, midwifery, and genetic counseling, including almost 20 years working with families affected by Huntington Disease. In 2004 she was appointed as a Reader in Health Genetics at the University of Plymouth. She is now Deputy Head (for Research) of the School of Nursing and Community Studies. Since 2000, Dr. Skirton has been Director of the European Genetics Foundation course on genetic counseling and is a past president of the International Society of Nurses in Genetics (ISONG). Her research centers on professional education in genetics, the impact of genetic disease on families, and delivery of effective genetic healthcare. She continues to work as a voluntary counselor for the Huntington Disease Association. Dr. Skirton is the co-editor of two textbooks on practical genetic healthcare for nurses.

Ida J. Spruill, PhD, MSN, RN, LIWS
Post-doctoral Fellow in Clinical Genetics at University of Iowa,
College of Nursing

Dr. Johnson-Spruill completed her PhD in Nursing at Hampton University School of Nursing in 2007; her research interest is ethno-cultural barriers to genetic literacy among rural African American families. Past research experiences included managing and directing a community-based genetic research study known as Project SuGar which was interested in isolating and identifying the genes responsible for the expression of diabetes and obesity in Gullah families of South Carolina. The project was successful in developing and implementing a recruitment strategy known as CPR (Community, Plan, and Reward) and enrolled over 600 African American families into the study.

Robert E. Taylor, MD, PhD, FACP, FCCP
Dean, Howard University College of Medicine

Dr. Taylor is a Professor of Pharmacology, Medicine, and Psychiatry; Chairman, Department of Pharmacology; and Director, Division of Clinical Pharmacology, Howard University Hospital. Board certified in Internal Medicine with an extensive record in research, he has received several National Institute on Alcohol Abuse and Alcoholism/National Institutes of Health (NIAAA/NIH) research grants. These have produced important studies on the clinical course and the genetics of alcoholism in African Americans. Dr. Taylor has served as member and/or chairman on numerous federal advisory committees and other special committees, task forces, and research review committees.

John G. Twomey, PhD, PNP
Massachusetts General Hospital Institute of Health Professions

Dr. Twomey is an Associate Professor at the Graduate Program in Nursing at the Institute of Health Professions at Massachusetts General Hospital in Boston. Having served on the ANA Task Force that rewrote the profession's code of ethics, he teaches bioethics and research and serves on several human subjects committees. In 2000, Dr. Twomey attended the Genetics Program for Nursing Faculty at the University of Cincinnati School of Nursing. He subsequently served on the Expert Panel that advised the Bureau of Nursing on genetics education priorities. From 2004 to 2006 he was a Post-Doctoral Fellow in Clinical Genetics in the T32 Fellowship in the College of Nursing at the University of Iowa. He does research in the area of the ethics of genetic testing of children and has authored several manuscripts about this topic.

Timikia Vaughn, MS
Genetics Counselor, Division of Medical Genetics,
Schneider Children's Hospital

Timikia Vaughn received her Bachelor's of Science in Biology and Master's of Science in Genetic Counseling from Howard University. She has presented her graduate work about the attitudes of muslims toward reproductive issues at the National Society of Genetic Counselors meeting in Los Angeles. She is working as a prenatal and pediatric genetics counselor at Schneider Children's Hospital, Division of Medical Genetics, in Manhasset, New York.

Janet K. Williams, PhD, RN, PNP, CGC, FAAN
Kelting Professor of Nursing, University of Iowa

Also Director of the University of Iowa's Clinical Genetics Nursing Research Post-doctoral Fellowship program and author of over 90 articles on genetic nursing topics, Dr. Williams has a clinical background that includes maternal child health nursing and genetic counseling. Educated as a Pediatric Nurse Practitioner, she earned a PhD in Educational Psychology. Since 1990, she has directed the integration of genetic concepts into coursework at all levels of nursing education at the University of Iowa. The Principal Investigator of a NIH/NINR funded study to describe health problems encountered by families of persons with Huntington Disease, Dr. Williams also directed an NIH/ELSI funded grant to develop a CD-ROM on Ethics and Genetic Testing for Nurses. She is a past president and founding member of the International Society of Nurses in Genetics (ISONG).

INDEX

A

AAPINA (Asian American/Pacific Islander Nurses Association), 227

Abbott, Margaret
about, 429
on mid-century medical genetics, xix

Abdul-Malik, Imam Johari
about, 429
on Muslim attitudes to genetics, 149–163

abortion. *See also* pregnancy
Christian beliefs, 172, 173, 175
Hindu beliefs, 120–121
Islamic beliefs, 158
Jewish beliefs, 134
Muslim beliefs, 155
Sikh beliefs, 120–121

Abyssinian Baptist Church Health Ministry, 225

Access Working Group, 34

access to genetic information, technologies, and testing, 34, 47, 245, 285

accuracy of genetic testing, 243

ACMG (American College of Medical Geneticists), 321

ACOG (American College of Obstetrics and Gynecology), 321

acronyms, 423–428

ACS (American Cancer Society) dietary guidelines, 379

AD. *See* Alzheimer's Disease (AD)

AD inheritance (autosomal dominant inheritance), 417

ADA (Americans with Disabilities Act) of 1990, 28, 68, 98

advanced directives
environments of care, 257–260
guiding principles, 256–257
historical perspectives, 253–256
overview, 251–252
parental requests for, 251–260
quality of life debate, 258–259

advanced level genetics nurses, 20

advocacy
education by nurses of clients and patients as, 287, 291
ethical aspects of, 8, 10, 11, 24
ethical provision for, 8
ethics standard and, 24
as core nursing ethic, 284–285, 410–411
as professional nursing competency, x

African Americans
definition and race, 214–215
education and community outreach, 225–227
ethnic and social issues, 228
family, 215–216
genetic discovery and utilization, 227–228
health disparities, 216–218
HGP and historical unethical research, 223–224
Human Genome Project (HGP), 219–222
inequality, equity, and inequity, 218–219
legal issues, 229
overview, 213–214
resistance to research studies, 223–224
risk of cystic fibrosis in, 320

Nature Genetics, 168
nature of persons, Christian beliefs,
167–171
Nazi Germany, 67, 170, 255
NBNA (National Black Nurses
Association), 226–227
NBS. *See* newborn screening (NBS)
NCEMNA (National Coalition of Ethnic
Minority Nurse Associations), 227
NCHPEG (National Coalition for Health
Professional Education in Genetics), xiv,
xvii, 6, 101, 361, 424, 426
Negotiating Control, 304, 309–311
Netherlands, global genetic counseling
training programs, 111*t*
newborn screening (NBS)
Catholic beliefs, 146
cystic fibrosis, 323–324, 326
Newman, Louis, "Woodchoppers and
Respirators: The Problem of
Interpretation in Contemporary Jewish
Ethics," 132
NHGRI (National Human Genome
Research Institute), vii–xi, 361, 417, 424
Nightingale, Florence, 7
NIH (National Institutes of Health), vii,
138, 332, 356
non-paternity ethical issue, 389, 391–392
non-steroidal anti-inflammatory drugs
(NSAIDs), 290
nondirectiveness, 335–336
nonmaleficence
Catholic beliefs, 144
defined, 144
in predictive testing for Huntington
Disease (HD), 337–338
principle of, 21, 284
Norway, global genetic counseling training
programs, 111*t*
NSAB (National Surgical Adjuvant Breast
and Bowel Project), 289
NSAIDs (Non-Steroidal Anti-
Inflammatory Drugs), 290
Nuremberg Code, 67
nurses. *See also* genetics and genomic
nursing practice
abundance of, 88
relationship with patients, 410–411
responsibilities in caring for families
and communities, 411–412
Nursing: Scope and Standards of Practice
(ANA), 18

*Nursing Care in the Genomic Era:
A Case-Based Approach* (Collins &
Guttmacher), ix
Nursing Pledge (Florence Nightingale), 7

O

Oath of Hippocrates, 53
Oberleitner, Melinda Granger
about, 438
on challenges of informed consent,
65–75
Odesina, Victoria
about, 438
sickle cell disease (SCD) case study,
359–367
Office of Management and Budget, on
race and Hispanic origin, 202
Olsen, Sharon J.
about, 439
on genetic inheritance, identity, and the
proper role of nursing, 79–92
Oncology Nursing Society (ONS), 386
Online Mendelian Inheritance in Man web
site, 427
online resources. *See* web sites
ONS (Oncology Nursing Society), 386
oral contraceptives, hereditary breast cancer
case study, 382
Out of Africa model, 167
outcomes identification, standard of
practice, 22
oversight of genetic technologies
overview, 45
policy considerations/efforts, 45–46

P

palliative care (pediatric), 252, 258
Paniagua, Carmen T.
about, 439
on Hispanic perspectives on genetics
and ethics, 201–209
parent-child ethics, 271
parental decision making, 266–268
Participation in Lifelong Surveillance,
Conceptual Method, 303–304, 305*f*
patents in genes and genetics, access issues
of, 31, 32, 33, 46–47
Native Americans and, 182, 183, 185
patient-centered decisions, 256–257
Patient Self-Determination Act of 1991
(PSDA), 257